Advances in the Prevention and Management of Obesity and Eating Disorders

Special Issue Editors

Amanda Sainsbury

Felipe Q. da Luz

MDPI • Basel • Beijing • Wuhan • Barcelona • Belgrade

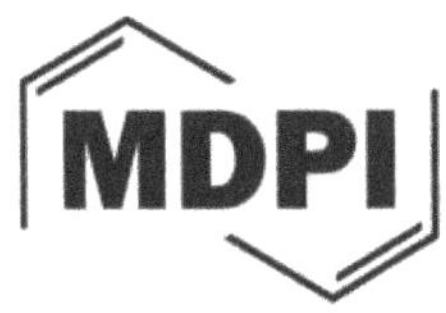

Special Issue Editors
Amanda Sainsbury
The University of Sydney
Australia

Felipe Q. da Luz
The University of Sydney
Australia

Editorial Office
MDPI
St. Alban-Anlage 66
Basel, Switzerland

This edition is a reprint of the Special Issue published online in the open access journal *Behavioral Sciences* (ISSN 2076-328X) in 2017 (available at: http://www.mdpi.com/journal/behavsci/special_issues/obesity_and_eating_disorders).

For citation purposes, cite each article independently as indicated on the article page online and as indicated below:

Lastname, F.M.; Lastname, F.M. Article title. *Journal Name* **Year**, *Article number*, page range.

First Editon 2018

ISBN 978-3-03842-853-4 (Pbk)
ISBN 978-3-03842-854-1 (PDF)

Table of Contents

About the Special Issue Editors v

Preface to "Advances in the Prevention and Management of Obesity and Eating Disorders" . vii

Felipe Q. da Luz, Amanda Sainsbury, Phillipa Hay, Jessica A. Roekenes, Jessica Swinbourne, Dhiordan C. da Silva and Margareth da S. Oliveira
Early Maladaptive Schemas and Cognitive Distortions in Adults with Morbid Obesity: Relationships with Mental Health Status
doi: 10.3390/bs7010010 1

Tracy Burrows, Janelle Skinner, Rebecca McKenna and Megan Rollo
Food Addiction, Binge Eating Disorder, and Obesity: Is There a Relationship?
doi: 10.3390/bs7030054 12

Henry Kewen Lu, Haider Mannan and Phillipa Hay
Exploring Relationships between Recurrent Binge Eating and Illicit Substance Use in a Non-Clinical Sample of Women over Two Years
doi: 10.3390/bs7030046 22

Ewelina M. Swierad, Lenny R. Vartanian and Marlee King
The Influence of Ethnic and Mainstream Cultures on African Americans' Health Behaviors: A Qualitative Study
doi: 10.3390/bs7030049 35

Michelle Harvie and Anthony Howell
Potential Benefits and Harms of Intermittent Energy Restriction and Intermittent Fasting Amongst Obese, Overweight and Normal Weight Subjects—A Narrative Review of Human and Animal Evidence
doi: 10.3390/bs7010004 55

Alice A. Gibson and Amanda Sainsbury
Strategies to Improve Adherence to Dietary Weight Loss Interventions in Research and Real-World Settings
doi: 10.3390/bs7030044 77

Claudia Harper and Judith Maher
Investigating Philosophies Underpinning Dietetic Private Practice
doi: 10.3390/bs7010011 88

Priyanka Thapliyal, Deborah Mitchison and Phillipa Hay
Insights into the Experiences of Treatment for An Eating Disorder in Men: A Qualitative Study of Autobiographies
doi: 10.3390/bs7020038 107

Camilla Lindvall Dahlgren and Kristin Stedal
Cognitive Remediation Therapy for Adolescents with Anorexia Nervosa—Treatment Satisfaction and the Perception of Change
doi: 10.3390/bs7020023 124

Clare E. Collins, Philip J. Morgan, Melinda J. Hutchesson, Christopher Oldmeadow, Daniel Barker and Robin Callister
Efficacy of Web-Based Weight Loss Maintenance Programs: A Randomized Controlled Trial Comparing Standard Features Versus the Addition of Enhanced Personalized Feedback over 12 Months
doi: 10.3390/bs7040076 . . . . **145**

Sarah Barakat, Sarah Maguire, Lois Surgenor, Brooke Donnelly, Blagica Miceska, Kirsty Fromholtz, Janice Russell, Phillipa Hay and Stephen Touyz
The Role of Regular Eating and Self-Monitoring in the Treatment of Bulimia Nervosa: A Pilot Study of an Online Guided Self-Help CBT Program
doi: 10.3390/bs7030039 . . . . **154**

Marcele Regine de Carvalho, Thiago Rodrigues de Santana Dias, Monica Duchesne, Antonio Egidio Nardi and Jose Carlos Appolinario
Virtual Reality as a Promising Strategy in the Assessment and Treatment of Bulimia Nervosa and Binge Eating Disorder: A Systematic Review
doi: 10.3390/bs7030043 . . . . **171**

About the Special Issue Editors

Amanda Sainsbury, With a Bachelor of Science from the University of Western Australia and a PhD from the University of Geneva, Switzerland, Professor Amanda Salis (publishing as Sainsbury) leads full-time research into dietary treatments for overweight and obesity at the University of Sydney's Boden Institute of Obesity, Nutrition, Exercise & Eating Disorders. Her translational research into hypothalamic control of appetite, eating behaviour, energy expenditure, body weight, and body composition spans transgenic mice, adults with overweight or obesity, as well as adult athletes. Her randomised controlled trials comparing the long-term effects of fast versus slow weight loss—using intermittent versus continuous energy restriction—are funded by a Senior Research Fellowship and Project Grants from the National Health and Medical Research Council (NHMRC) of Australia. She has authored two books about adult weight management that are available internationally in three languages and are used by consumers, community health centers/gyms, and healthcare professionals.

Felipe Q. da Luz started his career as a psychologist at the Diabetes and Endocrinology Centre in Salvador, Brazil. Following completion of a Master's degree in Clinical Psychology at the Pontifical Catholic University of Rio Grande do Sul in Porto Alegre in Brazil, he went on to complete a PhD in Psychology at the University of Sydney's Boden Institute of Obesity, Nutrition, Exercise & Eating Disorder in Australia, with a competitive scholarship from the CAPES Foundation. Felipe's research aims to find safe ways to treat overweight or obesity with co-morbid binge eating disorders. His research has led to several awards, notably, the 2017 Peter Beumont Young Investigator Award from the Australia & New Zealand Academy for Eating Disorders, the 2016 University of Sydney Postgraduate Research Prize for Outstanding Academic Achievement, as well as the 2016 University of Sydney School of Psychology Publication Prize.

Preface to "Advances in the Prevention and Management of Obesity and Eating Disorders"

Obesity and eating disorders remain major public health concerns worldwide. While we are far from having definitive solutions, scientific insights into the prevention and management of obesity and eating disorders have developed significantly in recent years. This research has been stimulated by the continuous challenge of reducing the global burden of obesity and its commonly associated health complications, as well as the life-threatening characteristics of eating disorders. While there are significant differences between obesity and eating disorders, and while these conditions are often treated and researched in isolation, there are also important similarities between them. For instance, people with obesity or eating disorders alike often engage in unhealthy eating behaviors and inappropriate levels of physical activity. Additionally, obesity and eating disorders often co-exist in the same person, and individuals with both of these conditions are at risk for severe medical and psychosocial complications. Looking towards better solutions for these pressing public health concerns, this book addresses recent scientific findings regarding the prevention and management of obesity and eating disorders. It reports on cognition and mental health in people with obesity, as well as on food addiction, co-morbidities of eating disorders, cultural aspects of eating, intermittent dietary energy restriction as a treatment for overweight or obesity, factors influencing the adherence to dietary treatments for overweight and obesity, philosophies underpinning dietary practices, treatment of eating disorders in men, cognitive remediation therapy for anorexia nervosa, and online or virtual interventions for weight management or bulimia nervosa—all drawing from culturally diverse findings from research groups around the world (e.g. Australia, UK, Norway, Brazil). With this book, we encourage healthcare professionals and researchers working primarily in the field of obesity to learn more about eating disorders, and vice-versa, so that knowledge in each field can be enriched by knowledge from the other, ultimately enabling the increasing numbers of people living with obesity and/or eating disorders to reap the benefits.

Amanda Sainsbury and Felipe Q. da Luz
Special Issue Editors

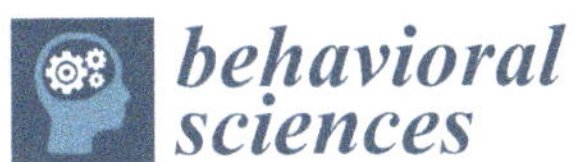

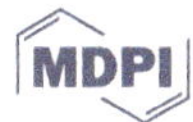

Article

Early Maladaptive Schemas and Cognitive Distortions in Adults with Morbid Obesity: Relationships with Mental Health Status

Felipe Q. da Luz [1,2,3,*], Amanda Sainsbury [1,2], Phillipa Hay [4], Jessica A. Roekenes [1], Jessica Swinbourne [1], Dhiordan C. da Silva [3] and Margareth da S. Oliveira [3]

1. The Boden Institute of Obesity, Nutrition, Exercise & Eating Disorders, Sydney Medical School, Charles Perkins Centre, The University of Sydney, NSW 2006, Australia; amanda.salis@sydney.edu.au (A.S.); jess.roekenes@gmail.com (J.A.R.); jessica.swinbourne@sydney.edu.au (J.S.)
2. School of Psychology, Faculty of Science, The University of Sydney, NSW 2006, Australia
3. Faculty of Psychology, Pontifical Catholic University of Rio Grande do Sul, Av. Ipiranga 6681, Porto Alegre/RS, CEP 90619-900, Brazil; dhiordanc@gmail.com (D.C.d.S.); marga@pucrs.br (M.d.S.O.)
4. Centre for Health Research and School of Medicine, The University of Western Sydney, Locked Bag 1797, Penrith NSW 2751, Australia; p.hay@westernsydney.edu.au

* Correspondence: felipe.quintodaluz@sydney.edu.au; Tel.: +61-02-8267-1961

Academic Editor: Scott J. Hunter
Received: 4 November 2016; Accepted: 24 February 2017; Published: 28 February 2017

Abstract: Dysfunctional cognitions may be associated with unhealthy eating behaviors seen in individuals with obesity. However, dysfunctional cognitions commonly occur in individuals with poor mental health independently of weight. We examined whether individuals with morbid obesity differed with regard to dysfunctional cognitions when compared to individuals of normal weight, when mental health status was controlled for. 111 participants—53 with morbid obesity and 58 of normal weight—were assessed with the Mini-Mental State Examination, Young Schema Questionnaire, Cognitive Distortions Questionnaire, Depression, Anxiety and Stress Scale, and a Demographic and Clinical Questionnaire. Participants with morbid obesity showed higher scores in one (insufficient self-control/self-discipline) of 15 early maladaptive schemas and in one (labeling) of 15 cognitive distortions compared to participants of normal weight. The difference between groups for insufficient self-control/self-discipline was not significant when mental health status was controlled for. Participants with morbid obesity showed more severe anxiety than participants of normal weight. Our findings did not show clinically meaningful differences in dysfunctional cognitions between participants with morbid obesity or of normal weight. Dysfunctional cognitions presented by individuals with morbid obesity are likely related to their individual mental health and not to their weight.

Keywords: obesity; morbid obesity; psychology; dysfunctional cognition; mental health

1. Introduction

Schema Theory proposes that some individuals can develop dysfunctional patterns of beliefs and unhelpful perceptions of the world and themselves [1]. These beliefs and perceptions usually develop during childhood or adolescence as a result of psychologically harmful experiences involving family members or other significant individuals, and for this reason are referred to as early maladaptive schemas. According to this theory, early maladaptive schemas develop in response to unmet core emotional needs, namely: secure attachment to others, autonomy/competence, freedom to express emotions, spontaneity, and realistic limits/self-control. It was previously suggested that as a result of this process, people can develop different types of psychological disorders and engage in a continuum of dysfunctional behaviors [1].

There is some evidence that early maladaptive schemas can relate to dysfunctional eating behaviors. For example, the unhealthy eating behaviors seen in patients with eating disorders were found to be associated with the presence of early maladaptive schemas [2]. One study [3] evaluated the presence of early maladaptive schemas in participants with obesity and found that they showed more severe early maladaptive schemas than participants of normal weight, notably the early maladaptive schemas of social isolation/alienation and defectiveness/shame. Another study [4] found that the early maladaptive schemas of isolation/alienation, emotional inhibition, abandonment/instability and unrelenting standards/hypercriticalness negatively influenced aspects of identity amongst individuals with obesity. Additionally, a higher presence of the following early maladaptive schemas were found amongst adolescents with overweight or obesity in comparison to adolescents of normal weight: social isolation/alienation, defectiveness/shame, emotional deprivation, failure to achieve, dependence/incompetence, and subjugation [5], as well as emotional deprivation, abandonment/instability, subjugation and insufficient self-control/self-discipline [6]. Additionally, another study [7] involving adolescents with overweight found that those who experienced a loss of control over eating had a greater severity of the early maladaptive schemas of social isolation/alienation, abandonment/instability, unrelenting standards/hypercriticalness, mistrust/abuse, failure to achieve and subjugation, in contrast with those that did not experience loss of control over eating.

Another set of dysfunctional cognitive processes, named cognitive distortions, plays an important role in maintaining the negative core beliefs that form early maladaptive schemas, through the perceptual distortion of facts [1]. Cognitive distortions are common thoughts that happen quickly, involuntarily, and in a distorted manner [8]. Some specific types of cognitive distortions have been suggested to be experienced by individuals with obesity [9]. These distorted thoughts occur, for example, when someone thinks that the desire to eat is irresistible ("magnification"), that they are "losers" because they are obese ("labeling") or that people reject them because they are overweight ("mind reading"). One study found that dichotomous thinking (a type of cognitive distortion) about food, weight and eating was predictive of weight regain, and that a general dichotomous thinking pattern (not necessarily related to food, weight or eating) was an even better predictor of weight regain [10]. Two other studies [11,12] assessed vulnerability to a specific cognitive distortion, namely thought-shape fusion, in participants with obesity and participants of normal weight. This type of cognitive distortion occurs when the imagination of the consumption of high-energy food generates the feeling of being fat and negative moral judgment. In these studies, individuals with obesity were less vulnerable to thought-shape fusion than individuals of normal weight, thus revealing differences in cognitive processes between groups. Studies have further examined the correlation of cognitive distortions with binge eating disorder. A small ($n = 42$) exploratory study [13] reported that participants with obesity, whether or not they had binge eating disorder, showed more cognitive distortions than participants of normal weight. In contrast, another study [14] found that individuals with obesity and comorbid binge eating disorder were more affected by dichotomous thinking than individuals with obesity but without binge eating disorder. The studies above suggest that individuals with obesity, especially those with comorbid binge eating disorder, experience more of some types of cognitive distortions than individuals of normal weight.

Other studies, however, emphasize the relationship between dysfunctional cognitions and mental health status independently of the occurrence of eating or weight disorders. For example, there is evidence that early maladaptive schemas predict depression [15], are associated with complex cases of mood and anxiety disorders [16], and are vulnerability factors for the development of symptoms of depression and anxiety amongst individuals experiencing stressful situations [17]. There are also indications that early maladaptive schemas predict occupational stress [18]. Both early maladaptive schemas and cognitive distortions were found to be significantly associated with emotional problems, namely depression and anxiety [19]. In regards to cognitive distortions specifically, a study found that participants with depression showed strong negative interpretations of metaphors [20]. Cognitive distortions also predict depression and anxiety amongst children and adolescents [21]. Additionally, the cognitive model proposes that cognitive distortions, together with neurobiological correlates, influence how people cope with stressful situations and develop depression [22]. All of the studies discussed in this paragraph show a clear association of the occurrence of dysfunctional cognitions and mental health problems, irrespective of the weight of the participants. Therefore, it is possible that the observation that individuals with obesity experience more early maladaptive schemas or cognitive distortions than individuals of normal weight could be mediated by the fact that participants with obesity frequently experience symptoms of mental illness [23], and not because of their elevated weight.

In summary, dysfunctional thinking styles, known as early maladaptive schemas and cognitive distortions, have been found in individuals with eating disorders, overweight or obesity. However, it is possible that these findings are associated with the mental health status of the participants and not necessarily with their obesity. Our study thus aimed to further examine this issue. Therefore, we sought to clarify whether individuals with morbid obesity show higher levels of dysfunctional cognitions than individuals of normal weight, and if so, if this is related to their individual mental health condition. Ultimately, this understanding could aid in the development of effective psychological and behavioral assessments and subsequent interventions, tailored specifically for individuals with morbid obesity.

2. Methods

2.1. Ethical Considerations

The study was conducted in accordance with the Declaration of Helsinki. This project was approved by the Research Ethics Committees of the Pontifical Catholic University of Rio Grande do Sul (Brazil) (CAAE: 07888612.4.0000.5336) and the Conceição Hospital Group where the participants were assessed. Informed consent was obtained from participants.

2.2. Participants

Participants were included if they had morbid obesity (BMI $\geq$ 40 kg/m^2) or normal weight (BMI: 18.5–24.9 kg/m^2) [24], were aged between 18 and 65 years, and had at least five years of education. The exclusion criterion was low cognitive performance (score $\leq$ 23) as assessed by the Mini Mental State Examination (MMSE) [25], as this could compromise comprehension and hence the accuracy in answering questionnaires. Two potential participants were excluded from the study because of this criterion.

There were 111 participants in this study, 53 (47.7%) with morbid obesity and 58 (52.3%) of normal weight. Participants with morbid obesity were recruited from the hospital bariatric surgery clinic and were classified as such by the medical team. Participants of normal weight were recruited through advertisements within the hospital. Participants' weight and height were recorded based on self-report. The groups were comparable with regards to sex, age, education, marital status and economic criteria of participants (see Table 1). Participants were not compensated for their participation in this research.

Table 1. Demographic details and body mass index of the participants with morbid obesity versus participants of normal weight.

Variables	Group				p
	Morbid Obesity (n = 53)		Normal Weight (n = 58)		
	n	%	n	%	
Sex					
Female	41	77.4	45	77.6	>0.999 $^{\Phi}$
Male	12	22.6	13	22.4	
Age (years)					
Mean ± standard deviation (range)	42.3 ± 9.6 (25–59)		38.7 ± 13.9 (18–65)		0.072 $^{£}$
Median (interquartile range)	42.0 (35.0–42.5)		38.5 (26.0–52.0)		
Highest education completed					

Table 1. *Cont.*

Variables	Group				p
	Morbid Obesity (n = 53)		Normal Weight (n = 58)		
	n	%	n	%	
Primary	24	45.3	24	41.4	0.678 ¶
Secondary/Tertiary	29	54.7	34	58.6	
Marital status					
Single	12	22.6	18	31.0	
Married	36	67.9	36	62.1	0.580 ¶
Separated/Divorced/Widowed	5	9.4	4	6.9	
Brazilian economic criteria					
Highest affluence	24	45.3	36	62.1	0.089 ¶
Lowest affluence)	29	54.7	22	37.9	
Body mass index (kg/m^2)					
Mean ± standard deviation	48.9 ± 6.3		22.1 ± 1.8		

Φ: Pearson's chi-square test with continuity correction; £: Students t-test for independent groups; ¶: Fisher's Exact Test for Monte Carlo simulation.

2.3. *Questionnaires and Interviews*

All questionnaires and interviews were conducted or overseen by the first author, in the bariatric surgery clinic of the hospital. The assessments of participants with morbid obesity occurred before bariatric surgery.

2.3.1. Mini Mental State Examination (MMSE)

The MMSE was used to assess mental state and cognitive deficits in potential participants [25]. The questions in this examination are divided into seven categories to assess specific cognitive functions: time orientation, place orientation, attention, basic calculation, word recognition and memorization, language and visual ability. The scores for examination can range from 0 to 30 points, with scores equal to or higher than 24 indicating normal cognition [25].

2.3.2. Young Schema Questionnaire (YSQ)

The YSQ is a self-report questionnaire that aims to identify the occurrence of early maladaptive schemas. This questionnaire has been used for research into core beliefs associated with psychological disturbances [26]. It is available in both a long and short version (205 and 75 items, respectively). Both versions of the YSQ have good psychometric properties, as indicated by statistically significant internal consistency [1]. Indeed, Cronbach's alpha is greater than 0.80 for each of the subscales on both versions [27]. The questionnaire's short form (YSQ-S2) was validated for use in Brazil (Cronbach's alpha = 0.95) [28] and was used in this study. The YSQ-S2 consists of a 75-item questionnaire assessing 15 types of early maladaptive schemas (groups of 5 items assess each of the 15 schemas). Participants are asked to answer the degree that they emotionally feel that the statements describe them according to the following options: 1—Completely untrue of me; 2—Mostly untrue of me; 3—Slightly more true than untrue; 4—Moderately true of me; 5—Mostly true of me and 6—Describes me perfectly. High scores in the items that relate to a specific early maladaptive schema indicate greater severity.

2.3.3. Cognitive Distortions Questionnaire (CD-Quest)

The CD-Quest is a self-report questionnaire that assesses a combination of the last week's frequency (no, occasional, much of the time or almost all of the time) and intensity (no, a little, much or very much) with which participants engaged in 15 common types of cognitive distortions [29]. Participants can score from 0 to 5 in each cognitive distortion, with higher scores indicating greater occurrence of the cognitive distortion. This instrument has been validated in Brazil and was found to have robust psychometric properties (Cronbach's alpha = 0.85) [30].

2.3.4. Depression, Anxiety and Stress Scale (DASS-21)

The DASS-21 measures symptoms of depression, anxiety and psychological stress in clinical and nonclinical groups. It has good internal consistency and concurrent validity [31]. In the current study, the short version with 21 items was used. This instrument has adequate internal consistency, with a Cronbach's alpha of 0.94 for the depression scale, 0.87 for the anxiety scale and 0.91 for the stress scale [31]. The DASS-21 has been validated for use in Brazil and the following Cronbach's alpha values were found for the depression, anxiety and stress scales, respectively: 0.92, 0.86 and 0.90 [32]. The DASS-21 provides specific scores for depression, anxiety and stress. Higher scores indicate greater severity of the symptoms.

2.3.5. Demographic and Clinical Questionnaire

Demographic and clinical features were assessed by a structured interview developed for this study. Questions included date of birth, marital status, education level, economic status, and use of psychiatric medications. The Brazilian Economic Criteria were used to classify economic status according to the following categories (highest to lowest affluence): A, B, C, D and E [33], computed from quantification of household assets and income.

2.4. Statistical Analysis

Descriptive statistics were used to describe the results in terms of absolute and relative distribution, as well as central tendency and variability measures. Age distribution was compared using the Kolmogorov-Smirnov test [34].

For bivariate analysis of categorical variables, the Pearson's chi-square test ($\chi 2$) was used. Fisher's exact test was performed in contingency tables where at least 25% of cell values presented an expected frequency of less than 5. Monte Carlo simulation was used when at least one variable had polytomous characteristics. For correlational analysis of continuous variables, the Spearman ranked correlations test (Spearman rho, r_s) was employed because of non-normality of data. For between-group comparisons of non-parametric ordinal or continuous variables, the Mann-Whitney U test was used.

On data inspection, all early maladaptive schemas and cognitive distortions correlated significantly with levels of depression, anxiety and stress as measured with the DASS-21 (all $r_s > 0.40$, all $p > 0.001$). Thus, Multivariable logistic regression analysis was applied to test the strength of association between the dependent variable (obesity, using binary yes/no, with the reference category being 'participants with obesity') and independent variables (early maladaptive schemas and cognitive distortions) that were found to be significant or approaching significance at a level of 5% when univariate tests were performed and adjusted for levels of depression, anxiety and stress. A significance level of $p < 0.05$ was employed for all tests. Analyses were conducted using the SPSS for Windows version 20 (Armonk, NY, USA).

3. Results

3.1. Early Maladaptive Schemas in Participants with Morbid Obesity Versus Participants of Normal Weight

As shown in Table 2, scores for the early maladaptive schema of insufficient self-control/self-discipline were significantly higher in participants with morbid obesity compared to participants of normal weight, as assessed using the YSQ-S2. High scores on this early maladaptive schema indicate beliefs of insufficient control over emotions or impulses and beliefs of not having enough capacity to deal with boredom or frustration in order to complete tasks [1]. There were no other statistically significant differences between participants with morbid obesity and participants of normal weight with respect to scores on early maladaptive schemas (see Table 2).

Table 2. Early maladaptive schemas as assessed by the YSQ-S2 in participants with morbid obesity versus participants of normal weight.

YSQ-S	Groups						p §
	Morbid Obesity (n = 53)			Normal Weight (n = 58)			
	Mean	Standard Deviation	Median	Mean	Standard Deviation	Median	
Emotional deprivation	2.5	1.5	2.0	2.0	1.3	1.5	0.08
Abandonment/instability	2.6	1.6	2.0	2.5	1.6	1.6	0.44
Mistrust/abuse	2.4	1.5	2.0	2.2	1.3	1.8	0.58
Social isolation/alienation	2.0	1.4	1.4	1.9	1.3	1.3	0.57
Defectiveness/shame	1.5	1.2	1.0	1.3	0.8	1.0	0.77
Failure	1.7	1.2	1.2	1.6	1.0	1.2	0.72
Dependence/incompetence	1.7	1.1	1.2	1.5	0.7	1.4	0.91
Vulnerability to harm	2.0	1.2	1.6	2.1	1.3	1.6	0.86
Enmeshment	1.7	1.0	1.2	2.0	1.2	1.7	0.16
Subjugation	1.8	1.1	1.4	1.8	1.2	1.2	0.53
Self-sacrifice	4.1	1.5	4.2	3.7	1.6	3.9	0.29
Emotional inhibition	2.5	1.6	1.8	1.9	1.2	1.6	0.11
Unrelenting standards	3.1	1.5	3.0	2.7	1.1	2.5	0.15
Entitlement/grandiosity	2.6	1.4	2.4	2.3	1.2	1.8	0.22
Insufficient self-control/self-discipline	2.5	1.4	2.4	2.0	1.2	1.6	0.01

YSQ-S: Young Schema Questionnaire—short form. §: Values compared using the Mann-Whitney U test.

3.2. Cognitive Distortions in Participants with Morbid Obesity Versus Participants of Normal Weight

Participants with morbid obesity showed a statistical trend ($p = 0.05$) for higher scores on the cognitive distortion of labeling in comparison with participants of normal weight (see Table 3). Labeling is a type of cognitive distortion that occurs when someone gives derogatory or demeaning names to themselves or others (e.g., "I am a failure") [29]. There were no other statistically significant differences between participants with morbid obesity and participants of normal weight, with respect to scores on cognitive distortions.

Table 3. Cognitive distortions as assessed by the CD-Quest in participants with morbid obesity versus participants of normal weight.

CD-Quest (¥)	Group						p §
	Morbid Obesity (n = 53)			Normal Weight (n = 58)			
	Mean	Standard Deviation	Median	Mean	Standard Deviation	Median	
All-or-nothing thinking	1.5	1.9	0.0	1.3	1.7	0.0	0.60
Fortune-telling	1.2	1.7	0.0	1.1	1.5	0.0	0.91
Disqualifying	0.5	1.0	0.0	0.5	1.2	0.0	0.45
Emotional reasoning	1.9	2.0	1.0	1.8	1.8	1.0	0.93
Labeling	1.4	1.7	1.0	0.8	1.3	0.0	0.05
Magnification/minimization	0.8	1.3	0.0	0.7	1.3	0.0	0.67
Mental filter	0.9	1.5	0.0	1.1	1.5	0.0	0.22
Mind reading	1.3	1.5	1.0	1.1	1.6	0.0	0.39
Overgeneralization	1.0	1.5	0.0	1.2	1.6	0.0	0.37
Personalization	0.8	1.4	0.0	0.8	1.2	0.0	0.58
Should statements	2.4	1.9	2.0	1.9	1.7	2.0	0.21
Jumping to conclusions	1.4	1.8	1.0	1.4	1.6	1.0	0.69
Blaming	1.6	1.9	1.0	1.3	1.7	0.0	0.45
What if...?	1.4	1.9	0.0	1.8	1.9	1.0	0.30
Unfair comparisons	1.2	1.8	0.0	1.0	1.5	0.0	0.98
CD-Quest Total	19.1	15.7	16.0	17.7	14.4	15.0	0.74

CD-Quest: Cognitive Distortions Questionnaire. §: Values compared using the Mann-Whitney U test; ¥: Asymmetrically distributed variable.

3.3. Depression, Anxiety and Stress Symptoms in Participants with Morbid Obesity Versus Participants of Normal Weight

No significant differences between groups were found on scores of symptoms of depression or stress. However, participants with morbid obesity showed significantly higher scores on anxiety symptoms in comparison to participants of normal weight (see Table 4). Median and interquartile range were used (instead of mean and standard deviation) to analyze differences between participants with morbid obesity and participants of normal weight, because data on levels of depression, anxiety and stress were highly skewed.

Table 4. Levels of depression, anxiety and stress scores on the DASS-21 in participants with morbid obesity compared to participants of normal weight.

DASS-21	Group		Z, p
	Morbid Obesity (n = 53)	Normal Weight (n = 58)	
Depression			
Mean ± standard deviation	9.7 ± 10.2 (0–40.0)	7.3 ± 9.9 (0–42.0)	
Median (interquartile range)	6.0 (2.0–14.0)	4.0 (0–10.5)	−1.58, 0.14
Anxiety			
Mean ± standard deviation (range)	12.6 ± 11.9 (0–42.0)	8.1 ± 10.1 (0–42.0)	
Median (interquartile range)	8.0 (2.0–23.0)	4.0 (0–12.5)	−2.37, 0.018
Stress			
Mean ± standard deviation (range)	16.1 ± 13.4 (0–42.0)	13.1 ± 11.1 (0–42.0)	
Median (interquartile range)	14.0 (4.0–30.0)	9.0 (3.5–20.0)	−0.953, 0.34

Z = Z score from the Mann-Whitney U test, conducted on the non-parametric median and interquartile range statistics.

3.4. Comparative Analysis by Binary Logistic Regression to Predict Morbid Obesity

Logistic regression analysis revealed that the difference in scores of the early maladaptive schema of insufficient self-control/self-discipline between participants with morbid obesity and participants of normal weight was no longer significant when adjustment was made for levels of depression, anxiety and stress. The difference in scores of the cognitive distortion of labeling between participants with morbid obesity and participants of normal weight however was significant when adjustment was made for levels of depression, anxiety and stress (see Table 5).

Table 5. Results of multivariable (logistic regression) analysis with presence or absence of morbid obesity as dependent variable * (Model Nagelkerke R^2 = 0.15).

Predictor (Independent) Variable	Exp (B)	95% Confidence Interval	p
Early maladaptive schema: insufficient self-control/self-discipline	0.70	0.47; 1.05	0.09
Cogntive distortion: Labelling	0.69	0.49; 0.96	0.03
Anxiety	0.92	0.85; 0.99	0.03
Depression	1.05	0.97; 1.13	0.25
Stress	1.06	0.99; 1.13	0.10

* The reference category (specified as 'participants with obesity') is such that a value of Exp (B) (also referred to as the odds ratio) of less than 1 implies that the predictor variable is higher in participants with obesity.

3.5. Psychiatric Medication Use in Participants with Morbid Obesity Versus Participants of Normal Weight

Data from the demographic and clinical questionnaire showed that the group of participants with morbid obesity had a significantly higher number of users of psychiatric medication at the time of the assessment in comparison to participants of normal weight (28 out of 53 or 54% of participants with morbid obesity versus 8 out of 58 or 14% of the participants of normal weight, χ^2 = 19.98, p < 0.001).

4. Discussion

The main aim of this study was to compare the occurrence of early maladaptive schemas and cognitive distortions in participants with morbid obesity versus those of normal weight, and to examine if mental health status could influence potential differences between groups in the occurrence of these dysfunctional cognitions. Higher occurrences of the early maladaptive schema of insufficient self-control/self-discipline and a statistical trend towards higher occurrence of the cognitive distortion of labeling were found in participants with morbid obesity compared to participants of normal weight. However, after controlling for symptoms of depression, of anxiety, and stress, participants with morbid obesity and participants of normal weight did not differ statistically in regards to scores on early maladaptive schemas. These findings support a previous study that found that an individual's responses in the YSQ-S are influenced by their emotional state while completing the questionnaire [35].

Furthermore, even before controlling for mental health status, the statistical differences of early maladaptive schemas and cognitive distortions found amongst participants with morbid obesity compared to participants of normal weight were small (1 out of 15 types of early maladaptive schemas and 1 out of 15 types of cognitive distortions). These are slight differences that may have been found due to chance. These findings do not indicate significant clinical differences in the occurrence of dysfunctional cognitions between those with morbid obesity and those of a normal weight.

We did not find statistically significant differences between participants with morbid obesity and participants of normal weight in regards to symptoms of depression and stress. However, significant differences were found in the presence of anxiety symptoms between groups. These findings contradict a systematic review and meta-analysis that found an association between obesity and depression, particularly amongst women [36]. The levels of depression symptoms in the participants with morbid obesity in our sample were possibly low since more than half (54%) of our participants with morbid obesity were being treated with psychiatric medication at the time of the assessment. Although stress-induced eating habits seem to have an important role in the development of obesity [37], in our study, no differences in the level of stress symptoms were found between groups. Our findings regarding the higher anxiety symptoms amongst participants with morbid obesity are consistent with the outcomes from a systematic review and meta-analysis that found a positive association between anxiety disorders and obesity [38]. A previous study found that individuals with obesity, especially those with comorbid binge eating disorders, tend to eat in response to unpleasant emotional states [39].

An additional finding of our study is that the participants with morbid obesity used significantly more psychiatric medication than the participants of normal weight. This may have been influenced by the fact that the participants with morbid obesity were patients of the bariatric surgery clinic and therefore were regularly seen by the medical team, and such medical attention did not necessarily occur for participants of normal weight. This finding is compatible with a previous study [40] that found high psychiatric medication use amongst individuals with morbid obesity (40.7% of their sample). A controversial issue regarding the prescription of psychiatric medication for individuals with morbid obesity is the effect of these medicines on weight. A recent systematic review reported that body fat accumulation is a common side effect of psychotropic medication [41]. Therefore, it is possible that the higher use of psychiatric medication contributed to the excess weight of the participants with morbid obesity, albeit this was not the focus of the current study.

The current findings have relevance to clinical practice. Lifestyle interventions aimed at promoting healthy eating habits and appropriate levels of physical activity are routinely recommended for people with morbid obesity, due to their role in reducing the medical complications related to morbid obesity and in improving psychological health [42]. However, further psychological therapy may be required for some individuals with morbid obesity. Their mental health status should be assessed, and those with depression, anxiety and/or psychological distress may be considered for further assessment of early maladaptive schemas and cognitive distortions and these (if present) may need to be addressed with specific psychotherapy, such as cognitive and/or schema therapy [1,8].

Limitations of this study include the use of self-report assessment of early maladaptive schemas and cognitive distortions, as some people may have difficulty identifying their own dysfunctional thoughts [43]. A second limitation is that participants with morbid obesity may have tried to express socially desirable responses in an attempt to allay social stigma [44], or for fear of a psychological evaluation that could deny or delay their referral for bariatric surgery [45] (although they were told that their responses would be confidential). A third limitation of this study is that types of psychiatric medication used by the participants, psychotherapeutic treatment and psychiatric diagnosis were not assessed. Future research in this field should include participants with obesity that are not seeking treatment, and examine causal effects of anxiety symptoms and use of psychiatric drugs amongst individuals with morbid obesity.

5. Conclusions

In conclusion, higher occurrence of dysfunctional cognitions (the early maladaptive schema of insufficient self-control/self-discipline and the cognitive distortion of labeling) amongst participants with morbid obesity in comparison to participants of normal weight was small and the early maladaptive schema of insufficient self-control/self-discipline was no longer statistically significant once symptoms of depression, anxiety and stress were controlled for. Dysfunctional cognitions presented by individuals with morbid obesity are probably related to their individual mental health status and not to their weight disorder.

Acknowledgments: This work was supported by the CAPES Foundation, Ministry of Education of Brazil, via scholarships to Felipe Quinto da Luz and via the National Health and Medical Research Council (NHMRC) of Australia via a Project Grant and Senior Research Fellowship to Amanda Sainsbury. Our thanks also go to Sanja Lujic for statistical advice.

Author Contributions: Felipe Quinto da Luz and Margareth da Silva Oliveira conceived and designed the study. Felipe Quinto da Luz collected the data. Felipe Quinto da Luz, Amanda Sainsbury, Phillipa Hay, Jessica Ann Roekenes, Jessica Swinbourne, Dhiordan Cardoso da Silva and Margareth da Silva Oliveira analyzed the data and wrote the paper.

Conflicts of Interest: Amanda Sainsbury has received payment from Eli Lilly, the Pharmacy Guild of Australia, Novo Nordisk and the Dietitians Association of Australia for seminar presentation at conferences, and has served on the Nestlé Health Science Optifast®VLCD™ Advisory Board since 2016. She is also the author of The Don't go Hungry Diet (Bantam, Australia and New Zealand, 2007) and Don't go Hungry for Life (Bantam, Australia and New Zealand, 2011). Phillipa Hay receives royalties from Hogrefe and Huber and McGrawHill Publishers.

References

1. Young, J.E.; Klosko, J.S.; Weishaar, M.E. *Schema Therapy: A Practitioner's Guide*; Guilford Publications: New York, NY, USA, 2003.
2. Unoka, Z.; Tölgyes, T.; Czobor, P. Early Maladaptive Schemas and Body Mass Index in Subgroups of Eating Disorders: A Differential Association. *Compr. Psychiatry* **2007**, *48*, 199–204. [CrossRef] [PubMed]
3. Anderson, K.; Rieger, E.; Caterson, I. A Comparison of Maladaptive Schemata in Treatment-Seeking Obese Adults and Normal-Weight Control Subjects. *J. Psychosom. Res.* **2006**, *60*, 245–252. [CrossRef] [PubMed]
4. Poursharifi, H.; Bidadian, M.; Bahramizadeh, H.; Salehinezhad, M.A. The Relationship between Early Maladaptive Schemas and Aspects of Identity in Obesity. *Procedia Soc. Behav. Sci.* **2011**, *30*, 517–523. [CrossRef]
5. Vlierberghe, L.V.; Braet, C. Dysfunctional Schemas and Psychopathology in Referred Obese Adolescents. *Clin. Psychol. Psychother.* **2007**, *14*, 342–351. [CrossRef]
6. Turner, H.M.; Rose, K.S.; Cooper, M.J. Schema and Parental Bonding in Overweight and Nonoverweight Female Adolescents. *Int. J. Obes. Relat. Metab. Disord.* **2005**, *29*, 381–387. [CrossRef] [PubMed]
7. Vlierberghe, L.V.; Braet, C.; Goossens, L. Dysfunctional Schemas and Eating Pathology in Overweight Youth: A Case–Control Study. *Int. J. Eat. Disord.* **2009**, *42*, 437–442. [CrossRef] [PubMed]
8. Beck, J.S. *Cognitive Therapy: Basics and Beyond*; Guilford Press: New York, NY, USA, 1995.
9. Beck, J.S. *The Beck Diet Solution: Train Your Brain to Think Like a Thin Person*; Oxmoor House, Inc.: New York, NY, USA, 2012.
10. Byrne, S.M.; Cooper, Z.; Fairburn, C.G. Psychological Predictors of Weight Regain in Obesity. *Behav. Res. Ther.* **2004**, *42*, 1341–1356. [CrossRef] [PubMed]
11. Coelho, J.S.; Jansen, A.; Bouvard, M. Cognitive Distortions in Normal-Weight and Overweight Women: Susceptibility to Thought-Shape Fusion. *Cognit. Ther. Res.* **2012**, *36*, 417–425. [CrossRef]
12. Coelho, J.S.; Siggen, M.J.; Dietre, P.; Bouvard, M. Reactivity to Thought–Shape Fusion in Adolescents: The Effects of Obesity Status. *Pediatr. Obes.* **2013**, *8*, 439–444. [CrossRef] [PubMed]
13. Volery, M.; Carrard, I.; Rouget, P.; Archinard, M.; Golay, A. Cognitive Distortions in Obese Patients with or without Eating Disorders. *Eat. Weight Disord.* **2006**, *11*, 123–126. [CrossRef]
14. Ramacciotti, C.E.; Elisabetta, C.; Bondi, E.; Burgalassi, A.; Massimetti, G.; Dell'Osso, L. Shared Psychopathology in Obese Subjects with and without Binge-Eating Disorder. *Int. J. Eat. Disord.* **2008**, *41*, 643–649. [CrossRef] [PubMed]

15. Halvorsen, M.; Wang, C.E.; Eisemann, M.; Waterloo, K. Dysfunctional Attitudes and Early Maladaptive Schemas as Predictors of Depression: A 9-Year Follow-up Study. *Cognit. Ther. Res.* **2010**, *34*, 368–379. [CrossRef]
16. Hawke, L.D.; Provencher, M.D. Early Maladaptive Schemas: Relationship with Case Complexity in Mood and Anxiety Disorders. *J. Cogn. Psychother.* **2013**, *27*, 359–369. [CrossRef]
17. Cámara, M.; Calvete, E. Early Maladaptive Schemas as Moderators of the Impact of Stressful Events on Anxiety and Depression in University Students. *J. Psychopathol. Behav. Assess.* **2012**, *34*, 58–68. [CrossRef]
18. Bamber, M.; McMahon, R. Danger-Early Maladaptive Schemas at Work!: The Role of Early Maladaptive Schemas in Career Choice and the Development of Occupational Stress in Health Workers. *Clin. Psychol. Psychother.* **2008**, *15*, 96–112. [CrossRef] [PubMed]
19. Leung, P.W.L.; Poon, M.W.L. Dysfunctional Schemas and Cognitive Distortions in Psychopathology: A Test of the Specificity Hypothesis. *J. Child Psychol. Psychiatry* **2011**, *42*, 755–765. [CrossRef]
20. Bartczak, M.; Bokus, B. Cognitive Representations (Metaphorical Conceptualizations) of Past, Future, Joy, Sadness and Happiness in Depressive and Non-Depressive Subjects: Cognitive Distortions in Depression at the Level of Notion. *J. Psycholinguist. Res.* **2015**, *44*, 159–185. [CrossRef] [PubMed]
21. Weems, C.F.; Berman, S.L.; Silverman, W.K.; Saavedra, L.M. Cognitive Errors in Youth with Anxiety Disorders: The Linkages between Negative Cognitive Errors and Anxious Symptoms. *Cognit. Ther. Res.* **2001**, *25*, 559–575. [CrossRef]
22. Beck, A.T. The Evolution of the Cognitive Model of Depression and Its Neurobiological Correlates. *Am. J. Psychiatry* **2008**, *165*, 969–977. [CrossRef] [PubMed]
23. Müller, A.; Mitchell, J.E.; Sondag, C.; de Zwaan, M. Psychiatric Aspects of Bariatric Surgery. *Curr. Psychiatry Rep.* **2013**, *15*, 1–8. [CrossRef] [PubMed]
24. World Health Organization. *Obesity: Preventing and Managing the Global Epidemic: Report of a WHO Consultation*; World Health Organization Technichal Report Series: Geneva, Switzerland, 2000.
25. Folstein, M.F.; Folstein, S.E.; McHugh, P.R. "Mini-Mental State". A Practical Method for Grading the Cognitive State of Patients for the Clinician. *J. Psychiat. Res.* **1975**, *12*, 189–198. [CrossRef]
26. Renner, F.; Lobbestael, J.; Peeters, F.; Arntz, A.; Huibers, M. Early Maladaptive Schemas in Depressed Patients: Stability and Relation with Depressive Symptoms over the Course of Treatment. *J. Affect. Disord.* **2012**, *136*, 581–590. [CrossRef] [PubMed]
27. Waller, G.; Meyer, C.; Ohanian, V. Psychometric Properties of the Long and Short Versions of the Young Schema Questionnaire: Core Beliefs among Bulimic and Comparison Women. *Cognit. Ther. Res.* **2001**, *25*, 137–147. [CrossRef]
28. Cazassa, M.; Oliveira, M. Validação Brasileira Do Questionário De Esquemas De Young: Forma Breve. *Estud. Psicol.* **2012**, *29*, 23–31. [CrossRef]
29. De Oliveira, I.R. *Trial-Based Cognitive Therapy: A Manual for Clinicians*; Routledge: London, UK, 2014; pp. 28–35.
30. De Oliveira, I.R.; Seixas, C.; Osório, F.L.; Crippa, J.A.S.; Abreu, J.N.; Menezes, I.G.; Pidgeon, A.; Sudak, D.; Wenzel, A. Evaluation of the Psychometric Properties of the Cognitive Distortions Questionnaire (Cd-Quest) in a Sample of Undergraduate Students. *Innov. Clin. Neurosci.* **2015**, *12*, 20–27. [PubMed]
31. Antony, M.M.; Bieling, P.J.; Cox, B.J.; Enns, M.W.; Swinson, R.P. Psychometric Properties of the 42-Item and 21-Item Versions of the Depression Anxiety Stress Scales in Clinical Groups and a Community Sample. *Psychol. Assess.* **1998**, *10*, 176–181. [CrossRef]
32. Vignola, R.C.B.; Tucci, A.M. Adaptation and Validation of the Depression, Anxiety and Stress Scale (Dass) to Brazilian Portuguese. *J. Affect. Disord.* **2014**, *155*, 104–109. [CrossRef] [PubMed]
33. Associação Brasileira de Empresas de Pesquisa. Critério De Classificação Econômica Brasil. Available online: www.abep.org/Servicos/Download.aspx?id=07 (accessed on 3 November 2016).
34. Everitt, B.; Dunn, G. *Applied Multivariate Data Analysis*; Wiley: London, UK, 1991.
35. Stopa, L.; Waters, A. The Effect of Mood on Responses to the Young Schema Questionnaire: Short Form. *Psychol. Psychother.* **2005**, *78*, 45–57. [CrossRef] [PubMed]
36. De Wit, L.; Luppino, F.; van Straten, A.; Penninx, B.; Zitman, F.; Cuijpers, P. Depression and Obesity: A Meta-Analysis of Community-Based Studies. *Psychiatry Res.* **2010**, *178*, 230–235. [CrossRef] [PubMed]
37. Dallman, M.F. Stress-Induced Obesity and the Emotional Nervous System. *Trends Endocrinol. Metab.* **2010**, *21*, 159–165. [CrossRef] [PubMed]

38. Gariepy, G.; Nitka, D.; Schmitz, N. The Association between Obesity and Anxiety Disorders in the Population: A Systematic Review and Meta-Analysis. *Int. J. Obes.* **2010**, *34*, 407–419. [CrossRef] [PubMed]
39. Zeeck, A.; Stelzer, N.; Linster, H.W.; Joos, A.; Hartmann, A. Emotion and Eating in Binge Eating Disorder and Obesity. *Eur. Eat. Disord. Rev.* **2011**, *19*, 426–437. [CrossRef] [PubMed]
40. Mitchell, J.E.; Selzer, F.; Kalarchian, M.A.; Devlin, M.J.; Strain, G.W.; Elder, K.A.; Marcus, M.D.; Wonderlich, S.; Christian, N.J.; Yanovski, S.Z. Psychopathology before Surgery in the Longitudinal Assessment of Bariatric Surgery-3 (Labs-3) Psychosocial Study. *Surg. Obes. Relat. Dis.* **2012**, *8*, 533–541. [CrossRef] [PubMed]
41. Dent, R.; Blackmore, A.; Peterson, J.; Habib, R.; Kay, G.P.; Gervais, A.; Taylor, V.; Wells, G. Changes in Body Weight and Psychotropic Drugs: A Systematic Synthesis of the Literature. *PLoS ONE* **2012**, *7*, e36889. [CrossRef] [PubMed]
42. Stanton, R.; Reaburn, P. Exercise and the Treatment of Depression: A Review of the Exercise Program Variables. *J. Sci. Med. Sport* **2014**, *17*, 177–182. [CrossRef] [PubMed]
43. Beck, A.T. *Cognitive Therapy of Depression*; Guilford Press: New York, NY, USA, 1979.
44. Lee, L.; Shapiro, C.M. Psychological Manifestations of Obesity. *J. Psychosom. Res.* **2003**, *55*, 477–479. [CrossRef]
45. Ambwani, S.; Boeka, A.G.; Brown, J.D.; Byrne, T.K.; Budak, A.R.; Sarwer, D.B.; Fabricatore, A.N.; Morey, L.C.; O'Neil, P.M. Socially Desirable Responding by Bariatric Surgery Candidates During Psychological Assessment. *Surg. Obes. Relat. Diseas.* **2013**, *9*, 300–305. [CrossRef] [PubMed]

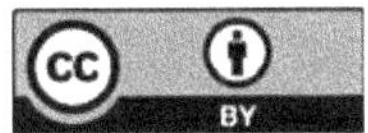

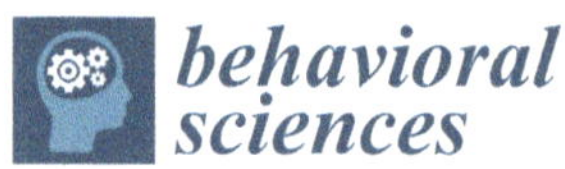
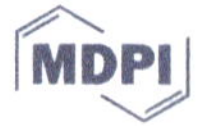

Article

Food Addiction, Binge Eating Disorder, and Obesity: Is There a Relationship?

Tracy Burrows [1,2,*], Janelle Skinner [1,2], Rebecca McKenna [1,2] and Megan Rollo [1,2]

1 School of Health Sciences, Faculty of Health and Medicine, University of Newcastle, Callaghan 2308, Australia; Janelle.skinner@uon.edu.au (J.S.); Rebecca.Mckenna@uon.edu.au (R.M.); megan.rollo@newcastle.edu.au (M.R.)
2 Priority Research Centre for Physical Activity and Nutrition, University of Newcastle, Callaghan 2308, Australia
* Correspondence: tracy.burrows@newcastle.edu.au; Tel.: +61-2-49215514

Received: 26 June 2017; Accepted: 9 August 2017; Published: 14 August 2017

Abstract: Existing research suggests that there is an overlap between binge eating disorder (BED) and the construct of 'food addiction' (FA). The objective of this study was to determine the overlapping features of BED and FA through a comparison of the individual scales of commonly used tools including the Binge Eating Scale (BES) and the Yale Food Addiction Scale (YFAS) in a sample of Australian adults. Adults (>18 years of age) were invited to complete an anonymous online survey on FA. Binge eating was assessed through the BES and addictive eating behaviours were assessed through the YFAS (n = 1344). The prevalence and severity of both FA and binge eating increased across weight categories. The overall correlation between the total score from the BES and FA symptoms was $r = 0.76$, $p < 0.001$; for females it was $r = 0.77$, $p < 0.001$, and for males it was $r = 0.65$, $p < 0.001$. Total BES score and the BES emotion factor were most often associated with FA symptoms, as was demonstrated to produce stronger correlations with FA symptoms. In contrast, the BES behaviour factor was less strongly associated to FA with the majority of correlations <0.6. This study demonstrates the overlap between BED and FA, and highlights the possible unique differences between the forms of disordered eating.

Keywords: binge eating; food addiction

1. Introduction

'Food addiction' (FA) presents as a contentious construct, which has yet to gain scientific acceptance due to an overall lack of high quality research [1]. There is scientific debate about the appropriateness of terminology, with 'eating addiction' previously proposed to be more reflective rather than 'food addiction', given the uncertainty of whether addictive eating behaviours more closely align to substance-based addictions, like drug and alcohol addictions, or with behavioural addictions, such as gambling addiction [2]. Addictions to drugs, alcohol, and gambling are formally recognised in the Diagnostic Statistics Manual, version 5 (DSM-5) [2]. However, FA is currently not a recognised condition in DSM and instead is characterised through the assessment and endorsement of addiction-like symptoms through self-report tools or surveys. The most commonly used tool is the Yale Food Addiction Scale (YFAS). Originally developed in 2009 and revised in 2016, the YFAS 2.0 maps to the criteria used to classify substance dependence [3]. The YFAS tool assesses 11 symptoms of addiction, as well the level of distress associated with them, which parallel other addiction symptoms in DSM such as tolerance and craving. In addition, the tool can determine the level of severity of addiction ranging from mild to severe [4].

There has been previous suggestion that FA may be a sub-type of disordered eating, and that the FA construct is an indicator of higher eating disorder severity [5]. Research suggests that FA does show overlap with several disordered eating phenotypes, with the majority of existing research investigating binge eating disorder (BED) and bulimia nervosa rather than other disordered eating categories such as anorexia nervosa [6,7].

BED is classified by the DSM-5 as the recurrent, periodic, and uncontrolled consumption of large quantities of food without compensatory behaviours (e.g., purging, laxative use) to control weight [8]. It has been estimated that BED affects approximately 2% of the global population [9], while FA affects approximately 20%, with both conditions found to be more common in females [1,10]. The prevalence of FA in two existing studies of individuals with diagnosed BED was 41.5% and 56.8% [11,12]. The prevalence of FA in individuals with a current diagnosis of bulimia nervosa was 83.6% and 100%, and 30% of individuals with a history of bulimia nervosa met the diagnostic criteria for FA [13,14]. In a more recent study of individuals with clinical BED assessed through an objective clinical interview rather than self-report, those with BED were also identified with FA (33.8%). Existing research suggests an overlap between these conditions, often through cross-sectional studies, which show that the overlap between BED and FA varies between 0.59 and 0.78) [1]. The overlap between BED and FA however is not 100%, and while binge eating is a key eating disorder feature, the association between FA and disordered eating behaviour is unclear. It is acknowledged that the symptoms of general psychological distress found to be associated with FA are strongly associated with binge eating and other eating disorder symptoms [15,16].

Similarities in symptomology that exist between FA and BED include the consumption of larger amounts of food than intended, reduced control over eating and continued use despite negative consequences [13,17], intense cravings [18], emotional dysregulation, and increased impulsivity [5,6,19]. Due to these similarities, it is not unusual that BED and FA are often highly correlated. A meta-analysis also reported that YFAS symptom scores were positively associated with binge eating behaviours [1].

Existing research has investigated FA specifically in binge eating populations and individuals seeking bariatric surgery, and identified similarities in the specific characteristics of both conditions when assessed by validated surveys [20,21]. In addition, recent research highlights the associations between patterns of compulsive overeating, including binge eating with 'food addiction' [22]. However, these conditions have not been investigated at the scale, factor, or item level of common assessment scales. Instead previous research has explored associations in absolute scores that indicate the overall severity of FA or BED. Investigating factor levels for these constructs may provide important information about where the overlapping features exist and whether there are factors which separate these conditions. Strong correlations would be expected between subscales that may map to the same attribute, and lower correlations between subscales from different attributes. Therefore, the current study aims to determine the overlapping features of BED and FA through a comparison of the individual constructs of the Binge Eating Scale (BES) and YFAS in a sample of Australian adults.

2. Materials and Methods

Participants aged 18 years or above and living in Australia were invited to complete an anonymous online survey on FA. The survey took approximately 20 min to complete. Exclusion criteria included being pregnant/currently lactating and being unable to comprehend English. Recruitment was undertaken over a three month period in 2016. The study was advertised through University of Newcastle media releases and promoted via a variety of social media platforms (i.e., Facebook, Twitter). The advertisements contained a link to the survey, and participants provided informed consent before completing the survey. Survey completers were invited to enter a prize draw to win 1 of 10 shopping vouchers ($50 value). This study was approved by The University of Newcastle Ethics Committee.

The survey comprehensively assessed a range of measures relating to diet and mental health which has been previously reported [15]. The current study is a secondary analysis relating specifically to FA and BED status. Demographic information was assessed through 10 items and included information on gender, age, ethnicity, marital status, postcode, highest level of education, height, and weight, which was converted into body mass index (BMI) using standardised equations. Participants' BMI was then classified according to World Health Organisation classifications [23]. Postcode was used to determine the Index of Relative Socioeconomic Advantage and Disadvantage (ISRAD), where postcode is rated from one (most disadvantage/least advantage) to 10 (least disadvantaged/most advantaged).

FA was assessed using the 35-item YFAS 2.0 [4]. Each question offers a participant an option of eight responses ranging from 'never' to 'every day'. Each symptom is considered met when one or more of the relevant questions for each criteria meet a predefined threshold. It provides a 'diagnosis' of FA which, depending on the number of symptoms endorsed, can be classified as 'mild', 'moderate' or 'severe'. A mild diagnosis score is given when 2–3 symptoms are reported, moderate when 4–5 symptoms are present, and severe when 6 or more symptoms. Symptoms include tolerance, withdrawal, and loss of control with respect to eating behaviour. The YFAS 2.0 asks participants to think of specific foods such as highly processed foods; however, participants in this study were asked to consider all food. In the current study, the Cronbach alpha for this tool was 0.95, indicating acceptable internal consistency.

Binge eating was assessed through the standardised BES, which comprises 16 questions. Each question requires a response consisting of three to four possible responses, reflecting a range of severity. The total score is tallied to give a score out of 46, with higher scores representing increased binge status. Based on the total score, individuals can be classified as 'no binge eating' if the score is ≤ 17, 'mild to moderate binge eating' if the score is 18–26, and 'severe binge eating' if the score is >27. The BES has been previously shown to have a two-factor structure, which was originally demonstrated by Gormally et al. [24] and confirmed more recently by Kelly et al. [25]. These factors relate to (1) behavioural manifestations (eight items) including factors such as eating large amounts of food, and (2) feelings and cognitions (eight items) surrounding a binge eating episode including guilt, fear of not being able to stop eating, and preoccupation with eating. For the current study, in addition to the total score, the two-factor scores were also determined according to author instructions. The BES is not designed as a direct measure of BED [26]. In the current, study the Cronbach alpha for this tool was 0.92, indicating acceptable internal consistency.

Statistics: Descriptive statistics were undertaken, *t*-tests were used to examine differences between groups (food addicted vs. non-food addicted or females vs. males). ANOVA were used to determine differences in addiction severity (mild, moderate, severe). Correlation matrices for the scales for both YFAS and BES were undertaken. Also, Spearman and Pearson correlations were determined in the cases where data distribution was not normal. Both correlations produced similar results; associations between factors of the BES and between symptoms of the YFAS are presented using Pearson correlations. Correlations were determined as small (0.1–0.2), medium (0.3–0.5), or large (>0.6). The correlation analysis between scales used for this study has been undertaken in previous health research [27]. The results presented are for complete cases, with 869 of the 1344 respondents who started the survey having answered all questions. A missing value analysis was undertaken, and the demographics of those with missing values were compared, with no patterns identified. Therefore, there was no imputation of data for missing values. Due to the multiple statistical tests completed as part of this analysis, data were adjusted using a Bonferroni correction with a lower statistical threshold, and a statistical significance of $p < 0.01$. Data was analysed using SPSS version 22.0 (SPSS Inc., Chicago, IL, USA).

3. Results

3.1. Participants

The survey recruited $n = 1344$ individual; 80.7% were female and 19.3% were male. The demographic details can be found in Table 1. The mean ISRAD score was 6.2 ± 2.9, reflecting a moderate socioeconomic status; however, this value varied from 1–10, reflecting a moderately diverse population group. A total of 44.3% of the sample were married, 27% were never married, and 14.5% had been married but were without a current partner. The population comprised 1.6% with a trade/apprenticeship, 20% with a certificate/diploma, 36% with a university degree, and 31% with a higher education including masters, Ph.D.

3.2. Food Addiction and Binge Eating

Across the whole sample, the prevalence of FA was found to be 22.2% (n = 228). This differed significantly by gender, with females (24.4%) having a higher prevalence than males (13.3%; $p < 0.001$). According to the YFAS 2.0 categorisations of severity, the majority of individuals classified as severely food addicted 18.9% (n = 194), while 2.6% (n = 27) were moderately addicted, and <1% were classified as mild. The prevalence and severity of both FA and binge eating increased across weight categories (Table 2).

Table 1. Demographic details of samples according to food addiction status.

Demographic	NFA Male (n = 176)	FA Male (n = 27)	p Value	NFA Female (n = 624)	FA Female (n = 201)	p Value
	Mean ± SD	Mean ± SD		Mean ± SD	Mean ± SD	
Age (years)	42.0 ± 13.2	46.0 ± 16.4	0.531	39.6 ± 13.1	40.1 ± 13.0	0.407
Height (cm)	178.8 ± 0.1	179.7 ± 0.1	0.629	166.0 ± 0.1	165.9 ± 0.1	0.935
Weight (kg)	87.4 ± 15.4	113.7 ± 28.3	<0.01	70.0 ± 16.7	88.4 ± 22.9	<0.01
BMI * (kg/m^2)	27.4 ± 4.8	35.4 ± 8.8	<0.01	25.5 ± 6.0	32.7 ± 13.1	<0.01
	n = 149	n = 22		n = 517	n = 183	
BES total	7.4 ± 5.8	20.1 ± 6.1	<0.01	8.5 ± 6.5	22.8 ± 8.1	<0.01

Note: Statistically significant differences between sex determined by t-tests. NFA, non-food addicted; FA, food addicted; BES, Binge Eating Survey. BMI body mass index

Table 2. Comparison of food addiction (FA) and Binge Eating (BE) according to BMI category [a].

Condition	Underweight (n = 14)	Healthy (n = 439)	Overweight (n = 263)	Obese (n = 286)	p Value
Food Addiction (FA)	%	%	%	%	
NFA	85.7	92.5	78.7	53.8	<0.001
Mild FA	0.0	0.9	0.4	0.7	0.368
Moderate FA	7.1	1.6	3.4	3.5	0.07
Severe FA	7.1	5.0	17.5	42.0	<0.001
Binge Eating (BE)					
Non-bingeing	90.0	89.3	74.8	50.6	<0.001
Moderate	10.0	7.5	19.5	30.4	<0.001
Severe	0.0	3.2	5.8	19.0	<0.001

Note: Data are shown as percentages within each group. Statistical significance was determined using ANOVA between weight categories [a] BMI categories (kg/m^2): Underweight ≤18.50, Healthy = 18.50–24.99, Overweight = 25.00–29.99, Obese ≥30.00. FA, food addiction; NFA, non-food addicted.

For those who had completed the BES, the mean BES score was 11.9 ± 9.3 (range 0–42). For males the mean BES scores was 9.2 ± 7.4 (range 0–36), and for females the mean score was 12.6 ± 9.6 (range 0–42). The mean values for each sex were significantly different ($p < 0.01$). For the BES, severity for the total group was determined, with 74% of individuals classified as non-binge eaters (n = 660), 17.4% (n = 155) moderate binge eaters, and 8.7% (n = 78) severe binge eaters. Differences in BES severity were determined by sex, and significant differences were found between males and females. Among non-binge eaters, males accounted for 86.2% vs. females 70.9%, among moderate binge eaters it was males 12.1% vs. females 18.6%, and among severe binge eaters it was males 1.7% vs. females 10.4%, all $p < 0.01$. Individuals with FA reported significantly higher on the BES total, emotions, and behavioural scales than those who were non-food addicted (Table 3). Of those with FA, 72.7% reported scores of either moderate (41%) or severe (31.7%) bingeing compared with only 9.9% in the non-food addicted group. A significant correlation was found between the two-factor scores of behaviours and emotions of the BES: $r = 0.82$, $p < 0.001$ (Table 4).

Table 3. Comparison of BES scores and categories according to food addiction status.

Condition	NFA ($n = 666$)	FA ($n = 205$)	p Value
	Mean ± SD	Mean ± SD	
BES total	8.23 ± 6.35	22.56 ± 7.93	<0.001
BES emotions	4.05 ± 3.71	12.76 ± 4.44	<0.001
BES behaviours	4.72 ± 3.66	11.56 ± 4.75	<0.001
	%	%	
Non-bingeing	90.1	27.3	<0.001
Moderate bingeing	9.0	41.0	0.046
Severe bingeing	0.9	31.7	<0.001
Total	100.0	100.0	

Note: BES, Binge Eating Survey; NFA, Non-food addicted; FA, food addicted. Differences in BES scores determined by independent samples t-tests, differences in proportions for BES category determined by chi squares.

Table 4. Pearson correlation coefficients between the BES factors and YFAS symptoms ($n = 953$).

Measure	BES Total	BES Emotions	BES Behaviours
Binge Eating			
1. BES total	-		
2. BES emotions	0.95 ***	-	
3. BES behaviours	0.96 ***	0.82 ***	-
Food Addiction			
4. Total FA symptoms	0.76 ***	0.75 ***	0.71 ***
5. Consumed more than planned	0.24 ***	0.21 ***	0.25 ***
6. Unable to cut down or stop	0.61 ***	0.62 ***	0.55 ***
7. Great deal of time spent	0.58 ***	0.55 ***	0.56 ***
8. Activities given up or reduced	0.61 ***	0.61 ***	0.56 ***
9. Continued use despite physical/emotional consequences	0.67 ***	0.67 ***	0.60 ***
10. Tolerance	0.54 ***	0.54 ***	0.50 ***
11. Withdrawal	0.52 ***	0.52 ***	0.48 ***
12. Continued use despite social consequences	0.52 ***	0.51 ***	0.48 ***
13. Fail to fulfil roles and obligations	0.53 ***	0.53 ***	0.48 ***
14. Use in physically hazardous situations	−0.49 ***	−0.50 ***	−0.44 ***
15. Craving	0.65 ***	0.64 ***	0.59 ***
16. Impairment or distress	0.68 ***	0.70 ***	0.61 ***

*** $p < 0.001$. Shading indicates correlations that are > $r = 0.6$, BES, Binge Eating Survey; YFAS, Yale Food Addiction Scale.

3.3. Relationships between Food Addiction and Binge Eating

The overall correlation between the total score from the BES and FA symptoms was $r = 0.76$, $p < 0.001$; for females it was $r = 0.77$, $p < 0.001$, and for males it was $r = 0.65$, $p < 0.001$ (Figure 1). Total BES score and BES emotion factor were more strongly associated with FA symptoms, as evidenced by the majority of correlations ($n = 7$) with values >0.6. In contrast, the BES behaviour factor was less strongly associated to FA, as evidenced by smaller correlation values, with only three correlations classified as large ($r > 0.6$, $p < 0.001$). Of the 11 individual FA symptoms and clinical impairments, correlations with BES factors and the FA symptoms 'consumed more than planned' were small, with the majority being <0.3, while 'use in physically hazardous situations' produced significant negative correlations.

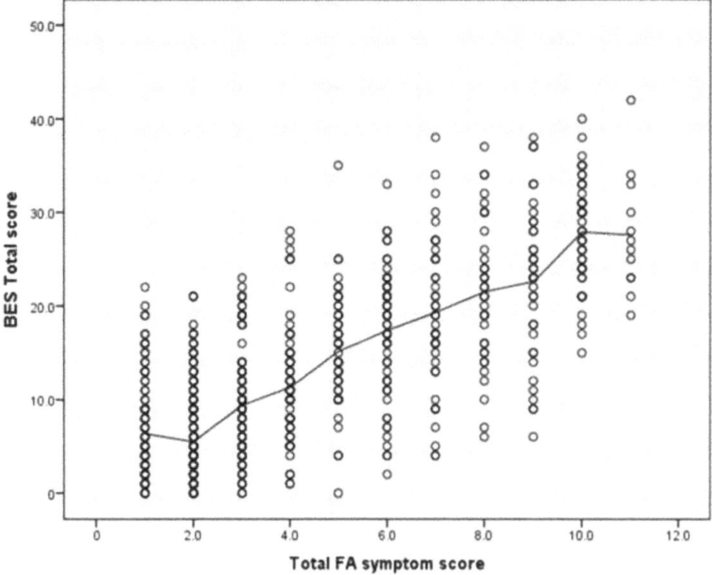

Figure 1. Correlation between BES total scores and YFAS symptom scores.

4. Discussion

This study investigated the overlap in symptoms of FA and BED as measured by the YFAS 2.0 and the BES's emotional and behavioural factors. It was found that substantial overlap (r = 0.76) exists between the commonly used assessment tools in a sample of Australian adults from a wide age range, which concurs with existing research [28,29]. However, this is the first study to demonstrate that the strongest overlap occurred with the BES emotion factor, while less overlap was observed with the BES behaviour factor. This was evidenced by larger correlation values with the BES emotion factor, compared with very few strong correlations (greater than 0.6) with the BES behaviour factor. The behaviour factor relates to behavioural expressions surrounding a binge eating episode which showed small to moderate correlations with the majority of the 11 symptoms assessed by the YFAS 2.0 tool. These correlations are not unexpected, as previous findings indicate that individuals with co-existing FA and BED experience significantly higher levels of depression, negative affect, poorer emotion dysregulation, and lower self-esteem [11]. This would seem to indicate that high levels of emotional and psychosocial distress accompany both eating pathologies. Research has demonstrated that, in the context of binge eating, emotions and behaviour rarely occur exclusively [30] and are correlated as shown in this study. For this reason, it would be expected that both features be present and it is unsurprising that these symptoms would co-occur in FA. However, strong evidence for the cognitive and behavioural aspects of BED is lacking, and further investigations into BED and behaviour are warranted.

It is important to attempt to articulate the unique features that may set the construct of FA apart from BED, given that previous overlaps have been shown, although these are not in entirety or not 100% overlapping. In this study, it appears that several symptoms are unique to FA, as evidenced by lower correlation valueswith BES. Specifically, small associations were found with FA symptoms of 'consumed more than planned' or 'use in physically hazardous situations'; the latter symptom in this study actually showed significant negative relationships. The symptom of 'use in physically hazardous situations' has previously been debated as a difficult factor to interpret in relation to food, given that food in its true sense is needed for survival. Recent studies assessing FA using the YFAS 2.0 tool have found the endorsement of 'use in physically hazardous situations' symptom in three non-clinical samples (n = 1900) to have low endorsement rates ranging from 9.1% to 24.8%; with two of the studies reporting the endorsement rate in FA individuals (n = 109) as 37.0% and 68.3%, respectively [4,28,31]. However, in the context of FA, this symptom can be described as causing impairment to performance, such as eating while driving, or impairment to health that is hazardous. In the context of obesity and related metabolic syndrome risk factors, this could include the consequences of individuals with diabetes, dyslipidaemia, or hypertension overconsuming foods containing excessive amounts of sugar, fat, or sodium [32]. However, this symptom may not have been well-reported by participants with this rationale in mind nor understood in terms of addiction by the participants completing the surveys, thus influencing the results because the questions did not ask participants to consider this aspect of the symptom. Existing public views suggest that individuals believe some foods are addictive and that addiction can cause obesity [33]. Future qualitative work on FA is warranted to better understand how the symptoms are experienced and if they differ for each individual, particularly as this field is still emerging.

The FA symptom of "loss of control with respect to eating behaviour" overlaps with that of "loss of control over eating", the latter being a core eating disorder behaviour and a diagnostic criterion for the eating disorders bulimia nervosa and binge eating disorder [32]. The symptoms of FA as assessed by the YFAS were determined with mapping to the DSM–5. However, it is noted that when considering some of these symptoms at a broader population level, with increasing prevalence rates of overweight and obesity, some symptoms or traits presently being assessed overlap with general dieting practices undertaken by many individuals. FA symptoms measured by the YFAS, specifically 'repeated attempts to cut down food', may not be unique to FA, but apply to the population in general.

In the current analysis of those individuals with FA, 72.7% also had reported BES scores which related to either moderate or severe bingeing. While not directly comparable due to the use of different tools and methods to assess the disordered eating status, the value in the current study is higher than that previously reported by Gearhardt et al., who found in a sample of overweight individuals with BED, determined by clinical interview, that 57% met the classification for FA [11]. In a more racially diverse sample of obese, treatment-seeking adults with BED (n = 96) as assessed by an alternate tool, The Eating Disorder Examination Questionnaire (EDEQ), the findings were similar, with 42% of participants meeting the classification for FA [12]. In both studies, YFAS scores were also significant predictors of binge eating frequency. In an additional study, Ivezaj et al. [34] examined the eating and health-related behaviours of overweight/obese adults (n = 502), and found that 61.7% of adults meeting BED criteria as assessed by the EDEQ also met FA criteria. Adults with co-occurring BED and FA had significantly higher BMI and depression scores, combined with greater disturbances on most impulsivity and self-control measures relative to the control group [35]. A strong association between FA and BE severity (r = 0.78, p = 0.0045) as well as a moderate association between FA and measures of general psychopathology were reported. A similar relationship between FA and BE has also been shown to exist in younger adolescent populations [35].

Rates of FA among those with BED is higher in individuals with obesity than in those who are not obese [36]; this was also shown in the current study across increasing weight status of healthy, overweight, and obese participants. Individuals who meet the criteria for both BED and FA tend to exhibit more frequent binge eating episodes, experience stronger cravings for food, and elevated levels of impulsivity and depressive symptoms than those with only BED [5,12,13]. It has been suggested the co-occurrence of BED and FA may represent a more severe BED subgroup characterised by greater eating disorder psychopathology and associated pathology [11].

Recent evidence suggests altered reward sensitivity may contribute to the pathophysiology of disordered eating behaviours. A review of neuroimaging studies (n = 15) in BED found that the alterations in corticostriatal circuitry were similar to those observed in substance abuse, including altered function of prefrontal, insular, and orbitofrontal cortices and the striatum [37]. Preliminary evidence by Gearhardt et al. suggests that reward dysfunction may also be a relevant mechanism in the FA construct [38]. Human genetics and animal studies suggest that changes in neurotransmitter networks, including dopaminergic and opioidergic systems, are associated with compulsive-eating behaviours [37,39].

This study has several limitations which should be considered when interpreting the findings: the survey was collected online and is based on self-report measures and was analysed using correlation analysis only. However, it is noted that for food addiction and binge eating, the majority of measures used for these eating behaviours are based on self-report, and self-reported height and weight have been shown previously to be a valid measure of weight status [40]. It could be likely that individuals who are motivated by food may have been more likely to complete the survey. The study sample had a majority of participants who were female, so results may not be generalisable to the broader population or to other ethnicities. The findings of this study have some clinical implications, as they provide a further understanding of the underlying aetiology of co-occurring FA and BED, to progress and tailor treatment options as FA appears to be more physiological than behavioural in nature.

5. Conclusions

This is one of the first studies to investigate the potential overlap between the common tools used to assess BED and FA and their individual constructs, particularly with reference to the YFAS 2.0 tool which maps to current DSM criteria. This study demonstrates the overlap between BED and FA, and highlights the possible unique differences between the forms of disordered eating.

Acknowledgments: T.B. is supported by a UON Brawn research fellowship.

Author Contributions: T.B. conceived, designed and conducted the study; T.B. analysed the data; T.B. developed initial draft of paper, and J.S., R.M. and M.R. contributed to and approved the final version of the manuscript.

Conflicts of Interest: The authors declare no conflict of interest.

References

1. Pursey, K.M.; Stanwell, P.; Gearhardt, A.N.; Collins, C.E.; Burrows, T.L. The Prevalence of Food Addiction as Assessed by the Yale Food Addiction Scale: A Systematic Review. *Nutrients* **2014**, *6*, 4552–4590. [CrossRef] [PubMed]
2. Hebebrand, J.; Albayrak, Ö.; Adan, R.; Antel, J.; Dieguez, C.; de Jong, J.; Leng, G.; Menzies, J.; Mercer, J.G.; Murphy, M.; et al. "Eating addcition" rather than "food addcition" better captures addictive like eating behaviour. *Neurosci. Biobehav. Rev.* **2014**, *47*, 295–306. [CrossRef] [PubMed]
3. Gearhardt, A.; Corbin, W.; Brownwell, K.D. Preliminary validation of the Yale Food Addiction Scale. *Appetite* **2009**, *52*, 32–36. [CrossRef] [PubMed]
4. Gearhardt, A.N; Corbin, W.R; Brownwell, K.D. Development of the Yale Food Addiction Scale Version 2.0. *Psychol. Addict. Behav.* **2016**, *30*, 113–121. [CrossRef] [PubMed]
5. Davis, C. From Passive Overeating to "Food Addiction": A Spectrum of Compulsion and Severity. *ISRN Obes.* **2013**, 1–20. [CrossRef] [PubMed]
6. Schulte, E.M.; Grilo, C.M.; Gearhardt, A.N. Shared and unique mechanisms underlying binge eating disorder and addictive disorders. *Clin. Psychol. Rev.* **2016**, *44*, 125–139. [CrossRef] [PubMed]
7. Hilker, I.; Sánchez, I.; Steward, T.; Jiménez-Murcia, S.; Granero, R.; Gearhardt, A.N.; Rodríguez-Muñoz, R.C.; Dieguez, C.; Crujeiras, A.B.; Tolosa-Sola, I.; et al. Food Addiction in Bulimia Nervosa: Clinical Correlates and Association with Response to a Brief Psychoeducational Intervention. *Eur. Eat. Disord. Rev.* **2016**, *24*, 482–488. [CrossRef] [PubMed]
8. American Psychiatric Association. *Diagnostic and Statistical Manual of Mental Disorders*, 5th ed.; American Psychiatric Publishing: Arlington, TX, USA, 2013.
9. Kessler, R.; Berglund, P.A.; Chiu, W.T.; Deitz, A.C.; Hudson, J.I.; Shahly, V.; Aguilar-Gaxiola, S.; Alonso, J.; Angermeyer, M.C.; Benjet, C.; Bruffaerts, R.; et al. The Prevalence and Correlates of Binge Eating Disorder in the World Health Organization World Mental Health Surveys. *Biol. Psychiatry* **2013**, *73*, 904–914. [CrossRef] [PubMed]

10. Preti, A.; de Girolamo, G.; Vilagut, G.; Alonso, J.; de Graaf, R.; Bruffaerts, R.; Demyttenaere, K.; Pinto-Meza, A.; Haro, J.M.; Morosini, P.; et al. The epidemiology of eating disorders in six European countries: Results of the ESEMeD-WMH project RSS. *J. Psychiatr. Res.* **2009**, *43*, 1125–1132. [CrossRef] [PubMed]
11. Gearhardt, A.N.; White, M.A.; Masheb, R.M.; Morgan, P.T.; Crosby, R.D.; Grilo, C.M. An Examination of the food addcition construct in obese patients with binge eating disorder. *Int. J. Eat. Disord.* **2012**, *45*, 657–663. [CrossRef] [PubMed]
12. Gearhardt, A.; White, M.A.; Masheb, R.M.; Grilo, C.M. An examination of food addiction in a racially diverse sample of obese patients with binge eating disorder in primary care settings. *Compr. Psychiatr.* **2013**, *54*, 500–505. [CrossRef] [PubMed]
13. Gearhardt, A.N.; Boswell, R.G.; White, M.A. The association of "food addiction" with disordered eating and body mass index. *Eat. Behav.* **2014**, *15*, 427–433. [CrossRef] [PubMed]
14. Meule, A.; von Rezori, V.; Blechert, J. Food addiction and bulimia nervosa. *Eur. Eat. Disord. Rev.* **2014**, *5*, 33. [CrossRef] [PubMed]
15. Burrows, T.; Hides, L.; Brown, R.; Dayas, C.V.; Kay-Lambkin, F. Differences in Dietary Preferences, Personality and Mental Health in Australian Adults with and without Food Addiction. *Nutrients* **2017**, *9*, 285. [CrossRef] [PubMed]
16. Heatherton, T.; Baumeister, R. Binge eating as escape from self-awareness. *Psychol. Bull.* **1991**, *110*, 86–108. [CrossRef] [PubMed]
17. Gearhardt, A.; White, M.; Potenza, M. Binge Eating Disorder and Food Addiction. *Curr. Drug Abuse Rev.* **2011**, *43*, 201–207. [CrossRef]
18. Potenza, M.N.; Grilo, C.M. How relevant is food craving to obesity and its treatment? *Front. Psychiatry* **2014**, *5*, 164. [CrossRef] [PubMed]
19. Pivarunas, B.; Conner, B.T. Impulsivity and emotion dysregulation as predictors of food addiction. *Eat. Behav.* **2015**, *19*, 9–14. [CrossRef] [PubMed]
20. Clark, S.; Saules, K. Validation of the yale Food Addiction Scale among a weight loss surgery population. *Eat. Behav.* **2013**, *14*, 216–219. [CrossRef] [PubMed]
21. Meule, A.; Heckel, D. Correlates of food addiction in obese individuals seeking bariatric surgery. *Clin. Obes.* **2014**, *4*, 228–236. [CrossRef] [PubMed]
22. Davis, C. A commentary on the associations among 'food addiction', binge eating disorder, and obesity: Overlapping conditions with idiosyncratic clinical features. *Appetite* **2017**, *115*, 3–8. [CrossRef] [PubMed]
23. WHO (The World Health Organisation). BMI Classifcation. Available online: http://apps.who.int/bmi/index.jsp?introPage=intro_3.htm (accessed on 25 July 2017).
24. Gormally, J.; Black, S.; Daston, S.; Rardin, D. The assessment of Binge Eating Severity among obese. *Addict. Behav.* **1982**, *7*, 47–55. [CrossRef]
25. Kelly, N.R.; Mitchell, K.S.; Gow, R.W.; Trace, S.E.; Lydecker, J.A.; Bair, C.E.; Mazzeo, S. An evaluation of the reliability and construct validity of eating disorder measures in white and black women. *Psychol. Assess.* **2012**, *24*, 608–617. [CrossRef] [PubMed]
26. Grupski, A.E.; Hood, M.M.; Hall, B.J.; Azarbad, L.; Fitzpatrick, S.L.; Corsica, J.A. Examining the binge eating scale in screening for binge eating disorder with bariatric surgery candidates. *Obes. Surg.* **2013**, *23*, 1–6. [CrossRef] [PubMed]
27. Santor, D.A.; Haggerty, J.L.; Lévesque, J.-F.; Burge, F.; Beaulieu, M.-D.; Gass, D.; Pineault, R. An Overview of Confirmatory Factor Analysis and Item Response Analysis Applied to Instruments to Evaluate Primary Healthcare. *Healthc. Policy* **2011**, *7*, 79–92. [CrossRef] [PubMed]
28. Brunault, P.; Courtois, R.; Gearhardt, A.N.; Gaillard, P.; Journiac, K.; Cathelain, S.; Réveillère, C.; Ballon, N. Validation of the French Version of the DSM-5 Yale Food Addiction Scale in a Nonclinical Sample. *Can. J. Psychiatry* **2017**, *62*, 199–210. [CrossRef] [PubMed]
29. Imperatori, C.; Fabbricatore, M.; Vumbaca, V.; Innamorati, M.; Contardi, A.; Farina, B. Food Addiction: definition, measurement and prevalence in healthy subjects and in patients with eating disorders. *Riv. Psichiatr.* **2016**, *51*, 60–65. [PubMed]
30. Kittel, R.; Brauhardt, A.; Hilbert, A. Hilbert A. Cognitive and emotional functioning in binge-eating disorder: A systematic review. *Int. J. Eat. Disord.* **2015**, *48*, 535–554. [CrossRef] [PubMed]

31. Hauck, C.; Weiß, A.; Schulte, E.M.; Meule, A.; Ellrott, T. Prevalence of 'Food Addiction' as Measured with the Yale Food Addiction Scale 2.0 in a Representative German Sample and Its Association with Sex, Age and Weight Categories. *Eur. J. Obes.* **2017**, *10*, 12–24. [CrossRef] [PubMed]
32. Meule, A.; Gearhardt, A.N. Food addiction in the light of DSM-5. *Nutrients* **2014**, *6*, 3653–3671. [CrossRef] [PubMed]
33. Ruddock, H.; Hardman, C. Food Addiction Beliefs Amongst the Lay Public: What Are the Consequences for Eating Behaviour? *Curr. Addict. Rep.* **2017**, *4*, 110–115. [CrossRef] [PubMed]
34. Ivezaj, V.; White, M.A.; Grilo, C.M. Examining binge-eating disorder and food addiction in adults with overweight and obesity. *Obesity* **2016**, *24*, 2064–2069. [CrossRef] [PubMed]
35. Ahmed, A.Y.; Sayed, A.M.; Alshahat, A.A.; Abd Elaziza, E.A. Can food addiction replace binge eating assessment in obesity clinics? *Egypt. J. Med. Hum. Genet.* **2017**, *18*, 181–185. [CrossRef]
36. Long, C.; Blundell, J.; Finlayson, G. A Systematic Review of the Application and Correlates of YFAS-Diagnosed 'Food Addiction' in Humans: Are Eating-Related 'Addictions' a Cause for Concern or Empty Concepts? *Obes. Facts* **2015**, *8*, 386–401. [CrossRef] [PubMed]
37. Kessler, R.M.; Hutson, P.H.; Herman, B.K.; Potenza, M.N. The neurobiological basis of binge-eating disorder. *Neurosci. Biobehav. Rev.* **2016**, *63*, 223–238. [CrossRef] [PubMed]
38. Gearhardt, A.N.; Yokum, S.; Orr, P.T.; Stice, E.; Corbin, W.R.; Brownell, K.D. Neural correlates of food addiction. *Arch. Gen. Psychiatry* **2011**, *68*, 808–816. [CrossRef] [PubMed]
39. Schrieber, L.; Odlaug, B.; Grant, J. The overlap between binge eating disorder and substance use disorders: Diagnosis and neurobiology. *J. Behav. Addict.* **2013**, *2*, 191–198. [CrossRef] [PubMed]
40. Pursey, K.; Burrows, T.L.; Stanwell, P.; Collins, C.E. How accurate is web-based self-reported height, weight and body mass index in young adults? *J. Med. Internet Res.* **2014**, *16*, e4. [CrossRef] [PubMed]

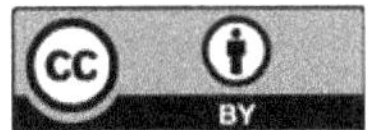

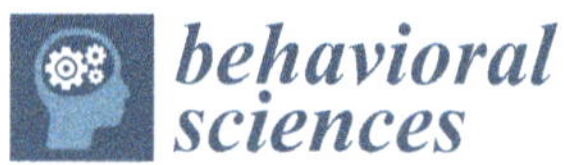
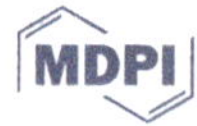

Article

Exploring Relationships between Recurrent Binge Eating and Illicit Substance Use in a Non-Clinical Sample of Women over Two Years

Henry Kewen Lu [1], Haider Mannan [1,2] and Phillipa Hay [2,*]

[1] School of Medicine, Western Sydney University, Penrith NSW 2751, Australia; 17812812@student.westernsydney.edu.au (H.K.L.); H.Mannan@westernsydney.edu.au (H.M.)

[2] Translational Health Research Institute (THRI), School of Medicine, Western Sydney University, Penrith NSW 2751, Australia

* Correspondence: p.hay@westernsydney.edu.au; Tel.: +61-412-330-428

Received: 24 April 2017; Accepted: 3 July 2017; Published: 18 July 2017

Abstract: (1) Background: With the new edition of the Diagnostic and Statistical Manual of Mental disorders, 5th Edition (DSM-5), numerous parallels have been drawn between recurrent binge eating (RBE) and substance use disorders, with many authors examining RBE or binge eating disorder (BED) as a "food addiction". The present study aims to clarify the relationship between recurrent binge eating (RBE) and illicit substance use (ISU) through investigating the temporal association between the two problems. (2) Methods: This study was embedded within a larger longitudinal study of non-clinical adult women recruited from Australian tertiary institutions. Participants responded at year 2 and year 4 of follow-up to the Eating Disorder Examination—Questionnaire. ISU was measured using a modified questionnaire taken from the Australian Longitudinal Study on Women's Health. (3) Results: RBE and ISU co-morbidity was 5.88% in this non-clinical sample, and having one condition increased the likelihood of the other. The two conditions had a different trajectory over two years whereby ISU participants had significant risk of developing RBE in addition to or in place of their ISU but the reverse was not found for RBE participants. (4) Conclusion: This unidirectional relationship suggests that in spite of the similarities of RBE and ISU they may be distinct with respect to their co-morbidity over time.

Keywords: recurrent binge eating; illicit substance use; binge eating disorder; longitudinal; co-morbidity; symptom trajectory

1. Introduction

1.1. Background

Binge eating disorder (BED) is characterised by recurrent episodes of binge eating (RBE)—defined by an objective overconsumption of food and a sense of loss of control—without the compensatory behaviours which define bulimia nervosa. BED has an estimated lifetime prevalence between 1.9% and 2.8% depending on the population surveyed, making it the most common eating disorder [1–3]. It is categorised within the Feeding and Eating Disorder (ED) chapter of the Diagnostic and Statistical Manual of Mental disorders, Fifth Edition (DSM-5), and is thus distinct from substance use disorders (SUDs). However, parallels have been drawn between BED and SUDs by a number of authors, many of them examining BED as a "food addiction" [1–4]. Criterion A for SUD within the DSM-5 may be divided into groupings of "impaired control, social impairment, risky use and pharmacological criteria" [5]. These are comparable to the BED criteria of "a sense of a lack of control", eating alone due to embarrassment, ongoing overeating despite negative consequences, and eating large amounts of food when not physically hungry.

BED and SUD also share a number of psychological, neurobiological and genetic correlates. Factors such as neuroticism, impulsivity, sensation seeking and mood dysregulation are associated with both BED and SUD [6–8]. Animal models also support the theory that both BED and SUD follow from dysregulation of the same dopaminergic pathways [9,10] and have likewise been able to produce somatic withdrawal symptoms with sucrose cessation [11].

1.2. Co-Morbidity

Literature regarding the co-morbidity shared between RBE/BED and SUD supports the idea that there is an underlying shared pathology between the two conditions. In examining the literature, there are a number of classification issues leading to variability in reported rates of co-morbidity and prior to its recognition in the DSM-5 [5], BED was included as a type of Eating Disorders Not Otherwise Specified (EDNOS) [12]. Complicating matters further, numerous studies either have failed to specify the type of ED they had studied or have classified participants with inconsistent criteria [13]. For many studies RBE has been used to represent BED. For example, in a US national face-to-face survey of 9282 adults, 23% of those who had BED—which was defined as having 3 months or more of RBE—suffered also from a type of SUD [14]. The WHO World Mental Health Surveys support these findings, in which 23.7% of those with BED would have some form of SUD [15]. In exploring the prevalence of SUD, it is noted that the classification of substance abuse is similarly difficult; research in this field varies not only in the scope of substance abuse, ranging from a focus on a single substance to looking at SUDs collectively, but also the severity of substance abuse, studying one-time use as well as physiological dependence [13,16]. Harrop & Marlatt's review [13] reflects these classification inconsistencies with co-morbidity prevalence ranging from 17–46% depending on ED and SUD types.

Illicit Substance Use (ISU) appears to be more common in ED populations than healthy controls; however, more information is needed to clarify the relationship between different types of illicit drugs and ED subgroups [16]. Cannabis [17,18] and opiate [17] use have found to be increased in those with an ED (subgroups combined) compared to controls. Evidence regarding amphetamine usage is inconsistent; one author reports associations of amphetamine usage with dieting and purging behaviour (without binging) [19,20] whilst another did not find increased use of amphetamines when comparing an ED group with the general population [17]. These findings may suggest that amphetamine usage may be associated with dieting and purging rather than with binging behaviour [16].

1.3. Longitudinal Predictors

On the other hand, longitudinal studies seem to suggest that however many similarities there may be between RBE/BED and ISU, they seem to differ in illness trajectories. A five-year longitudinal study of adolescent girls found that depressive symptoms were predictive of higher future levels of eating pathology and substance abuse (broadly defined and including alcohol use); eating pathology itself also predicted increased future substance abuse, with the inverse not being true [21]. Similarly, an Australian cohort study of adolescents and young adults found that even partial anorexia nervosa (AN)/bulimia nervosa (BN) diagnosis (where a participant satisfied two of four or three criteria for AN/BN) was predictive of amphetamine use [22]. The Growing Up Today Study has found that overeating (without a loss of control (LOC)) and RBE (overeating with a sense of a LOC) were both predictors for ISU; however, overeating alone was a stronger predictor for this outcome [23].

Fewer longitudinal papers have focused on predictors of RBE. Vogeltanze-Holm et al., found that the main factors predicting BED (strictly defined) was ISU in the past 12 months (odds ratio (OR) = 5.77, 95% CI = 1.64, 20.34) and more occasions of alcohol use until intoxication in the past 12 months (OR = 1.38, 95% CI = 1.03, 1.85) [24].

Finally, a five-year longitudinal study documenting the natural history of a variety of behavioural addictions over this period found a central effect of time on the problem behaviours, where the prevalence of the behaviours decreased and often resolved without intervention [25]. Excessive eating (examined over four years only) was found to decrease in prevalence at the same rate as comorbid substance use (broadly defined), with a mean 11.7% (SD = 2.3) suffering from comorbid SUD during the four-year time period.

These findings—in particular, that RBE/BED and ISU/SUD may not mutually predict risk for each other—suggest that perhaps distinct higher-order factors are mediating the relationship between RBE/BED and ISU/SUD rather than being controlled by the same underlying factor [13]. In a review of the phenomenology and treatment of behavioural addictions, Grant et al. hypothesises the opposite [26], claiming that one neurobiological dysfunction could give rise to multiple behavioural symptoms. The support for this theory comes from "consummatory cross-sensitisation" where prolonged intake and sensitisation with one substance can lead to increased consumption of another [4]. As a result of this cross-sensitisation, opiate- and stimulant-dependent individuals may have a cross-substitutability of preference for highly palatable foods, leading to reported cravings and binges [9,27].

Although there have been these studies of outcomes and putative symptoms substitution, it is notable that there have been few studies of the impact of comorbidity on other clinical features such as overall psychological distress, health-related quality of life and/or body weight, and findings have been mixed or inconsistent [28]. This may be of clinical importance if co-morbidity was found to be associated with poorer mental health and/or increased likelihood of obesity.

1.4. Aim and Hypotheses

In this study, we aimed to elucidate the nature of co-morbidity by (1) characterising the extent of the overlap of these two features within a non-clinical population, and (2) examining the trajectories of participants with regard to RBE and ISU over a period of two years' time. We hypothesised that there would be significant co-morbidity between the two problems and, furthermore, that participants with RBE and those with ISU will have differing illness trajectories without mutual substitution between the two behaviours. We did not have specific hypotheses in regard to examining general psychological distress or health-related quality of life as these have been little studied in regard to the comorbidity of ISU and RBE.

2. Materials and Methods

2.1. Participants

Participants were 794 women initially recruited in 2004/2005 who were assessed repeatedly over a nine-year period (T0–T9). Any one follow-up assessment was not contingent on having competed any other follow-up. They were recruited through advertisements in four regional universities and vocational colleges (including adult students) in the Australian states of Queensland and Victoria for the purpose of a longitudinal study of community (non-clinical) women with and without eating disorder symptoms. Some participants were recruited via email and responded to the questionnaire online, whilst others were directly approached on campus locations and given hard-copy questionnaires and reply-paid envelopes. Due to these recruitment methods, characteristics of non-responders and overall response rate could not be measured.

ISU was only assessed in T2 and T4 of the longitudinal study. As such, the present study comprises of participants who responded in T2 (n = 357) and those who responded in T4 who also responded in T2 (n = 268). Respondents who had no data for measures of binge eating or substance use in T2 (n = 4) or T4 (n = 9) were excluded. Figure 1 shows the participant flow through T1, T2 and T4 of the longitudinal study.

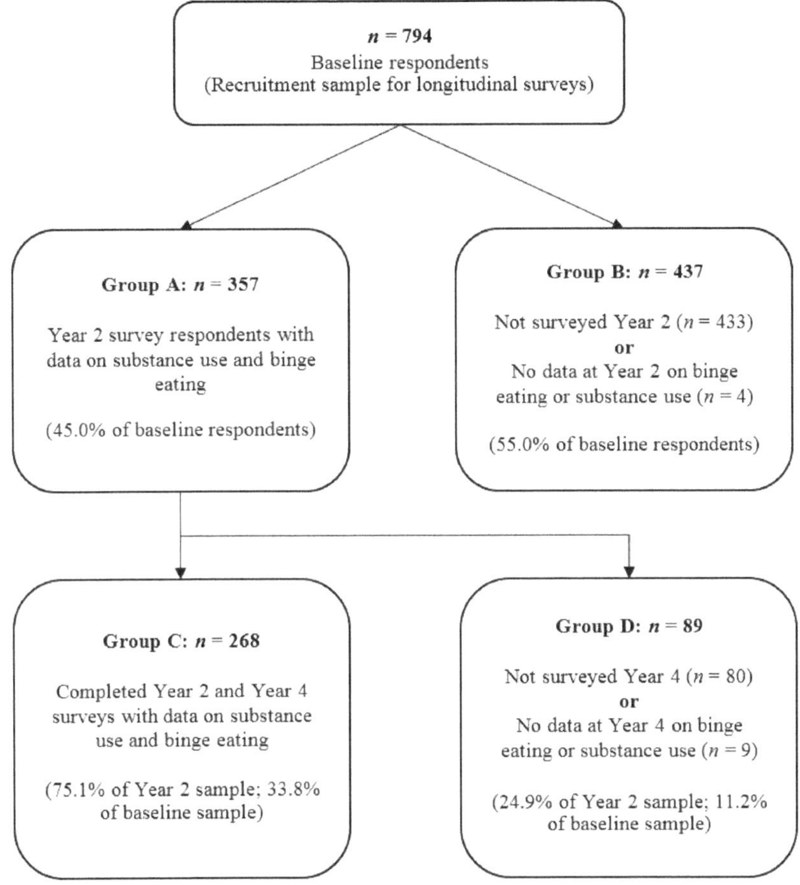

Figure 1. Participant flow from the beginning of the survey.

2.2. Procedures

The study was approved by the human research ethics committees (HREC) of the universities involved, with the Western Sydney University as lead HREC (Approval number 07/240). All participants completed written informed consent forms and there were no children requiring consent from a parent or guardian.

2.3. Measures

2.3.1. Binge Eating

The Eating Disorder Examination Questionnaire (EDE-Q), a self-report questionnaire based on the Eating Disorder Examination (EDE) interview was used in order to assess eating disorder psychopathology. The EDE-Q has been validated in both community and clinical samples of patients with eating disorders and demonstrates close agreement with the EDE overall [29]. However, with regard to the complex features involved with binge eating behaviours the EDE-Q consistently generated higher levels of disturbance relative to the EDE [30].

Four items in the questionnaire targeted binge eating behaviours. The first two assessed objective binge eating (OBE), asking if the respondent had ever consumed what other people would regard as an unusually large amount of food, with a sensation of loss of control, and if so, how many times that had occurred over the past 28 days. This correlates with the DSM-5 criteria for recurrent binge eating episodes (Criterion A) but does not specify a discrete time period [5]. The second two assessed subjective binge eating (SBE), asking if the respondent had consumed a normal amount of food for the circumstances but had experienced a loss of control, and if yes, the number of times that had occurred. This is consistent with binge eating criteria being considered for the incoming International Classification of Diseases, 11th revision (ICD-11) [31], on the basis that people with subjective episodes have similar levels of impairment and distress related to binge eating as well as other psychopathology as do people with objective episodes [32,33]. As such, binge eating was coded as "present" if they had reported "yes" to either an objective or subjective binge for more than four episodes in the past 28 days and is used as the measure in this study of RBE. At the end of the EDE-Q there was a question asking current weight and height from which body mass index (BMI; kg/m^2) scores were derived.

2.3.2. Illicit Substance Use (ISU)

The questionnaire assessed frequency and amount of use of the following illicit substances: cannabis, amphetamines, hallucinogens, barbiturates, "ecstasy/designer drugs/cocaine", "inhalants" and heroin. Participants were asked if they had used any of the illicit substances listed above in the past year, and if yes, the frequency of their current use over a one-month period. These questions were modified from the Australian Longitudinal Study on Women's Health (ALSWH), where their frequency of use was categorised into scores of: 1 = less than monthly, 2 = monthly, 3 = weekly, 4 = two to three times per week, and 5 = daily [34]. The ordinal data gathered by this questionnaire allowed the creation of a new variable for the present study measuring overall ISU, which was calculated by taking the sum of the scores for each of the seven drug categories. A score of zero indicated no ISU, whilst the maximum score of thirty-five indicated that the participant was taking illicit drugs in all seven categories every single day of the week. The score is therefore influenced both by the range of illicit drugs consumed, as well as their frequency. For the purpose of this study, ISU was coded as present if the score was greater than 0, i.e., 1 or more.

2.3.3. Psychological Distress

This was assessed with the Kessler-10 item distress scale (K-10) which was designed to detect cases of anxiety and affective disorders in the general population [35]. It is a 10-item instrument with an ordinal 5-point response to each question. It measures the level of distress and severity associated with psychological symptoms of depression and anxiety. The K10 is extensively used internationally, including in the WHO World Mental Health Survey and by government organizations in Australia, Spain, Colombia and Peru [36]. The advantages of the K-10 are its brief nature and its strong psychometric properties. It focuses on the previous 28 days thus is comparable in time-frame to the EDE-Q.

2.3.4. Health-Related Quality of Life (HRQoL)

HRQoL was assessed with the well-validated 12-item Short Form-12 Health Status Questionnaire (SF-12) [37]. The SF-12 measures the impact of physical and mental ill-health on role limitations. It has been used extensively in research assessing impairment associated with physical and mental health conditions, and has robust psychometric properties, including in an Australian population sample [37,38]. It is a 12-item questionnaire that generates two weighted scales, a Physical Component Summary Scale (PCS) and a Mental Component Summary Scale (MCS), with each a mean of 50 and standard deviation of 10 in normative samples. Higher scores indicate higher levels of functioning.

2.4. Statistical Methods

Data were inspected for normality. Descriptive statistics were employed to report frequencies of socio-demographic variables, general symptoms, binge eating and substance use. Between-group differences were compared using ANOVA with post-hoc Tukey analyses for continuous normal data and Kruskal–Wallis and Mann–Whitney U tests for continuous non-normal data. The chi-squared test was utilised to test differences in distribution between categorical groups and ordinal data. Fisher's exact test was utilised to calculate the p-value for the contingency tables given the small sample size. To determine whether a trajectory based on a transition from year 2 to year 4 was statistically significant, we tested the significance of estimated marginal probability for each trajectory based on the multinomial logistic regression of a multi-category outcome containing all possible combinations of RBE & ISU measured at year 4 conditional on the same outcome at year 2, while controlling for age and mental health-related quality of life both being measured at year 2. While assessing the relationship between a multi-category outcome containing all possible combinations of RBE & ISU measured at year 2 & the same outcome measured at year 4, both the control variables were found to be confounders. Listwise deletion of missing data was applied to the data at year 4 because the percentage missing at time 4 out of a total of 359 cases at time 2 who had any of the four possible RBE & ISU conditions was very low (3.06%), and hence complete case analysis would introduce very little bias. A significance level of $p < 0.05$ was employed for all tests. Analyses were conducted using IBM SPSS Statistics for Windows, version 22.

3. Results

3.1. Participant Features

Of the 357 participants who completed the follow-up survey at T2 (45.0% of baseline respondents), the median age (at T2) was 25 (Interquartile Range (IQR) = 15), 58.0% were unmarried or separated and 52.9% lived with family, friends or alone. The sample was well educated, with 33.9% achieving at least year 12, and 48.5% attaining a bachelor's degree or higher. A large minority of the sample studied full-time (41.5%). Participants with symptoms were overrepresented in this study sample; compared to a previous general population study of Australian women, their Mental Health-Related Quality of Life scores (Short-Form 12 Mental Health Component Scores or SF-12 MCS) were lower and their EDE-Q subscale and global scores were higher, although lower than in clinical samples [39]. (See Section 2.3 for descriptors of these assessment measures.) ISU occurred in 20% (n = 72) of participants. Cannabis (n = 59, 82%) was the most frequently used substance followed by ecstasy/designer drugs/cocaine (n = 40, 56%). Other demographic and clinical features of the 357 participants at T2 can be found in Table 1.

Table 1. Descriptive data of 357 study participants in the present study.

	n	Mean	Standard Deviation	Median	Interquartile Range
Age/years at year 2	354	30.7	11.4	25	15
Body Mass Index (kg/m^2)	342	24.8	5.5	23.5	5.3
Eating Disorder Examination—Questionnaire					
Weight concern subscale	353	2.04	1.54	1.80	2.60
Eating concern subscale	350	0.953	1.18	0.400	1.20
Shape concern subscale	346	2.37	1.58	2.13	2.63
Restraint subscale	352	1.57	1.43	1.20	2.00
Global Score	336	1.74	1.29	1.44	1.95
Illicit substance use frequency [1]	357	0.65	1.72	0	0
Kessler 10 Psychological Distress Scale	351	17.5	6	16	7
Short Form-12 [2] Physical Component Score	348	52.1	8.2	54.5	8.3
Short Form-12 Mental Component Score	348	44.9	11.3	48.6	16.7

[1] Illicit substance use frequency (range none to daily use) was a summed score of the seven drug categories. [2] The Short Form-12 is a measure of Health-Related Quality of Life.

Table 2 compares key characteristics of the four subgroups within the longitudinal study to assess if respondents were significantly different from non-respondents at T2 and T4. These are divided by response status and availability of RBE and ISU data. These groups are also outlined in Figure 1.

Year 2 respondents (Group A) were significantly older (MD = 2.23, SE = 0.74) than those who responded at baseline but were lost to follow-up (Group B), but were not significantly different in the other measures of body mass index (BMI (kg/m^2)) and RBE characteristics. Participants who followed up at both year 2 and year 4 (Group C) were also significantly older (MD = 3.79, SE = 1.38) than their counterparts who did not respond in year 4 (Group D) and similarly, were not significantly different in BMI, RBE or ISU behaviours.

Table 2. Participant characteristics of subgroups within the study.

Feature	Group A [1]	Group B [2]		Group C [3]	Group D [4]	
	Mean (SD) *n*		*t*, *p*	Mean (SD) *n*		*t*, *p*
Age	28.7 (11.4) *354*	26.5 (10.5) *426*	−2.85, 0.005	31.7 (12.02) *266*	27.9 (8.54) *88*	−2.74, 0.006
Body Mass Index (kg/m^2)	24.3 (5.23) *336*	23.7 (5.52) *409*	−1.59, 0.11	24.91 (5.62) *254*	24.5 (5.17) *88*	−6.1, 0.545
	Median (IQR) *n*		*z*, *p*	Median (IQR) *n*		*z*, *p*
OBE/month	0 (0–1) *340*	0 (0–0) *408*	−3.34, 0.001	0 (0–0) *268*	0 (0–0) *89*	−0.62, 0.534
SBE/month	0 (0–2) *340*	0 (0–0) *408*	−2.75, 0.01	0 (0–2) *267*	0 (0–2) *89*	−0.09, 0.928
ISU	n.a. (ISU not assessed at baseline)			0 (0–0) *267*	0 (0–1) *89*	−1.70, 0.089

[1] Participants who responded at T2 (with BE and ISU data), *n* = 357; [2] Participants who responded at baseline, but not at T2 *or* had no BE or ISU data at T2, *n* = 437; [3] Participants who responded at T2 *and* T4 (with BE and ISU data), *n* = 268; [4] Participants who responded at T2 but *not* at T4 *or* had no BE or ISU data at T4, *n* = 94; OBE = objective binge eating episodes; SBE = subjective binge eating episodes; ISU = illicit substance use; BE = binge eating; IQR = Interquartile Range.

3.2. Co-Morbid ISU and RBE in the T2 Cohort

At T2, 226 of 357 (63.3%) respondents had neither RBE nor ISU behaviours; 55 (15.4%) had episodes of RBE *only*; the same number (*n* = 55, 15.4%) engaged in ISU *only*, whilst 21 participants (5.88%) in T2 admitted to engaging in both behaviours.

The majority of participants who were identified as having a problem (either RBE or ISU) had one problem only and not the other (55/76, 72.4%) and this finding was not significant ($\chi^2 = 2.32$, df = 1; $p = 0.09$). As shown in Table 3 it was determined that those who had RBE had significantly higher frequency of ISU compared to those without RBE, and similarly, those who had ISU had significantly higher frequency of RBE compared to those without ISU.

Table 3. Comparative levels of illicit substance use (ISU) and recurrent binge eating (RBE) in participants with and without either problem.

Level of Behaviour	Median, IQ Range, *n*		Mann–Whitney U *Z*, *p*
n = 357	RBE	No RBE	
ISU	1, 0–6, *73*	0, 0–2, *282*	−2.612, 0.009
	ISU	No. ISU	
RBE	0, 0–6, *76*	0, 0–2, *281*	−2.234, 0.026

Furthermore, participants with both ISU and RBE had the highest levels of eating disorder symptoms (global and subscale EDE-Q scores) and psychological distress (K-10 scores) and lowest levels of mental health HRQoL. These differences reached significance only for the findings of global EDE-Q scores compared to those with ISU alone, and K-10 scores compared to those with neither problem. Those with neither problem also had significantly lower EDE-Q global scores than all other groups and lower K-10 scores than those with RBE alone. These differences are shown in Table 4.

Table 4. Comparative clinical features of participants according to their RBE and ISU status.

	Neither [1]	**RBE** [2]	**ISU** [3]	**Both** [4]		**Post-Hoc Tests with $p < 0.05$**
Outcome	mean, SD, *n*				ANOVA F (df), *p*	Tukey test
EDE-Q Global	1.56, 1.21, 210	2.62, 1.38, 59	2.12, 1.43, 49	3.16, 1.23, 21	18.19 (3), <0.001	Neither ≠ Both, ISU, RBE; ISU ≠ Both
EDE-Q Restraint	1.17, 1.20, 219	2.59, 1.44, 59	1.46, 1.41, 50	2.87, 1.43, 23	27.33 (3), <0.001	Neither ≠ Both, RBE; ISU ≠ Both, RBE
EDE-Q Eating Concern	0.52, 0.74, 216	2.11, 1.29, 59	0.69, 0.73, 51	2.46,1.43, 23	70.62 (3), <0.001	Neither ≠ Both, RBE; ISU ≠ Both, RBE
EDE-Q Shape concern	1.86, 1.32, 210	3.82, 1.36, 59	2.01, 1.36, 53	3.89, 1.44, 23	44.24 (3), <0.001	Neither ≠ Both, RBE; ISU ≠ Both, RBE
EDE-Q Weight Concern	1.56, 1.28, 218	3.41, 1.42, 58	1.71, 1.24, 53	3.66, 1.43, 23	43.65 (3), <0.001	Neither ≠ Both, RBE; ISU ≠ Both, RBE
SF-12 MCS	45.94, 10.77, 219	43.04, 11.71, 59	44.31, 1.60, 52	41.09, 11.79, 23	2.13 (3), 0.096	n.a.
SF-12 PCS	52.61, 7.32, 291	51.24, 9.05, 59	53.15, 6.61, 52	51.20, 7.35, 23	0.89 (3), 0.45	n.a.
K-10 score	17.50, 6.23, 218	21.07, 7.65, 60	19.12, 7.8, 52	22.09, 7.99, 23	6.54 (3), <0.001	Neither ≠ RBE, Both
	median, IQ range, *n*				Kruskal–Wallis X^2 (df), *p*	Mann–Whitney U Z, *p*
Body Mass Index (kg/m^2)	23.6, 21.5–26.4 *211*	23.2, 20.8–29.2 *57*	23.5, 20.9–25.0 *50*	23.1, 20.2–25.0 *23*	1.924 (3), 0.588	n.a.

[1] Participants with neither RBE nor ISU features; [2] Participants with RBE only; [3] Participants with ISU features only; [4] Participants with both RBE and ISU features; RBE = Recurrent Binge Eating; ISU = illicit substance use; EDE-Q = Eating Disorder Examination—Questionnaire, SF-12 = Short-Form 12; MCS/PCS = Mental health/physical health component score; K-10 = Kessler 10-item questionnaire.

3.3. Participant Trajectories from T2 to T4

As shown in Table 5, the majority ($n = 139$, 82.2%) of participants with neither RBE nor ISU in T2 continued to have neither problem in T4, and 12% ($n = 21$) developed RBE. Almost half ($n = 6$, 46.2%) of those with both problems in T2 continued to have both problems in T4. Almost half ($n = 18$, 46.2%) of those with ISU in Year 2 continued to have ISU in year 4 and $n = 7$ (17.9%) developed an additional problem with RBE and $n = 5$ (12.8%) transitioned to RBE alone. The majority ($n = 26$, 57.8%) of those with RBE in T2 had neither problem in T4 and $n = 17$ (37.8%) continued to have RBE alone.

Table 5. Longitudinal movement of participants between groups ($n = 266$).

	Year 4 Participants			
	n (%)			
Year 2 Participants	**Neither**	**Both**	**ISU**	**RBE**
Neither [1]	139 (82.2)	2 (1.2)	7 (4.1)	21 (12.4)
Both [2]	2 (15.4)	6 (46.2)	3 (23.1)	2 (15.4)
ISU [3]	9 (23.1)	7 (17.9)	18 (46.2)	5 (12.8)
RBE [4]	26 (57.8)	1 (2.2)	1 (2.2)	17 (37.8)

[1] Participants with neither RBE *nor* ISU features; [2] Participants with both RBE and ISU features; [3] Participants with ISU features only; [4] Participants with RBE only; RBE = Recurrent Binge Eating ISU = illicit substance use.

As shown in Table 6, participants with neither RBE nor ISU at year 2: were significantly more likely ($p < 0.001$) to remain that way or have RBE only by year 4, were significantly more likely ($p < 0.01$) to have ISU only by year 4, but were not significantly more likely to have both RBE and ISU by year 4. The most likely trajectory for those who were neither RBE nor ISU at year 2 was to remain that way by year 4. Participants being both RBE and ISU at year 2: were significantly more likely ($p < 0.05$) to have ISU only or both RBE & ISU by year 4, but were not significantly more likely to have RBE only or neither RBE nor ISU by year 4. The most likely trajectory for those who were both RBE and ISU at year 2 was to remain that way by year 4. Participants being RBE only at year 2 on the contrary: were significantly more likely ($p < 0.05$) to have RBE only or neither RBE nor ISU by year 4, but were not significantly more likely to have ISU only or both RBE & ISU by year 4. The most likely trajectory for those who were RBE only at year 2 was to have neither RBE nor ISU by year 4. For participants being ISU only at year 2 all transitions to year 4 were statistically significant with the most likely trajectory being both ISU only at year 2 and year 4.

Table 6. Estimated marginal probability with 95% confidence interval for each trajectory from year 2 to year 4 based on multinomial logistic regression controlling for age and mental health-related quality of life.

	Year 4 Outcome Estimated Marginal Probability with 95% Confidence Interval			
	Neither RBE nor ISU	**Both RBE & ISU**	**RBE Only**	**ISU Only**
Year 2 Status				
Neither RBE nor ISU	0.825 [a] (0.764, 0.886)	0.009 (−0.005, 0.024)	0.120 [a] (0.068, 0.172)	0.045 [b] (0.012, 0.078)
Both RBE & ISU	0.213 (−0.556, 0.481)	0.334 [c] (0.009, 0.659)	0.139 (−0.052, 0.331)	0.314 [c] (0.007, 0.621)
RBE Only	0.587 [a] (0.432, 0.741)	0.012 (−0.013, 0.036)	0.363 [a] (0.211, 0.515)	0.038 (−0.016, 0.095)
ISU Only	0.270 [b] (0.116, 0.425)	0.137 [c] (0.012, 0.263)	0.116 [c] (0.014, 0.217)	0.477 [a] (0.299, 0.654)

Note: a is $p < 0.001$, b is $p < 0.01$, c is $p < 0.05$ RBE = recurrent binge eating; ISU = illicit substance use.

4. Discussion

The current study investigated the relationship between RBE and ISU in a sample of Australian non-clinical adult women. The co-occurrence of ISU and RBE was examined cross-sectionally and then longitudinally over two years.

4.1. Comorbid Psychopathology

The hypothesis that RBE and ISU co-occur in the setting of a broader community sample was confirmed. Our study found that those with RBE had a higher frequency of ISU as well as the inverse, i.e., those with ISU had higher frequency of RBE. This co-morbidity might be explained by common neurobiological pathways involved in the two conditions [3,4] or may be a reflection of a self-mediated attempt at regulating negative affect [40], as demonstrated by Killeen et al., who found that past 30 day opiate use was correlated with increased EDE-Q scores [41]. Furthermore, our findings support those of Grilo et al. [42], which found that patients with BED with another concurrent psychiatric disorder had elevated levels of eating disorder psychopathology, although in this study this did not reach significance possibly because of small numbers of those with both problems.

4.2. Participant Trajectories and Between-Group Associations

Results from comparing participant numbers as they moved through from year 2 to year 4 demonstrated that participants with ISU were more likely to develop RBE either in addition to, or in place of their ISU, whereas those with RBE were likely to remain unchanged or spontaneously resolve over time, supporting our hypothesis that the two conditions take unique temporal courses and are differentially predictive for each other. Whist our findings are theoretically supportive of the existing literature in distinguishing RBE/BED and ISU/SUD, there are some differences in results. Measelle et al.'s [21] longitudinal study was similar in part to the present study and focussed on a variety of psychiatric disorders in adolescent girls and the temporal associations between symptom domains; in their study they established that there was a unidirectional relationship between BED and SUD—however, in their case pre-existing eating pathology predicted future growth in substance abuse but not the reverse—the opposite conclusion to this present study. This difference might be because of the shorter duration of this study, that Measelle et al. studied substance use more broadly and included alcohol abuse, and that we were studying subthreshold syndromes. Our findings however support the longitudinal findings of Vogeltanz-Holm et al. [24] that the main predictors for BED are ISU and alcohol intoxication. Furthermore, cessation of drug abuse followed by hyperphagia and weight gain is an established phenomenon in human studies [43] and animal models [44], although whether or not this disordered eating persists and develops into RBE/BED is a matter requiring further investigation.

4.3. Strengths and Limitations

The main strengths of this study include the reasonable sample size (n = 268) for the trajectory analysis and a 75.1% rate of retention of participants over the two-year follow-up period. However, the low numbers of those with both ISU and RBE may have limited finding statistical significance. The longitudinal design of the paper adds robustness to the findings presented in the study. However, the voluntary nature of recruitment and follow-up resulted in only 33.8% of baseline respondents being included for analysis, possibly contributing to elevated findings of eating disorder and ISU. Notably, we did not have a full assessment of the criteria for either BED or SUD, or more detailed assessment of RBE over a longer time frame, and did not assess for legal SUDs. Thus, we turned our focus to ISU and did not include legal substances such as alcohol and tobacco on the presumption that the act of breaching the law and risking the consequences of such more strongly implicates disordered substance use. Another important limitation is the non-inclusion of men as they have significantly higher rates of alcohol and drug use disorders; inclusion might produce altered co-morbidity rates and differing trajectories [45]. Further limitations include the single follow-up, self-report assessments of symptoms and BMI.

4.4. Clinical Implications

The key take-away from this study is that many participants with ISU went on to develop RBE, whilst those with RBE had a tendency for their behaviour to resolve over time. This is a relevant piece of information for clinicians in practice as it suggests that early assessment, monitoring and appropriate early intervention is important for individuals with ISU, and that this occurred despite the low threshold for defining ISU in this research. Finally, despite the stated differences between RBE and ISU, taking an addiction framework towards BED may improve current interventions or instigate the development of new treatments [8].

4.5. Future Directions

Studies investigating predictors for binge eating and its temporal associations are limited and, as such, further mixed-gender longitudinal studies conducted over longer periods of time would be warranted to clarify the associations between RBE and ISU. Other relevant aspects inviting possible future study include the investigation of alcohol or tobacco usage and binge eating behaviour as these commonplace drugs are also frequently consumed in excess. As a final point of interest, within the DSM-5, gambling and other behavioural addictions have been included within the same section as SUDs [46]. Given the co-morbidity between BED and SUD, it would be relevant to also consider the possible neurobiological and symptomatic correlates between full-threshold BED and other addictive disorders. It should be kept in mind as well that BED may be a construct distinct from the entity of "food addiction" which may present more similarities with SUD, and as such, further research is required in this area.

5. Conclusions

In this study, RBE and ISU have been found to be comorbid conditions in a non-clinical sample of young adult women, and furthermore, each condition increased the frequency of episodes of the other. Despite their similarities, the two conditions had a diverse trajectory over time, whereby ISU participants had higher likelihood of later developing RBE co-morbidly or in substitution but the reverse was not found for RBE participants. Further studies are indicated of full-spectrum BED and SUDs.

Acknowledgments: The longitudinal research was funded by a grant from the Australian Rotary Health Research Fund to P.H. and colleagues. H.K.L. was supported by a summer research scholarship from the School of Medicine, Western Sydney University.

Author Contributions: H.K.L. and P.H. contributed to the conception, design and aims of the study. H.K.L., H.M. and P.H. conducted the data analysis. H.K.L. drafted the manuscript. All authors read and approved the final manuscript.

Conflicts of Interest: H.K.L. declares no conflict of interest. P.H. receives sessional fees and lecture fees from the Australian Medical Council, Therapeutic Guidelines publication, and New South Wales Institute of Psychiatry and royalties from Hogrefe and Huber, McGraw Hill Education, and Blackwell Scientific Publications, and she has received research grants from the NHMRC and ARC. She is Deputy Chair of the National Eating Disorders Collaboration steering committee in Australia (2012–2017).

References

1. Cassin, S.E.; von Ranson, K.M. Is binge eating experienced as an addiction? *Appetite* **2007**, *49*, 687–690. [CrossRef] [PubMed]
2. Gearhardt, A.N.; White, M.A.; Potenza, M.N. Binge eating disorder and food addiction. *Curr. Drug Abuse Rev.* **2011**, *4*, 201–207. [CrossRef] [PubMed]
3. Schreiber, L.R.; Odlaug, B.L.; Grant, J.E. The overlap between binge eating disorder and substance use disorders: Diagnosis and neurobiology. *J. Behav. Addict.* **2013**, *2*, 191–198. [CrossRef] [PubMed]

4. Smith, D.G.; Robbins, T.W. The neurobiological underpinnings of obesity and binge eating: A rationale for adopting the food addiction model. *Biol. Psychiatry* **2013**, *73*, 804–810. [CrossRef] [PubMed]
5. American Psychiatric Association. Feeding and Eating Disorders. In *Diagnostic and Statistical Manual of Mental Disorders*, 5th ed.; American Psychiatric Association: Washington, DC, USA, 2013.
6. Grant, J.E.; Potenza, M.N.; Weinstein, A.; Gorelick, D.A. Introduction to behavioral addictions. *Am. J. Drug Alcohol. Abuse* **2010**, *36*, 233–241. [CrossRef] [PubMed]
7. Ferriter, C.; Ray, L.A. Binge eating and binge drinking: An integrative review. *Eat Behav.* **2011**, *12*, 99–107. [CrossRef] [PubMed]
8. Schulte, E.M.; Grilo, C.M.; Gearhardt, A.N. Shared and unique mechanisms underlying binge eating disorder and addictive disorders. *Clin. Psychol. Rev.* **2016**, *44*, 125–139. [CrossRef] [PubMed]
9. Avena, N.M.; Rada, P.; Hoebel, B.G. Evidence for sugar addiction: Behavioral and neurochemical effects of intermittent, excessive sugar intake. *Neurosci. Biobehav. Rev.* **2008**, *32*, 20–39. [CrossRef] [PubMed]
10. Johnson, P.M.; Kenny, P.J. Dopamine D2 receptors in addiction-like reward dysfunction and compulsive eating in obese rats. *Nat. Neurosci.* **2010**, *13*, 635–641. [CrossRef] [PubMed]
11. Avena, N.M.; Rada, P.; Hoebel, B.G. Sugar and fat bingeing have notable differences in addictive-like behavior. *J. Nutr.* **2009**, *139*, 623–628. [CrossRef] [PubMed]
12. American Psychiatric Association. Feeding and Eating Disorders. In *Diagnostic and Statistical Manual of Mental Disorders*, 4th ed.; American Psychiatric Association: Washington, DC, USA, 1994.
13. Harrop, E.N.; Marlatt, G.A. The comorbidity of substance use disorders and eating disorders in women: Prevalence, etiology, and treatment. *Addict. Behav.* **2010**, *35*, 392–398. [CrossRef] [PubMed]
14. Hudson, J.I.; Hiripi, E.; Pope, H.G., Jr.; Kessler, R.C. The prevalence and correlates of eating disorders in the National Comorbidity Survey Replication. *Biol. Psychiatry* **2007**, *61*, 348–358. [CrossRef] [PubMed]
15. Kessler, R.C.; Berglund, P.A.; Chiu, W.T.; Deitz, A.C.; Hudson, J.I.; Shahly, V.; Aguilar-Gaxiola, S.; Alonso, J.; Angermeyer, M.C.; Benjet, C.; et al. The prevalence and correlates of binge eating disorder in the World Health Organization World Mental Health Surveys. *Biol. Psychiatry* **2013**, *73*, 904–914. [CrossRef] [PubMed]
16. Gregorowski, C.; Seedat, S.; Jordaan, G.P. A clinical approach to the assessment and management of co-morbid eating disorders and substance use disorders. *BMC Psychiatry* **2013**, *13*, 289. [CrossRef] [PubMed]
17. Calero-Elvira, A.; Krug, I.; Davis, K.; Lopez, C.; Fernandez-Aranda, F.; Treasure, J. Meta-analysis on drugs in people with eating disorders. *Eur. Eat. Disord. Rev. J. Eat. Disord. Assoc.* **2009**, *17*, 243–259. [CrossRef] [PubMed]
18. Root, T.L.; Pisetsky, E.M.; Thornton, L.; Lichtenstein, P.; Pedersen, N.L.; Bulik, C.M. Patterns of co-morbidity of eating disorders and substance use in Swedish females. *Psychol. Med.* **2010**, *40*, 105–115. [CrossRef] [PubMed]
19. Piran, N.; Robinson, S.R. Associations between disordered eating behaviors and licit and illicit substance use and abuse in a university sample. *Addict. Behav.* **2006**, *31*, 1761–1775. [CrossRef] [PubMed]
20. Piran, N.; Robinson, S.R. Patterns of associations between eating disordered behaviors and substance use in two non-clinical samples: A university and a community based sample. *J. Health Psychol.* **2011**, *16*, 1027–1037. [CrossRef] [PubMed]
21. Measelle, J.R.; Stice, E.; Hogansen, J.M. Developmental trajectories of co-occurring depressive, eating, antisocial, and substance abuse problems in female adolescents. *J. Abnorm. Psychol.* **2006**, *115*, 524–538. [CrossRef] [PubMed]
22. Patton, G.C.; Coffey, C.; Carlin, J.B.; Sanci, L.; Sawyer, S. Prognosis of adolescent partial syndromes of eating disorder. *Br. J. Psychiatry* **2008**, *192*, 294–299. [CrossRef] [PubMed]
23. Sonneville, K.R.; Horton, N.J.; Micali, N.; Crosby, R.D.; Swanson, S.A.; Solmi, F.; Field, A.E. Longitudinal associations between binge eating and overeating and adverse outcomes among adolescents and young adults: Does loss of control matter? *JAMA Pediatr.* **2013**, *167*, 149–155. [CrossRef] [PubMed]
24. Vogeltanz-Holm, N.D.; Wonderlich, S.A.; Lewis, B.A.; Wilsnack, S.C.; Harris, T.R.; Wilsnack, R.W.; Kristjanson, A.F. Longitudinal predictors of binge eating, intense dieting, and weight concerns in a national sample of women. *Behav. Ther.* **2000**, *31*, 221–235. [CrossRef]
25. Konkoly Thege, B.; Woodin, E.M.; Hodgins, D.C.; Williams, R.J. Natural course of behavioral addictions: A 5-year longitudinal study. *BMC Psychiatry* **2015**, *15*, 4. [CrossRef] [PubMed]
26. Grant, J.E.; Schreiber, L.R.; Odlaug, B.L. Phenomenology and treatment of behavioural addictions. *Can J. Psychiatry* **2013**, *58*, 252–259. [CrossRef] [PubMed]

27. Cowan, J.; Devine, C. Food, eating, and weight concerns of men in recovery from substance addiction. *Appetite* **2008**, *50*, 33–42. [CrossRef] [PubMed]
28. Long, C.G.; Blundell, J.E.; Finlayson, G. A Systematic Review of the Application And Correlates of YFAS-Diagnosed 'Food Addiction' in Humans: Are Eating-Related 'Addictions' a Cause for Concern or Empty Concepts? *Obes. Facts* **2015**, *8*, 386–401. [CrossRef] [PubMed]
29. Fairburn, C.G.; Beglin, S.J. Assessment of eating disorders: Interview or self-report questionnaire? *Int. J. Eat. Disord.* **1994**, *16*, 363–370. [PubMed]
30. Wilfley, D.E.; Schwartz, M.B.; Spurrell, E.B.; Fairburn, C.G. Assessing the specific psychopathology of binge eating disorder patients: Interview or self-report? *Behav. Res. Ther.* **1997**, *35*, 1151–1159. [CrossRef]
31. Al-Adawi, S.; Bax, B.; Bryant-Waugh, R.; Claudino, A.M.; Hay, P.; Monteleone, P.; Norring, C.; Pike, K.M.; Pilon, D.J.; Herscovici, C.R.; et al. Revision of ICD—Status update on feeding and eating disorders. *Adv. Eat. Disord.* **2013**, *1*, 10–20. [CrossRef]
32. Grilo, C.M.; White, M.A. A controlled evaluation of the distress criterion for binge eating disorder. *J. Consult. Clin. Psychol.* **2011**, *79*, 509–514. [CrossRef] [PubMed]
33. Wolfe, B.E.; Baker, C.W.; Smith, A.T.; Kelly-Weeder, S. Validity and utility of the current definition of binge eating. *Int. J. Eat. Disord.* **2009**, *42*, 674–686. [CrossRef] [PubMed]
34. Womens Health Australia. *The Australian Longitudinal Study on Women's Health: Data Book*, 2nd ed.; Womens Health Australia: Newcastle, UK, 1997.
35. Andrews, G.; Slade, T. Interpreting scores on the Kessler Psychological Distress Scale (K10). *Aust. N. Z. J. Public Health* **2001**, *25*, 494–497. [CrossRef] [PubMed]
36. Vargas Terrez, B.E.; Villamil Salcedo, V.; Rodríguez Estrada, C.; Pérez Romero, J.; Cortés Sotres, J. Validación de la escala Kessler 10 (K-10) en la detección de depresión y ansiedad en el primer nivel de atención. Propiedades psicométricas. *Salud Ment.* **2011**, *34*, 323–331.
37. Ware, J., Jr.; Kosinski, M.; Keller, S.D. A 12-Item Short-Form Health Survey: Construction of scales and preliminary tests of reliability and validity. *Med. Care* **1996**, *34*, 220–233. [CrossRef] [PubMed]
38. Sanderson, K.; Andrews, G. The SF-12 in the Australian population: Cross-validation of item selection. *Aust. N. Z. J. Public Health* **2002**, *26*, 343–345. [CrossRef] [PubMed]
39. Mond, J.M.; Hay, P.J.; Rodgers, B.; Owen, C.; Beumont, P.J. Validity of the Eating Disorder Examination Questionnaire (EDE-Q) in screening for eating disorders in community samples. *Behav. Res. Ther.* **2004**, *42*, 551–567. [CrossRef]
40. Davis, C.; Carter, J.C. Compulsive overeating as an addiction disorder. A review of theory and evidence. *Appetite* **2009**, *53*, 1–8. [CrossRef] [PubMed]
41. Killeen, T.; Brewerton, T.D.; Campbell, A.; Cohen, L.R.; Hien, D.A. Exploring the relationship between eating disorder symptoms and substance use severity in women with comorbid PTSD and substance use disorders. *Am. J. Drug Alcohol. Abuse* **2015**, *41*, 547–552. [PubMed]
42. Grilo, C.M.; White, M.A.; Masheb, R.M. DSM-IV psychiatric disorder comorbidity and its correlates in binge eating disorder. *Int. J. Eat. Disord.* **2009**, *42*, 228–234. [CrossRef] [PubMed]
43. Edge, P.J.; Gold, M.S. Drug withdrawal and hyperphagia: Lessons from tobacco and other drugs. *Curr. Pharm. Des.* **2011**, *17*, 1173–1179. [CrossRef] [PubMed]
44. Orsini, C.A.; Ginton, G.; Shimp, K.G.; Avena, N.M.; Gold, M.S.; Setlow, B. Food consumption and weight gain after cessation of chronic amphetamine administration. *Appetite* **2014**, *78*, 76–80. [CrossRef] [PubMed]
45. Merikangas, K.R.; McClair, V.L. Epidemiology of substance use disorders. *Hum. Genet.* **2012**, *131*, 779–789. [CrossRef] [PubMed]
46. American Psychiatric Association. Substance-Related and Addictive Disorders. In *Diagnostic and Statistical Manual of Mental Disorders*, 5th ed.; American Psychiatric Association: Washington, DC, USA, 2013.

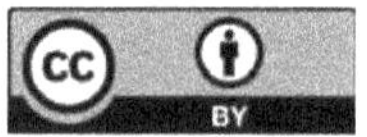

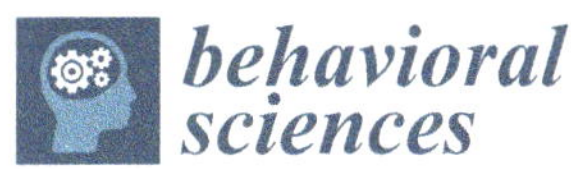
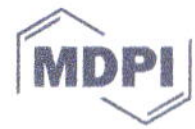

Article

The Influence of Ethnic and Mainstream Cultures on African Americans' Health Behaviors: A Qualitative Study

Ewelina M. Swierad [1], Lenny R. Vartanian [1,*] and Marlee King [2]

[1] School of Psychology, UNSW Sydney, Sydney, NSW 2052, Australia; e.swierad@psy.unsw.edu.au
[2] School of Social Sciences and Psychology, University of Western Sydney, Penrith 2751, Australia; Marlee.King@westernsydney.edu.au
* Correspondence: l.vartanian@unsw.edu.au; Tel.: +61-02-9385-8758

Academic Editors: Amanda Sainsbury and Felipe Q. da Luz
Received: 1 June 2017; Accepted: 2 August 2017; Published: 4 August 2017

Abstract: Background: Culture plays an important role in shaping individuals' health behaviors. This qualitative research examines the relationship between African Americans' ethnic and mainstream cultures and their health behaviors (i.e., food intake and physical activity). Methods: This study used in-depth semi-structured interview format with a group of 25 African Americans to examine the influence of ethnic and mainstream culture on African Americans' food intake and physical activity. Thematic analysis was used to identify common themes and patterns related to African Americans' health behaviors as well as to report these patterns within data. Results: The present study found that African Americans position both their ethnic and mainstream culture as important influences on their health behaviors pertaining to food intake and physical activity. Most participants reported taking advantage of "the best of both worlds" by engaging in *picking and choosing* healthy behaviors from both cultures to which they belong, and they perceived preparing *healthy makeovers* as a way to optimize their health. They also identified a range of practical considerations that can facilitate or hinder engagement in healthy eating and physical activity (e.g., affordability, social support). Participants discussed a number of other positive (e.g., resilience, spirituality) and negative (e.g., experience of discrimination) influences on health behaviors. Conclusions: African Americans consider both their ethnic and mainstream cultures important in shaping their health behaviors. These cultural influences need to be understood in the context of other psycho-socio-environmental factors that affect individuals' health behaviors. The current study has practical implications for designing health promotion programs for African Americans.

Keywords: culture; health; ethnic culture; mainstream culture; health behaviors; picking and choosing; healthy makeovers

---

1. Introduction

African Americans and members of other minority groups are disproportionately affected by overweight and obesity [1–4]. Recent data suggest that, although obesity rates in the US have stabilized in the general population, rates of obesity continue to increase among minority groups, specifically non-Hispanic black women and Mexican American women [3]. Obesity rates are highest among African Americans, affecting 45.0% of non-Hispanic Blacks, as compared to 36.8% of Mexican-Americans, and 30.6% of Whites [5]. Half of African American women and 37% of African American men are obese [6]. African Americans also have one of the lowest rates of physical activity among all ethnic groups in the US [7,8] and are also 38% less likely to meet recommendations for fruit and vegetable consumption as compared to White Americans [9]. Understanding the factors that contribute to these disparities in health and health behaviors is an important part of developing effective preventions. (Note that, in this paper, we use the term "health behaviors" to refer to the broad range of behaviors related to food intake and physical activity.)

It is widely recognized that culture can shape people's food intake and physical activity [10–12] because culture represents set of values, social norms, traditions, and ways of doing things and engaging with the world that are transmitted across generations and influence behaviors [13]. In particular, culture shapes health related values, norms, beliefs, and behaviors through people's connection to their social and physical environments [14]. Given that individuals' social and physical environments change, the influence of culture and culture itself can change as well. Thus, it is also important to recognize that culture embodies not only fixed but also fluid qualities [13]. Some aspects of culture are fixed (e.g., the collectivistic or individualistic focus of a given culture) in that they are transmitted over generations, but other aspects are fluid in that they evolve as the social environment becomes increasingly diverse (e.g., culturally preferred foods that evolve as immigrants come and bring their "own culture" to an existing culture) [15].

Most research in the area of culture and health has focused exclusively on the influence of individuals' ethnic culture on their health behaviors [16–18]. Here we consider ethnic culture to reflect a group of individuals of the same ethnic background sharing similar values, norms, and engaging in similar practices or behaviors. For instance, Airhihenbuwa et al. [16] explored African Americans' perceptions about positive and negative cultural food practices and the contexts in which they occur. Their participants reported that, not only does ethnic culture affect individuals' food choices, but culture also influences how the food is prepared and the context in which it is consumed by creating social norms surrounding these practices.

In addition to exploring the influence of individuals' ethnic culture, the health practices of African Americans also need to be also considered in the context of their mainstream culture (i.e., the most popularized or typical beliefs, norms, and practices—including health related trends surrounding food intake and physical activity—common within American culture). Because African Americans belong to both their ethnic and mainstream cultures, they are exposed to two sets of cultural norms surrounding food intake and physical activity. These multiple cultural norms can potentially have positive or negative influences on individuals' health behaviors. The negative influence is related to the idea that norms of different cultures can be in conflict with each other. Given that cultural norms affect health behaviors, bicultural groups, such African Americans, may be simultaneously exposed to discrepant cultural lifestyle-related norms, and these norms may adversely affect their food intake and physical activity. A few previous qualitative studies explored the relationship between cultural norm discrepancy and health behaviors [18–21]. For example, in one of these qualitative studies, participants reported feeling conflicted between culturally informed eating habits, body size image, and mainstream culture dietary guidelines [21]. Such conflicting norms can contribute to poor health behaviors [11]. For example, they may confuse individuals with regard to what constitutes healthy lifestyle and make it more difficult for them to actually follow any of the norms promoting healthy behaviors that each culture has to offer. Furthermore, the confusion caused by conflicting norms might itself trigger inaction. The exact processes involved in cultural norm conflict and health behaviors, however, are yet to be identified.

There is also a potential positive influence of ethnic and mainstream cultures on one's health, and this is related to the idea that bicultural individuals may have more access to, and more knowledge about, health behaviors that are valued in each of these cultures and that shape their health practices. To date, however, there is very little research examining the ways in which African Americans perceive positive aspects of both cultures influencing health and the ways in which they can capitalize on health enhancing qualities of each culture. Thus, it is important to expand the exploration of culture on health and health behaviors by examining the simultaneous influence of African Americans' ethnic and mainstream cultures, particularly in terms of the positive factors contributing to better health.

The idea that belonging to two different cultures can positively influence one's actions, such as health behaviors, is supported by research on Bicultural Identity Integration [16,22]. According to this construct, exposure to two cultures provides people with an opportunity to learn and benefit from their rich cultural environment [17,23]. Embracing both parts of one's culture can enhance people's lives [18,19,24,25]. For instance, bicultural identity integration was found to increase individuals' creativity [20,26] and their wellbeing [18,19,24,25]. In the context of health, exposure to two cultures affords individuals two sources of information about health trends and practices common in each culture, and these different sources of influence can shape individuals' own health behaviors. For example, one can be exposed to behaviors common in mainstream American culture such as the trend toward healthy eating, and behaviors common in ethnic African American culture such as consuming foods at home with one's family. As a result, individuals can have a broader range of healthy behaviors to choose from while pursuing their healthy lifestyle. These potential benefits of being exposed to two cultures highlights the value in examining the simultaneous influence of African Americans' ethnic and mainstream culture on their health behaviors.

Of course, the influence of culture on individuals' health behaviors cannot be separated from their immediate social context and broader physical environment [12]. For example, research has shown that, because African Americans value collectivism and togetherness, family and friends play an important role in shaping their health behaviors [27,28]. Furthermore, the health behaviors of African Americans are often the result of health and economic disparities among this cultural group. African Americans (and many other minority groups) are disproportionately more likely than White Americans to experience factors such as compromised access to healthy food [29,30], limited access to safe places for physical activity [31] and low affordability of healthy foods [32], and these factors can impact their likelihood of engaging in health behaviors. Thus, the health behaviors of African Americans need to be examined in the context of personal factors, individuals' immediate social environment, and their physical environment [33,34].

The Present Study

There are a few gaps in the previous research on culture and health that the current study attempted to address. First, previous studies have focused on the relationship between culture and African Americans' health behaviors only in the context of African Americans' ethnic culture [11,16]. These studies did not take into account the simultaneous influence of individuals' mainstream and ethnic cultures on their health practices. Given that African Americans are simultaneously exposed to both their ethnic and mainstream American cultures, the present study examined the role of both cultures in individuals' food intake and physical activity.

Second, there are relatively few studies directly examining the interplay between culture and other psycho-socio-environmental factors that collectively affect individuals' health practices [11,16,18]. Because the opportunities to engage in healthy behaviors among African Americans depend on the myriad of interconnected personal, social, and environmental factors, the present study explored the influence of culture on African Americans' food intake and physical activity in the context of these factors. Adopting a qualitative methodological approach can help develop a richer understanding of the role of culture and other psychological, social, and environmental factors in African Americans' health behaviors [11,16,17,35].

Third, most recent studies have focused exclusively on unhealthy norms related to food intake and physical activity, omitting the healthy aspects of individuals' cultures. This approach represents a "deficit model," which, according to previous research, can be counterproductive in health promotion programs [36]. Therefore, in addition to the examination of health compromising (or unhealthy) factors connected to individuals' cultures, the present study focused predominantly on healthy behaviors from both cultures that may optimize African Americans' health and explored how receptive African Americans are to the idea of *picking and choosing* healthy behaviors from their ethnic and mainstream cultures as a means of optimizing their health.

The specific goals of the present qualitative study were to examine: (1) what is the role of people's ethnic and mainstream culture in shaping their health behaviors; (2) how do individuals perceive the idea of *picking and choosing* healthy behaviors from their ethnic and mainstream culture to optimize their health; and (3) what psycho-socio-environmental factors optimize the positive influence of culture on African Americans' food intake and physical activity?

2. Methods

2.1. Research Design

This study used an in-depth semi-structured interview format to examine the influence of ethnic and mainstream cultures on African Americans' health behaviors. This approach was selected because qualitative research has been considered effective in exploring cross-cultural issues related to health, including food intake and physical activity [11,16,17,35]. Semi-structured interviews allow participants reflect freely on their own experiences and observations [37] in their own words rather than categorizing and quantifying of experiences of research participants on pre-established quantitative scales [38]. The interview format enables researchers to obtain detailed insight about participants' experiences, perceptions, beliefs, values, and behaviors [37], which can be particularly important in examining concepts that are relatively unexplored, such as the role of individuals' ethnic and mainstream cultures in their health behaviors.

2.2. Participants and Recruitment Strategies

Participants were 25 individuals recruited from Columbia University and from Harlem, New York, USA (a neighborhood near the university that is largely African American) to participate in individual interviews about "healthy lifestyle related behaviors". Study advertisement fliers were posted throughout the Columbia University campus, and also in churches and grocery stores in Harlem. To be eligible for the study, participants needed to self-identify as African American. Participants were paid USD $20 for their participation in the study.

The majority of the sample (18 participants) was recruited from Columbia University. The remaining seven participants were recruited from Harlem, and they were not associated with Columbia University. See Table 1 for detailed demographic characteristics of the sample. With regard to participants' cultural identification, participants were asked a single question about whether they identified more with their ethnic or mainstream culture. There was variability in the extent to which participants identified with their ethnic vs. mainstream culture (see Table 1).

Table 1. Demographics of the Sample in the Study.

Demographic Characteristics	*n*
Gender	
Female	20
Male	5
Education	
Completed high school	4
BA	2
MA	17
PhD	2
Cultural Identification, self-identified	
Identified more with their ethnic culture	6
Identified more with their mainstream culture	1
Identified equally with both cultures	14
Other	4

The results section of the study will refer to particular participants' responses designated by a participant number. See Appendix A for information on each participant's level of education and cultural identification.

2.3. Procedure

Commencing each interview, the researcher introduced herself and explained the broad purpose of the study. After providing informed consent and permission to audio record the interview, participants completed a brief questionnaire assessing their gender, level of education, and cultural self-identification. The researcher then read the interview questions in sequence, implementing a semi-structured interview format. This format involved using pre-determined probes, such as brief open-ended questions or clarification statements to help participants elaborate on some important themes. Interviews were held over a three-week period at Columbia University. The interview questions aimed to explore the cross-section of culture and health, and focused specifically on two research questions: (1) "culture, barriers to, and facilitators of, healthy lifestyle among African Americans"; and (2) "the simultaneous influence of both one's ethnic and mainstream cultures on African Americans' health behaviors". Interview questions (see Table 2) were developed based on a combination of complementary strategies which included: (1) literature review of qualitative studies related to health behaviors among African Americans [11,16,18]; (2) conversations with a four self-identified members of African American culture; and (3) consultation with an African American researcher in the field of psychology to ensure the cultural sensitivity of the questions. The interviews lasted on average 40 min.

2.4. Ethical Considerations

The study was approved by UNSW ethics committee, and the permission to recruit participants for the study was obtained from the Institutional Review Board at Columbia University.

2.5. Thematic Analysis

The interviews were transcribed by three independent transcribers and de-identified. Each participant was assigned a number (e.g., "Participant 1"). Interview transcripts were then imported into NVivo version 10 (QSR International, Melbourne, Australia) [39], a qualitative data analysis computer software package.

Thematic analysis [37] was used to identify common themes and patterns related to African Americans' health behaviors as well as to report these patterns within data. Thematic analysis recognizes language as a tool for storytelling that reflects people's broader social and physical environments [40]. In other words, this approach highlights the ways in which people make sense of their experiences that are informed by their social and environmental context [41]. Understanding the context of people's experiences, such as culture and the psycho-socio-environmental factors examined in this study, seems to be particularly important in the case of members of minority groups (i.e., African Americans in the context of this study) that are often discriminated against and overpowered by external, systemic forces affecting their lives [40]. Therefore, this method is well-suited to examine the perceptions and experiences of African Americans with regards to their health behaviors.

Following the thematic analysis guidelines created by Braun and Clarke [37], the first step was 'in-depth familiarization' of data by reading transcripts multiple times. This enabled the generation of initial codes, which involved organizing data into meaningful groups and identifying potentially important information within a data set. Codes were then organized into themes. This process started from analyzing the patterns between previously identified codes and considering how different codes may connect with each other forming an overarching theme [37]. Once the final thematic framework was established, the names of the themes were further refined so that they fit the story that the data were illustrating. During each stage of analysis, the analyses were initially conducted by the first author and were then discussed in detail with the second and third authors. This ensured that there was a consistency within patterns identified, and that the analysis was plausible.

Table 2. Interview Script, Questions, and Probes.

Please think for a moment about the values, strengths, and beliefs that are common in your African American culture. Also think about the behaviors that are common in your African American culture that relate to health and wellbeing (defined as the state of being comfortable, healthy, and happy). Now I want to ask you some questions related to the connection of these values and strengths to healthy lifestyle and wellbeing.	
1	In general, what do you think helps African Americans living in urban areas: (1) eat healthy; (2) be active; and (3) increase their wellbeing? (Probe: please think about specific behaviors, e.g., ways of preparing food, portion size, food labels, type of exercise etc.)
2	In general, what do you think makes it difficult for African Americans living in urban areas to: (1) eat healthy; (2) be active; and (3) increase their wellbeing? (Probe: please think about specific behaviors, e.g., ways of preparing food, portion size, food labels, type of exercise etc.)
3	Which cultural strengths, beliefs, or values do you think can help African Americans living in urban areas: (1) eat healthy; (2) be active; and (3) increase their wellbeing?
4	What can mainstream American culture learn from African Americans about healthy lifestyle, specifically regarding: (1) eating healthy; (2) being active; and (3) wellbeing? (Probe: Any specific behaviors you may think of?)
5	What can African Americans learn from mainstream American culture about healthy lifestyle specifically related to: (1) eating healthy; (2) being active; and (3) wellbeing? (Probe: Any specific behaviors you may think of?)
6	As someone living in the US, you are exposed to components of both your African American culture and to mainstream American culture. When you think about the healthy lifestyle behaviors that you engage in, would you say that these are more common in mainstream American culture, or more common in your African American culture? Do you *pick and choose*, so to speak, different health behaviors from both cultures?
7	Do you think that African Americans can *pick and choose* healthy behaviors and practices from both their mainstream and ethnic culture in order to optimize their health? Can they do so without compromising their cultural identity? (Probe: Would it be difficult? Or easy? Do you do it? Do you know people who do it? What's difficult about it, if anything? What is easy about it, if anything? What would make it easier for people to do it?)
8	What should members of mainstream American culture do more of to facilitate the improvement of health and wellbeing, specifically healthy eating, and exercise, of African American communities? (Probe: Think of health providers, individuals, and mainstream organizations such as schools or work places.)
Now, I want you to talk specifically about those people in your African American culture who try to lead a healthy lifestyle. Please think about specific person or a group of people you know.	
1	What do they typically do that helps them lead a healthy lifestyle? (Probe: Any specific behaviors you may think of related to (1) eating healthy; (2) being active; and (3) wellbeing?)
2	What helps them engage in these behaviors? (Probe: The role of other people, family friends?)
3	How does your family affect your healthy lifestyle choices related to: (1) eating healthy; (2) being active; and (3) wellbeing?
4	How do your friends affect your healthy lifestyle choices regarding: (1) eating healthy; (2) being active; and (3) wellbeing?
Is there anything else that you would like to add that could be important to understanding health behaviors and healthy lifestyles for African Americans?	

3. Results

Two broad themes were identified throughout the interviews: (Section 3.1) Culturally-derived barriers to and facilitators of a healthy lifestyle and (Section 3.2) Practical considerations beyond culture when adopting a healthier lifestyle.

Within the first primary theme, (Section 3.1) *Culturally-derived barriers to and facilitators of a healthy lifestyle*, a number of subthemes were identified, including: (Section 3.1.1) "It's a strength": Drawing upon ethnic culture to improve health behavior; (Section 3.1.2) Difficulties changing a culturally ingrained proclivity for "unhealthy" behaviors; (Section 3.1.3) The "healthy" individual: Aligning health beliefs and behaviors with that of mainstream culture; (Section 3.1.4) "The best of both worlds": Combining cultural and mainstream approaches to health; and (Section 3.1.5) The importance of support from the ethnic and mainstream community.

Within the second theme, (Section 3.2) *Practical considerations beyond culture when adopting a healthier lifestyle*, the responses were coded under the following subthemes: (Section 3.2.1) "It's is not worth it to eat healthy": The cost of having a healthy lifestyle; (Section 3.2.2) Access to healthy foods, healthy living and education, and (Section 3.2.3) Personal factors and motivation.

3.1. *Culturally-Derived Barriers to and Facilitators of a Healthy Lifestyle*

Within this theme, African Americans described how their ethnic culture and their mainstream culture was a source of strength and a source of weakness to their health behaviors, detailing culturally-derived barriers to and facilitators of a healthy lifestyle.

3.1.1. "It's a Strength": Drawing upon Ethnic Culture to Improve Health Behavior

When asked to describe what cultural values, norms, or beliefs help African Americans lead a healthy lifestyle, many people spoke of resilience as a culturally valued trait that historically has helped African Americans to deal with slavery, oppression, and discrimination. This ability to endure externally imposed pain and discomfort in order to improve one's life circumstances was identified as a beneficial characteristic that African Americans can apply to healthy lifestyle. For example, *Participant 19* described the importance of resilience in facilitating health behaviors saying:

> "I feel like, our strengths and determination have help with healthy lifestyle; we tend to be very determined in doing anything we want to do; and it it's a fight; it's a strength and a fight to stand through a lot of harsh stuff. I feel like that strength, if it can be just implemented into healthy living, then I think that determination to want to change lifestyle from eating the traditional, unhealthy, greasy, heavily salted, to healthy living can change a lot of things in the culture".

Evident in the excerpt above, *Participant 19* attributes African Americans' experience with adversity and their determination as a strength that assists them when faced with challenges such as changing a culturally embedded practice—eating some traditional unhealthy foods. This idea of collective resilience emphasizes the notion of strength and pride associated with African American values.

In the same vein, several participants indicated that resilience, or as *Participant 11* puts it "you can do-itness", can be a powerful source of healthy behaviors, helping people to explore creative ways of eating healthy and exercising. That is, resilience helps people overcome some of the barriers to healthy living common within African American communities. For example, *Participant 13* emphasized the importance of resilience by saying:

> "In terms of the strengths, I think the strengths we have is that we're a resilient people and we know that we have the potential within us to improve, but we just need ... we need to make it a culture of speaking and engaging with each other about the things that are relevant to our health and happiness. And our eating habits. And once we can spread that word we can make that become more of a culture in the black community in terms of what we eat. I think it will make a tremendous difference. There are traces of that starting already".

Evident in the above excerpt is the notion that resilience goes beyond strength and becomes more of an issue of awareness, connected to happiness and health. The concept of resilience was also apparent in *Participant 16's* account:

> "With the little that we some of us, many of us do have we've learnt to like stretch and make a lot of it. Even with like the food that we have a lot of our ethnic food came from like. Even back from when we were enslaved and we like, like we had like you know not the best portions of particular animal or, um but we learnt how to you know like make it really good".

The importance of church or spirituality was also discussed as a factor that helps people engage in healthy eating and physical activity. Many participants talked about "spiritual connection" or "religion" as essential support systems that facilitate healthy lifestyle. *Participant 6* explained the role of spirituality in enhancing African Americans health behaviors and talked about the ways in which church can help in promoting healthy living:

> "In my church they encourage you to eat healthy and if you're stressed out, church is an avenue where you can find some type of relief so I would say that church would be one of the biggest things that helps".

Similarly, *Participant 5* spoke about a church as a place that provides a sense of community in which people work together on common goals and inspire one another to lead better and healthier lives: "If you're part of a church and your church group goes walking every day you're more likely to go walking with a group so you could talk and socialize and work out".

According to some participants, spirituality may also provide guidelines for the way people should treat their bodies. *Participant 4* emphasized her belief that, "your body is your temple from God and you're supposed to take care of it." She further stated:

> "This is the body that God gave me and I need to make sure I'm doing the best I can with it to; taking care of myself honors God because you know, gluttony is a sin and you're not supposed to over-eat, you're not supposed to do all of this stuff. So it's the spirituality and the appreciation of the body and the understanding what when I eat healthy, I feel better".

Noteworthy is how *Participant 4* emphasized that perceiving overeating as a sin helps her eat healthy. Therefore, the role of spirituality in initiating health behaviors among African Americans is not only about perceiving one's body "as a temple", but also fearing engagement in "sinful" overindulgence.

Participants also broadly discussed dance and music as factors that are highly appreciated in African American culture and that facilitate healthy lifestyle. The appreciation of dance and movement highlights that exercise does not have to be hard or unenjoyable, it can be a fun activity and a very normal part of one's life. In describing the importance of dance in her life, *Participant 20* said:

> "We all love to dance. I love to dance, where I grew up dance was the exercise you went to; an African weekly dance class or any kind of dance class like we did, all kinds of dance, modern, hip-hop like, even Zumba that used to be my primary way of exercising".

Reflecting the importance of music and dance in shaping African Americans health, *Participant 13* stated:

> "[...] Music. I think one thing you know, we're trendsetters. That's, you know, um ... if given the opportunity, we're an active people [...] when we don't have the opportunity, we find a way sometimes to enjoy ourselves and dancing, you know, is a strong culture in the black community".

Participants indicated that they stay active through non-traditional means of physical activity such as dancing, a cultural activity embedded in the black community. Similarly, *Participant 4* emphasized the importance of dance saying:

> "[...] The music, the rhythm, and dance - it is all like a big healthy thing but it's not framed as that. Like when kids go to dance and you see them dancing, I mean their dances are very aerobic. You don't always think of it as them exercising but it is".

3.1.2. Difficulties Changing a Culturally Ingrained Proclivity for 'Unhealthy' Behaviors

While discussing cultural factors that influence health-compromising behaviors, the majority of participants focused on culturally preferred, traditional ethnic foods which they described as mostly "unhealthy". Cooking with fat, such as lard, seasoning heavily with spices and salt, eating pork meat frequently—all these food consumption practices, derived from long standing tradition within the culture, were described as impeding a healthy lifestyle within African American communities. Because these practices are deeply ingrained within the culture, they are perceived as difficult to change. As *Participant 14* explained:

> "Within our community we've always been like, "the greasier the food, the better". We still like cooking with lard and, you know, it is just ingrained [...] it's literally a passed down thing from one generation to another".

Several participants expressed that, although most African Americans realize that some aspects of their traditional cuisine are unhealthy, ethnic food is comforting and allows for connectedness, expression of one's cultural identity, and the connection to African American culture. As *Participant 13* noted:

> "It [traditional ethnic food] is a cultural connotation and it's also almost a spiritual thing. It's, you know [...] And a loving thing because it's a part of this joy in cooking, and there's that, you know, feeling of love you're preparing for your family".

However, people reported feeling conflicted between their desire to unite around their ethnic food, and their awareness of the fact that their traditional food may not always be the healthiest. For example, *Participant 8* said:

> "Soul food' is not the healthiest food; and the food people typically choose to eat, as a culture, isn't the most healthy. But there's strong family bonds that happen around this food. So it's kind of a disconnect. Family bonds are strong, but the nutrition typically isn't that great".

Noteworthy is how participants indicated that their traditional ethnic food strengthens bonds with their families and their culture, but this type of food is also unhealthy. The conflict surrounding African Americans traditional ethnic foods is evident in *Participant 4*'s words: "it's a comfort food because we've united around that but it's not healthy food. And how do you change that without feeling like you're somehow stepping away from your culture"?

3.1.3. The 'Healthy' Individual: Aligning Health Beliefs and Behaviors with that of Mainstream Culture

In describing healthy aspects of their mainstream culture, many participants indicated that the recent trend of promoting healthy lifestyle within their mainstream culture seems to be an important factor encouraging their healthy behaviors. Quite frequently participants mentioned that mainstream culture promotes "adapting more vegetarian lifestyle" (Participant 4), "controlling one's portion size" (*Participant* 3), "learning about healthy options" (*Participant* 9), and "eating in moderation" (*Participant 19*). According to participants, healthy lifestyle was more frequently promoted within their mainstream American culture than in their African American culture. *Participant 1* expressed this observation by saying:

> "I think there's a lot of values that Americans place on health that are really important; like it's more of a priority than in African American culture [...] I think health should be a priority to people".

Similarly, when asked what African Americans can learn from their mainstream culture that would help them lead healthy lifestyle, *Participant 16* pointed to a focus on taking care of one's body, physical health, and wellbeing, saying:

> "I feel like we can definitely learn a lot more about just caring for our bodies in general. Even just things like drinking more water, which some of us don't like to do haha. You know drinking more water and just taking care of like both emotionally and mentally and also physically our well-being. So for sure".

This sentiment of equating some aspects of mainstream American culture with a strong emphasis on health was echoed in *Participant 6's* account. She noted that "mainstream America seems to be more focused on health and mental health as well and wellbeing".

Another important salutogenic property of mainstream American culture that many participants focused on was the importance of being physically active. Participants commented that regular physical activity is promoted within their mainstream culture, and that being active may exemplify itself in many different forms. As *Participant 6* noted:

> "Mainstream American culture promotes that you exercise every day; and promotes staying active and keep moving; and even if today's not basketball today, still go outside and take a walk kind of a thing".

3.1.4. "The Best of Both Worlds": Combining Cultural and Mainstream Approaches to Health

Participants were directly asked to share their perspective on the possibility of *picking and choosing* typical healthy behaviors from both cultures in order to optimize their health. They were very receptive to the idea of *picking and choosing* and they had a lot to say about an issue. *Participant 19* described the benefits of this approach by stating:

> "Everything that's out there when it comes to healthy behaviors we can implement into our everyday lives and it could be the best of both worlds; it's something new and something refreshing and then it's been a part of you for generations; and putting them both together can be amazing".

The majority of participants indicated that they indeed incorporate different elements of their ethnic and their mainstream culture into their healthy lifestyle related practices; and that "it's important to integrate both cultures as there are aspects from each culture that is positive that we [African Americans] can all learn from" (*Participant 20*). *Participant 6*, for example, described her experience in taking advantage of being part of both her ethnic and mainstream cultures to improve her health:

> "I *pick and choose*. Okay let's go to food. So the first one would be not eating out too much, that's something I grew up with in my ethnic culture, try and cook your own food. But then one thing I adapted from mainstream culture is - like I said, I'm a vegetarian- eating more greens and stuff like that. My answer would be *pick and choose* because I choose what's good from my culture and I choose what's good in my mainstream America, and I try to combine it".

Illustrated in the quote above is the flexibility of belonging to both ethnic and mainstream cultures. People are not bound by African American traditions, and they can move between their mainstream and ethnic cultures. Taking advantage of these two cultures to which African Americans belong further highlights that African Americans are "agentic" (*Participant 20*), actively making decisions about their health.

Participant 14 echoed the opinion expressed above by stating that *picking and choosing* is a good way "to try new and different healthy things," "to embrace both ethnic and mainstream culture," "to inspire other people to lead healthy lifestyle," and "to avoid boredom". As she said: "I think it's best to be able to *pick and choose* things [healthy behaviors] from both cultures so you don't get bored doing the same repetitive things that you've been doing".

Although people mostly talked about *picking and choosing* within one specific domain (i.e., food or physical activity), sometimes *picking and choosing* healthy behaviors from both cultures involved the mix of food intake and physical activity. This selective choice of the best of both worlds seems to be apparent in *Participant 23's* words:

> "I would say that in terms of eating habits eating more fresh vegetables and fruits and stuff like that, it's probably more from mainstream American culture, and then more of a focus on athleticism as a woman comes from my African American culture".

Most participants agreed that *picking and choosing* can be or is (for those who already *pick and choose*) beneficial for their health as they believed that in order to acquire an optimum health, it is essential to incorporate health behaviors from different cultures to which they belong.

Preparing *healthy makeovers* of some of the unhealthy dishes was another commonly identified strategy to optimize one's health. *Participant 19* emphasized the importance of preparing *healthy makeovers* of some of the less healthy foods saying:

> "You can choose to, prepare your traditional meals but opt for a better healthier version. Um don't heavily season it, don't overcook it, or um implement different areas of this healthy kick into the foods you've loved since you were a kid, and try new things and see what works for you".

Consuming *healthy makeovers* of some of the less healthy foods without the necessity to give up one's favorite dishes was described as a valuable, and not overly complicated way to improve one's health. Some participants indicated that they can still, as *Participant 23* stated, "create foods that [...] are staples of African-American diet," but prepare them in a "healthier way". *Participant 13* described his experiences with *healthy makeovers* saying:

> "I'm going to have my chicken baked instead of fried, how is that? Maybe I'll have a baked potato instead of French fries. Small things like that. But they [people in the community] need to see that and they need to see other black folks doing it. So it's, it's a communal thing and it needs to be in their face".

Evident in the above extract is the notion that preparing healthy makeover is a gradual process that involves small steps and engages the entire community so that it becomes a "communal" phenomenon.

3.1.5. The Importance of Support from the Ethnic and Mainstream Community

When it comes to lack of social support and aversive social environment, the experiences of discrimination and distrust toward mainstream culture were two of the most commonly mentioned factors rooted in mainstream culture that negatively affect African Americans' health behaviors and wellbeing. In particular, many people spoke about current racial tension in the United States and their discomfort with regard to "anything mainstream," and about their vanishing faith in mainstream culture. In describing her thoughts associated with barriers to healthy lifestyle that hail from mainstream culture, *Participant 4* said:

> "With everything that's going on now, you see that well-being, your emotional and physical well-being is very much influenced by the way that you're treated within these urban environments. And I think there's a higher percentage of African Americans who are not just, not well, because we know that we kinda live in an anti-black society".

Similarly, when asked about the factors that compromise African Americans' health behaviors and wellbeing, *Participant 24* spoke about daily experiences of racism among many African Americans:

> "Let's start with systematic racism. I think it's different for every person. I was fortunate enough to be able to attend Colombia University so I have slipped through the cracks of oppression and been able to have this great education here. But not everyone can make it out and not everyone can have those opportunities to see past a bunch of negativity whether it be from racist employers or racist police or people who would judge you by your appearance and not know what's in your head. Um, so I think that's one thing that's a daily challenge to a lot of people".

This point of view was common among other participants. Some people gave a quite vivid and emotional account of the experiences of racism and discrimination that were deemed to be an unfortunate part of many people's lives and that prevent them from being healthy. Some participants, such as *Participant 4*, spoke about lack of support from mainstream culture of African Americans' health in general and described the notion that African Americans are seen as lesser within the wider mainstream culture:

> "I don't know, I have very little faith in mainstream America right now and I have very little faith that they care enough to do anything different for the African American community. I think, they would have to see us as human before they would even be able to help us be healthier and I just don't think that enough of them believe in our humanity".

Noteworthy is the sense of helplessness in the above account and the degree of dependency on mainstream America to assist African Americans to become healthier.

Just as negative social environment can be detrimental for African Americans' health, strong social support can enhance individuals' health behaviors. Evident in participants' responses is that their social environment, specifically their family and friends, can constitute a powerful catalyst for healthy behaviors. Some participants reported that their loved ones, family and friends often inspired them to eat healthy and exercise. For example, *Participant 5* commented on the influence of people's social environment on their engagement of health behaviors by saying that:

> "Having friends who do it [lead healthy lifestyle] can help – if you know that group of people [that] work out and run from Central Park and back, I feel like that you're more likely like to engage in that type of behavior if you know your friends are doing it".

Furthermore, *Participant 16* suggested friends often provide a necessary support that prevents people from indulging in unhealthy food, stating:

> "My friend and I really encouraged each other. So I would be like "oh I'm really dying for chicken wings" she would be like "No don't do it!". And so like having that support that is really great. She would be like "oh I was at work today and I'm thinking about having a donut" and I'm like "don't do it! You don't want to do it"!

Some participants mentioned the role of family in highlighting different concerns related to health, such as delayed financial burden that can be triggered by unhealthy lifestyle choices, or the preference for a lean body type. Delayed financial burden refers to future financial consequences of current unhealthy practices. For example, *Participant 2* stated:

> "One of the things that my family really pressures me to do this eat healthy now because of the financial burden that it brings on later. So like my dad who has high blood pressure and diabetes [...] and he has to pay about $900 a month for medicine because of the choices that he made earlier in life so he encourages me to eat healthy and have a healthy lifestyle because of the financial burden it's caused. My mom on the other hand, she favors having a small frame being lean, being skinny and she pressures me to eat healthy because of that".

Other family members may provide indirect motivation for one to stay healthy. Reflecting on the role of family in her health, *Participant 19* said:

> "Family members with high blood pressure, and, some family members with diabetes motivate me a little bit more to want to continue exercising and healthy eating just so I won't have those complications later on in life".

This suggests that pursuing healthy lifestyle African Americans may not only be inspired by healthy behaviors of their family members and friends, but they also can be influenced by fear that comes from their willingness to avoid poor health in the future.

Additionally, participants often talked about bi-directional, cross-generational influence of family members on one's health. It seems as though both older and younger members of one's family can contribute to the improvement of other family members' health. For example, *Participant 10* reflects on these bi-directional influences between younger and older generation and on the importance of positive modelling behavior saying:

> "My mum makes smoothies, she's tried juicing [...] And like she goes to the gym sometimes, but mostly if I'm with her, she's more motivated to go. So I guess that companionship helps her to be more inclined to work out [...] I think I do influence my family too. 'Cause I'm always talking about eating healthy and you know they joke around with me about like, oh you're eating this and it's not gluten free, like so they'll poke fun at me but I definitely influence them. I feel like they have made some improvement in their food options as far as leaning more toward the healthy side because of me, so .... ."

While it is important to understand African Americans' mainstream and ethnic cultures in the context of the facilitators of and barriers to healthy food intake and physical activity, it is equally important to examine factors that directly affect the influence of culture on individuals' health. In other words the ability of culture to influence people's health depends on other practical considerations beyond culture.

3.2. *Practical Considerations beyond Culture When Adopting a Healthier Lifestyle*

3.2.1. "It's is not worth it to eat healthy": The Cost of Having a Healthy Lifestyle

Most participants reported that being able to afford fresh fruits and vegetables would make it much easier for them to engage in a range of different health behaviors that are typical in both ethnic and mainstream cultures. Most participants indicated that "income" influences "what and how healthy" people eat within African American communities. Lack of affordable food and exercise options was one of the major barriers to healthy living for African Americans. Therefore, providing affordable options with regard to healthy eating and exercising was identified as one of the most important factors that can facilitate healthy food intake and physical activity, as *Participant 16* said:

> "I think having things that are affordable. That's number one. That's a pretty big issue. If it's something that's free in the neighborhood or it's more affordable for them [African Americans] I feel like that will make them more like "okay I can do this. I can afford $10 once a week". So I definitely feel like having more affordable options for fitness and for food is definitely would help us".

Several, participants spoke about "the cost-benefit analysis" that they engage in daily when making decisions about the type of food they purchase, explaining that they are often faced with a dilemma to either pay more and get smaller amount of healthy food or pay less and get larger amount of unhealthy food. *Participant 10* described this dilemma saying:

> "If you have a choice between an apple for $1 for a full meal for $1, that may not be the healthy choice but that's gonna make you full, you will choose the second option".

Similarly, *Participant 18* said: "Why go buy a tomato for four dollars when I can go get four burgers at McDonald's for four dollars too"?

In general, participants expressed the belief that, in order for African Americans to engage in healthy behaviors from both their ethnic and mainstream culture, the healthy choices need to be more affordable. That is, there needs to be economically reasonable alternatives to the unhealthy food options that are both easily accessible and affordable. This belief is exemplified by the following statement from *Participant 24*:

> "I think that people would consider eating healthy it if it was economically feasible, but you know if you have cheaper ingredients, if it's cheaper to use butter than it is to use olive oil, then they're going to use the butter".

This notion of "it is not worth it to eat healthy" was common among participants and was described as one of the reasons for poor health behaviors within their communities.

3.2.2. Access to Healthy Foods, Healthy Living, and Education

Several participants indicated that it is essential for African Americans to be able to afford healthy foods, but these options need to be readily available to them. Consistent with this notion, *Participant 15* stated:

> "If healthy food and wellness, and lifestyle was sitting right there in front of you, I don't think anybody's choosing unhealthy option. It's not like if presented with option A—a life of prosperity, happiness, wellness, healthy, long-life, longevity, and option B—devastation, terrible diet, health, diabetes, anyone would say "I think I want B", you know. So if it's not presented to you don't even know you can choose it".

Some participants explained that having access and exposure to healthy food can make a difference in many African American communities. This notion is exemplified by the following excerpt from *Participant 14*:

> "If we have the access ... to fruit stands and the stores and the, you know, the health foods stores that they tend to have in other areas, I think it would work; I just think that we have to actually be able to see it in the area, you know. 'Cause if we see it we're gonna to be intrigued by something new. So I think if you put it within the community I think it'll work because initially we do wanna live a long period of time I think like everyone else".

Another frequently identified factors that can help African Americans enhance their health behaviors was health education. Knowing what is considered healthy, how to prepare healthy meals, and where to find an affordable place to exercise were identified by participants as common concerns. For example, *Participant 16* summarized the importance of education in shaping community's health saying:

> "Education I feel like is number one. So for people to know exactly where to find healthier options for food, where to find your exercise programs or fitness programs within their community so you don't have to travel so far".

Participant 4 shared a similar thought:

> "Showing people how to incorporate different foods into your diets is important. And now I'm ordering cookbooks and stuff so I can see different foods and spices, but like for people who haven't ventured out to learn about different healthy foods, they don't know what they eat, or how food affects their body, or how to cook them. So education is a key".

In general, participants often discussed education in the context of awareness of what constitutes healthy lifestyle and in which creative ways African Americans can learn about healthy practices.

3.2.3. Personal Factors and Motivation

Many participants described personal motivation as an essential ingredient in the pursuit and maintenance of healthy lifestyle. For example, Participant 16 expressed his opinion about the role of motivation in pursuing healthy behaviors, saying:

> "I feel like it [healthy lifestyle] has to first start with you motivating yourself. Some people feel like maybe it's too late, I've gotten too far, I can't start now. So that self-doubt probably is already there".

Similarly, with physical activity, many people identified motivation as a factor that "helps them start and then keeps them going". Personal motivation and commitment to a healthy lifestyle were indicated as essential components of taking advantage of healthy behaviors people are exposed to in both their ethnic and mainstream cultures. As *Participant 8* said, "If someone is not motivated, it's hard to have them change [. . .] I think that's the biggest thing, you know, prioritizing yourself".

4. Discussion

The present study explored: (1) the role of people's ethnic and mainstream cultures in shaping their health behaviors; (2) how individuals perceive the idea of *picking and choosing* healthy behaviors from their ethnic and mainstream culture to optimize their health; and (3) psycho-socio-environmental factors that optimize the positive influence of culture on African Americans' food intake and physical activity. The findings illustrate the importance of both ethnic and mainstream cultures in African Americans' food intake [11,16] and physical activity [17]. In particular, the present study found that African Americans position both their ethnic and mainstream culture as important influences on their health behaviors. Thus, the present findings extend previous research by highlighting the simultaneous influences of both African Americans' ethnic culture and mainstream American culture on their food intake and physical activity and by emphasizing the importance of taking the advantage of "the best of both worlds" (that is, combining cultural and mainstream approaches to health).

With respect to their ethnic culture, and consistent with previous research, participants often mentioned resilience [33], reliance on spirituality [11,42], dance and music [43] and social support [28] as important health-enhancing qualities endorsed in their African American culture. In contrast, traditional "soul food" cuisine was reported as one of the most important cultural factors that compromises healthy food intake within African American communities [43]. This finding may explain why preparing *healthy makeovers* of some of the less healthy traditional African American dishes appealed to participants in the present study. The importance of *healthy makeovers* identified in this study is consistent with previous research [11,16] and suggests that African Americans may embrace the idea of preparing healthier versions of some of the unhealthy traditional dishes in order to improve their health yet maintain connect with their cultural traditions.

With respect to individuals' mainstream culture, participants indicated that "healthy lifestyle trends" popularized within their mainstream culture and the importance placed on physical activity are two the most important salutogenic qualities of their mainstream culture. In contrast, and consistent with previous research [44], the experience of discrimination within one's mainstream culture was reported as one of the biggest health compromising factor. All these findings suggest that ethnic and mainstream cultural norms and behaviors around food intake and physical activity can be important in shaping African Americans' health behaviors.

Given that African Americans belong simultaneously to their ethnic and their mainstream cultures, the current study also examined individuals' reactions to the idea of *picking and choosing*, that is incorporating the healthy elements of both cultures into their lives. Most participants reported engaging in *picking and choosing* healthy behaviors related to food intake and physical activity from both cultures to which they belong. They also perceived *picking and choosing* these behaviors as a way to optimize their health. The potential benefits of incorporating normative behaviors from one's ethnic and mainstream cultures is consistent with the concept of Bicultural Identity Integration [22], which is associated with greater wellbeing, creativity, problem solving, and coping strategies [23]. In the context of current study, one possible explanation as to why engaging in behaviors from both cultures may be beneficial for African Americans' health is that doing so provides individuals with a wider range of health behaviors to choose from as opposed to relying on just one source of information about health and wellbeing. Belonging to more than one culture exposes individuals to a broader range of norms, values, and beliefs on the basis of which they can govern their behaviors [13,22], including their health behaviors.

There are also a variety of practical considerations (environmental and personal factors) that participants described as influencing their opportunities to engage in healthy behaviors from both cultures. Consistent with previous research, participants in the current study reported that affordability [45], access to healthy food [30], health knowledge [46] and personal factors [47] are important in determining African American's health behaviors. The current study, however, builds on previous research by examining these psycho-socio-environmental factors in association with individuals' ability to incorporate healthy behaviors from both their ethnic and mainstream cultures (i.e., to *pick and choose* and to *consume healthy makeovers* of unhealthy dishes). For example, the willingness to consume fruits and vegetables, which are heavily promoted within mainstream culture, depends on a proper access to these types of foods. This finding suggests that the influence of ethnic and mainstream culture on African American's health behaviors should be examined in the relation to their broader psycho-socio-environmental context (consistent with ecological models of health behaviors, such as the PEN-3 model [10]).

The results of the present study may have some implications for planning and designing health promotion programs for African Americans. First, the fact that participants show favorable attitudes toward *picking and choosing* and toward *healthy makeovers* suggests that they are open to taking advantage of healthy behaviors promoted in both their ethnic and mainstream cultures. Although there is the potential for both positive and negative influence of ethnic and mainstream cultures on health, these findings further suggest that health interventions could focus on positive health enhancing behaviors already celebrated within individuals' cultures [12], rather than focusing solely on eliminating health-compromising behaviors. Shifting from a deficit model to a strength-based model empowers ethnic minority groups and validates their experiences without unnecessarily pathologizing their health practices [16]. Of course, research is needed to determine the extent to which incorporating practices from both cultures (including *picking and choosing* and *consuming healthy makeovers*) is an effective means of improving the health and wellbeing of African Americans. Additionally, given that cultural practices and norms can be in conflict with one another and contribute to unhealthy behaviors surrounding food intake and physical [18,19], future studies should simultaneously examine the impact of positive cultural influences, negative cultural influence, and cultural conflicts on individuals' health behaviors.

Second, by providing an opportunity for individuals to decide which behaviors are important to them, the *picking and choosing* approach resembles the "cultural tailoring" framework of health promotion [14]. This health promotion model is directed toward individuals and cultural subgroups, and acknowledges within-culture differences among people, taking into consideration personal choices and preferences. The autonomy and freedom to make a choice is one of the most fundamental human needs affecting individuals' performance, relationships, and wellbeing [48,49]. Being able to make a choice increases individuals' intrinsic motivation and self-efficacy, which further enhance adherence to behavioral change goals [50,51]. Overall, having the opportunity to choose health behaviors that individuals want to pursue is gratifying, desirable, and important from health promotion perspective.

Third, there were a number of psycho-socio-environmental factors that were associated with the likelihood of *picking and choosing*. Targeting these factors in health interventions for African Americans could potentially increase the effectiveness of these interventions. For example, health promotion programs could design interventions that teach individuals how to select or *pick and choose* healthy behaviors that both of their cultures have to offer. Such a self-efficacy building approach to health promotion is empowering, and fosters ownership of individuals' behaviors, which can further increase the likelihood that they will engage in a variety of healthy behaviors [52].

Finally, the effectiveness of tailoring dietary messages may depend on individuals' connection to their cultures [53] as well as on differences within the culture [54]. For African Americans, this means that their willingness to *pick and choose* health behaviors from their ethnic and mainstream cultures, and their willingness to *consume healthy makeovers*, could depend on their level of connection to both their ethnic and their mainstream cultures. As Kreuter et al. [54] noted, African American culture does not comprise of a monolithic cultural milieu, and people's relationship to their culture can vary [54]. Therefore, health promotion programs for African Americans need to consider these variations and individuals' connections to their culture in the design and delivery of effective health promotion programs. For instance, in order to optimize the effectiveness of such programs, the focus and the content of health intervention can be tailored to individuals' level of connection to their ethnic and mainstream cultures. Moreover, these programs should also target personal factors such as motivation for leading healthy lifestyle because these factors are potentially important in triggering healthy behaviors.

Although this study revealed some important insights regarding African Americans' food intake and physical activity, there are some limitations that should be considered. First, the convenience sample consisted of African American students or alumni from Columbia University, or community members predominantly living in the Columbia University area. The sample is, therefore, not representative of the entire African American population. Living in an urban area as opposed to in the rural community can affect African Americans health behaviors differently. For example, these two groups may differ substantially in their access to healthy food and recreational spaces, as well as socio-economic status affecting their health behavior choices. Second, the participants in the study consisted of predominantly educated individuals, and mostly women. Interviews with individuals representing different educational levels and with more men as well might have yielded different conclusions given that both of these characteristics can affect food intake and physical activity. Third, the way participants perceive their African American culture and their mainstream culture may be tied to their level of education and their socioeconomic status, which were relatively high among the research participants in this study. Individuals with higher socioeconomic status might be more connected to their mainstream culture and therefore more willing and able to engage in healthy lifestyle practices common in their mainstream culture. Unfortunately, we did not collect comprehensive demographic and socioeconomic data, which limits our ability to fully understand the sample characteristics and how they relate to participants' responses. Therefore, future studies should clarify how socioeconomic status affects African Americans' perceptions of food intake and physical activity common in their ethnic and mainstream cultures. Fourth, most questions designed for this study explored participants' perceptions of other African Americans' health behaviors in the context of their ethnic and mainstream cultures; many fewer questions addressed participants' perceptions of their own behaviors. Because different processes can be involved in perceiving one's own versus others health behaviors, it would be important for the future research to distinguish these two types of views—of one's own beliefs and behaviors and those of others. Finally, in terms of our conceptualization of the influence of culture on individuals' food intake and physical activity, the current study has focused on only two dimensions of this influence (i.e., barriers and facilitators of healthy lifestyle). The rationale for this choice of dimensions is that it reflects the study's research questions; it has not been examined before in the context of individuals' ethnic and mainstream cultures; and it has implications for health promotions programs. However, there are many other ways in which the influence of African Americans' culture on their food intake and physical activity could be conceptualized, and future research would benefit from exploring those dimensions. Despite these limitations, the present research contributes to broadening the understanding of how African Americans make sense of their own experiences in relation to food intake and physical activity.

5. Conclusions

Overall, the findings of the present study demonstrate the importance of both ethnic and mainstream cultures in shaping African Americans' health behaviors. These influences need to be understood in the context of other psycho-socio-environmental factors that affect individuals' health behaviors. Given that most minority groups are often disproportionately affected by overweight and obesity, and by poor health in general [1,2,4], it is important to examine ways in which people can optimize their health by taking advantage of the diverse values, beliefs, and practices that exist in their ethnic and mainstream cultures. Healthy food intake and physical activity also need to be considered and understood in the context of one's larger social and physical environment. These findings have implications for health promotion programs directed at African Americans.

Author Contributions: E.M.S. and L.R.V. conceived and design the study. E.M.S. conducted the interviews and coded the transcripts. M.K. assisted with the analysis. All authors contributed to the manuscript preparation.

Conflicts of Interest: The authors declare no conflict of interest.

Appendix A. Participants' Level of Education and Cultural Identification

Participants' Number #	Education	Cultural Identification
Participant #1	4	4
Participant #2	3	1
Participant #3	3	3
Participant #4	4	1
Participant #5	3	3
Participant #6	3	3
Participant #7	3	1
Participant #8	3	3
Participant #9	3	4
Participant #10	3	1
Participant #11	2	3
Participant #12	1	3
Participant #13	3	3
Participant #14	3	1
Participant #15	3	4
Participant #16	3	3
Participant #17	3	3
Participant #18	1	1
Participant #19	1	3
Participant #20	3	3
Participant #21	3	3
Participant #22	1	2
Participant #23	3	3
Participant #24	3	4
Participant #25	2	3

Note: **Education**: 1 = high school, 2 = BA, 3 = MA; 4 = PhD; **Cultural Identification**: 1 = Identified more with ethnic culture, 2 = Identified more with mainstream culture, 3 = Identified equally with both cultures, 4 = Other.

References

1. Bélanger-Ducharme, F.; Tremblay, A. Prevalence of obesity in Canada. *Obes. Rev.* **2005**, *6*, 183–186. [CrossRef] [PubMed]
2. Choi, J. Prevalence of overweight and obesity among US immigrants: Results of the 2003 New Immigrant Survey. *J. Immigr. Minor. Health* **2012**, *14*, 1112–1118. [CrossRef] [PubMed]
3. Flegal, K.M.; Carroll, M.D.; Kit, B.K.; Ogden, C.L. Prevalence of obesity and trends in the distribution of body mass index among us adults, 1999–2010. *JAMA* **2012**, *307*, 491–499. [CrossRef] [PubMed]
4. Rennie, K.L.; Jebb, S.A. Prevalence of obesity in Great Britain. *Obes. Rev.* **2005**, *6*, 11–12. [CrossRef] [PubMed]
5. Ogden, C.L.; Carroll, M.D.; Curtin, L.R.; McDowell, M.A.; Tabak, C.J.; Flegal, K.M. Prevalence of overweight and obesity in the United States, 1999–2004. *JAMA* **2006**, *295*, 1549–1555. [CrossRef] [PubMed]
6. Zhang, Q.; Wang, Y. Trends in the association between obesity and socioeconomic status in U.S. Adults: 1971 to 2000. *Obes. Rev.* **2004**, *15*, 1622–1632. [CrossRef] [PubMed]
7. Macera, C.A.; Jones, D.A.; Yore, M.M.; Ham, S.A.; Al, E. *Prevalence of Physical Activity, Including Lifestyle Activities among Adults—United States, 2000–2001*; Center for Disease Control: Atlanta, GA, USA, 2003.
8. Schoenborn, C.A.; Adams, P.F.; Barnes, P.M.; Vickerie, J.L.; Schiller, J.S. Health behaviors of adults: United States,1999–2001, National Center for Health Statistics. *Vital Health Stat.* **2004**, *10*, 1–79.
9. Casagrande, S.S.; Wang, Y.; Anderson, C.; Gary, T.L. Have Americans increased their fruit and vegetable intake?: The trends between 1988 and 2002. *Am. J. Prev. Med.* **2007**, *32*, 257–263. [CrossRef] [PubMed]
10. Iwelunmor, J.; Newsome, V.; Airhihenbuwa, C.O. Framing the impact of culture on health: A systematic review of the PEN-3 cultural model and its application in public health research and interventions. *Ethn. Health* **2014**, *19*, 20–46. [CrossRef] [PubMed]

11. James, D. Factors influencing food choices, dietary intake, and nutrition-related attitudes among African Americans: Application of a culturally sensitive model. *Ethn. Health* **2004**, *9*, 349–367. [CrossRef] [PubMed]
12. Kumanyika, S.; Taylor, W.C.; Grier, S.A.; Lassiter, V.; Lancaster, K.J.; Morssink, C.B.; Renzaho, A.M.N. Community energy balance: A framework for contextualizing cultural influences on high risk of obesity in ethnic minority populations. *Prev. Med.* **2012**, *55*, 371–381. [CrossRef] [PubMed]
13. Oyserman, D. Culture as situated cognition: Cultural mindsets, cultural fluency, and meaning making. *Eur. Rev. Soc. Psychol.* **2011**, *22*, 164–214. [CrossRef]
14. Airhihenbuwa, C.O. Of culture and multiverse: Renouncing "the universal truth" in health. *J. Health Educ.* **1999**, *30*, 267–273. [CrossRef]
15. Oyserman, D.; Lee, S.W.S. A situated cognition perspective on culture: Effects of priming cultural syndromes on cognition and motivation. In *Handbook of Motivation and Cognition across Cultures*; Sorrentino, R., Yamaguchi, S., Eds.; Academic Press: San Diego, CA, USA, 2008; pp. 237–265.
16. Airhihenbuwa, C.O.; Kumanyika, S.; Agurs, T.D.; Lowe, A.; Saunders, D.; Morssink, C.B. Cultural aspects of African American eating patterns. *Ethn. Health* **1996**, *1*, 245–260. [CrossRef] [PubMed]
17. Harley, A.E.; Odoms-Young, A.; Beard, B.; Katz, M.L.; Heaney, C.A. African American Social and Cultural Contexts and Physical Activity: Strategies for Navigating Challenges to Participation. *Women Health* **2009**, *49*, 84–100. [CrossRef] [PubMed]
18. Rowe, J. Voices from the Inside: African American Women's Perspectives on Healthy Lifestyles. *Health Educ. Behav.* **2010**, *37*, 789–800. [CrossRef] [PubMed]
19. Chapman, G.E.; Ristovski-Slijepcevic, S.; Beagan, B.L. Meanings of food, eating and health in Punjabi families living in Vancouver, Canada. *Health Educ. J.* **2011**, *70*, 102–112. [CrossRef]
20. Diaz, V.A.; Mainous, A.G.; Pope, C. Cultural conflicts in the weight loss experience of overweight Latinos. *In. J. Obes.* **2006**, *31*, 328–333. [CrossRef] [PubMed]
21. Ristovski-Slijepcevic, S.; Chapman, G.E.; Beagan, B.L. Engaging with healthy eating discourse(s): Ways of knowing about food and health in three ethnocultural groups in Canada. *Appetite* **2008**, *50*, 167–178. [CrossRef] [PubMed]
22. Benet-Martínez, V.; Haritatos, J. Bicultural Identity Integration (BII): Components and Psychosocial Antecedents. *J. Personal.* **2005**, *73*, 1015–1050. [CrossRef] [PubMed]
23. Mok, A.; Morris, M.W. Managing Two Cultural Identities: The Malleability of Bicultural Identity Integration as a Function of Induced Global or Local Processing. *Personal. Soc. Psychol. Bull.* **2010**, *38*, 233–246. [CrossRef] [PubMed]
24. Chen, S.X.; Benet-Martínez, V.; Wu, W.C.H.; Lam, B.C.P.; Bond, M.H. The Role of Dialectical Self and Bicultural Identity Integration in Psychological Adjustment. *J. Personal.* **2013**, *81*, 61–75. [CrossRef] [PubMed]
25. Downie, M.; Koestner, R.; ElGeledi, S.; Cree, K. The impact of cultural internalization and integration on well being among tricultural individuals. *Personal. Soc. Psychol. Bull.* **2004**, *30*, 305–314. [CrossRef] [PubMed]
26. Cheng, C.Y.; Sanchez-Burks, J.; Lee, F. Connecting the dots within: Creative performance and identity integration. *Psychol. Sci.* **2008**, *19*, 1177–1183. [CrossRef] [PubMed]
27. Tibbs, T.; Haire-Joshu, D.; Schechtman, K.; Brownson, R.C.; Nanney, M.S.; Houston, C.; Auslander, W. The relationship between parental modeling, eating patterns, and dietary intake among African-American parents. *J. Am. Diet. Assoc.* **2001**, *101*, 535–541. [CrossRef]
28. Zhylyevskyy, O.; Jensen, H.H.; Garasky, S.B.; Cutrona, C.E.; Gibbons, F.X. Effects of Family, Friends, and Relative Prices on Fruit and Vegetable Consumption by African Americans. *South. Econ. J.* **2013**, *80*, 226–251. [CrossRef]
29. Borders, T.F.; Rohrer, J.E.; Cardarelli, K.M. Gender-Specific Disparities in Obesity. *J. Community Health* **2006**, *31*, 57–68. [CrossRef] [PubMed]
30. D'Angelo, H.; Suratkar, S.; Song, H.J.; Stauffer, E.; Gittelsohn, J. Access to food source and food source use are associated with healthy and unhealthy food-purchasing behaviours among low-income African-American adults in Baltimore City. *Public Health Nutr.* **2011**, *14*, 1632–1639. [CrossRef] [PubMed]
31. Lavizzo-Mourey, R.; Cox, C.; Strumpf, N.; Edwards, W.F.; Lavizzo-Mourey, R.; Stinemon, M.; Grisso, J.A. Attitudes and beliefs about exercise among elderly African Americans in an urban community. *J. Natl. Med. Assoc.* **2001**, *93*, 475–480. [PubMed]

32. Zenk, S.N.; Schulz, A.J.; Hollis-Neely, T.; Campbell, R.T.; Holmes, N.; Watkins, G.; Odoms-Young, A. Fruit and vegetable intake in African Americans—Income and store characteristics. *Am. J. Prev. Med.* **2005**, *29*, 1–9. [CrossRef] [PubMed]
33. Kumanyika, S.; Whitt-Glover, M.C.; Gary, T.L.; Prewitt, T.E.; Odoms-Young, A.M.; Banks-Wallace, J.; Samuel-Hodge, C.D. Expanding the Obesity Research Paradigm to reach African American communities. *Prev. Chronic Dis.* **2007**, *4*, A112. [PubMed]
34. Robinson, T. Applying the Socio-ecological Model to Improving Fruit and Vegetable Intake among Low-Income African Americans. *J. Community Health* **2008**, *33*, 395–406. [CrossRef] [PubMed]
35. Hargreaves, M.K.; Schlundt, D.G.; Buchowski, M.S. Contextual factors influencing the eating behaviours of African American women: A focus group investigation. *Ethn. Health* **2002**, *7*, 133–147. [CrossRef] [PubMed]
36. Airhihenbuwa, C.O.; Liburd, L. Eliminating health disparities in the African American population: The interface of culture, gender, and power. *Health Educ. Behav.* **2006**, *33*, 488–501. [CrossRef] [PubMed]
37. Braun, V.; Clarke, V. Using thematic analysis in psychology. *Qual. Res. Psychol.* **2006**, *3*, 77–101. [CrossRef]
38. Ponterotto, J. Qualitative research methods: The fifth force in psychology. *Couns. Psychol.* **2002**, *30*, 394–406. [CrossRef]
39. *NVivo Qualitative Data Analysis Software*, version 10; QSR International Pty Ltd.: Melbourne, Australia, 2014.
40. Van Dijk, T.A. *Discourse as Social Interaction*; Sage: London, UK, 1997.
41. Sims-Schouten, W.; Riley, S.C.E.; Willig, C. Critical Realism in Discourse Analysis: A Presentation of a Systematic Method of Analysis Using Women's Talk of Motherhood, Childcare and Female Employment as an Example. *Theory Psychol.* **2007**, *17*, 101–124. [CrossRef]
42. Dodor, B. The Impact of Religiosity on Health Behaviors and Obesity among African Americans. *J. Hum. Behav. Soc. Environ.* **2002**, *22*, 451–462. [CrossRef]
43. Bovell-Benjamin, A.C.; Dawkin, N.; Pace, R.D.; Shikany, J.M. Use of focus groups to understand African-Americans' dietary practices: Implications for modifying a food frequency questionnaire. *Prev. Med.* **2009**, *48*, 549–554. [CrossRef] [PubMed]
44. Corral, I.; Landrine, H. Racial discrimination and health-promoting vs. damaging behaviors among African-American adults. *J. Health Psychol.* **2012**, *17*, 1176–1182. [CrossRef] [PubMed]
45. Zenk, S.N.; Horoi, I.; McDonald, A.; Corte, C.; Riley, B.; Odoms-Young, A.M. Ecological momentary assessment of environmental and personal factors and snack food intake in African American women. *Appetite* **2014**, *83*, 333–341. [CrossRef] [PubMed]
46. Lucan, S.C.; Barg, F.K.; Karasz, A.; Palmer, C.S.; Long, J.A. Concepts of Healthy Diet among Urban, Low-Income, African Americans. *J. Community Health* **2012**, *37*, 754–762. [CrossRef] [PubMed]
47. Doldren, M.A.; Webb, F.J. Facilitators of and barriers to healthy eating and physical activity for Black women: a focus group study in Florida, USA. *Crit. Public Health* **2013**, *23*, 32–38. [CrossRef]
48. Glasser, W. "Choice theory" and student success. *Educ. Dig.* **1997**, *63*, 16–21.
49. Ryan, R.; Deci, E. Self-regulation and the problem of human autonomy: Does psychology need choice, self-determination, and will? *J. Personal.* **2006**, *74*, 1557–1585. [CrossRef] [PubMed]
50. Bandura, A. Social cognitive theory: An agentic perspective. *Ann. Rev. Psychol.* **2001**, *52*, 1–26. [CrossRef] [PubMed]
51. Cordova, D.; Lepper, M. Intrinsic motivation and the process of learning: Beneficial effects of contextualization, personalization, and choice. *J. Educ. Psychol.* **1996**, *88*, 715–730. [CrossRef]
52. Stephens, T.T.; Resinicow, K.; Latimer-Sport, M.; Walker, L. Social cognitive predictors of dietary behavior among African Americans. *Am. J. Health Educ.* **2015**, *46*, 174–181. [CrossRef]
53. Resnicow, K.; Davis, R.; Zhang, N.; Tolsma, D.; Calvi, J.; Alexander, G.; Cross, W.E. Tailoring a fruit and vegetable intervention on ethnic identity: Results of a randomized study. *Health Psychol.* **2009**, *28*, 394–403. [CrossRef] [PubMed]
54. Kreuter, M.W.; Lukwago, S.N.; Bucholtz, D.C.; Clark, E.M.; Sanders-Thompson, V. Achieving cultural appropriateness in health promotion programs: Targeted and tailored approaches. *Health Educ. Behav.* **2003**, *30*, 133–146. [CrossRef] [PubMed]

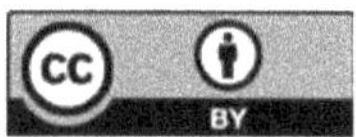

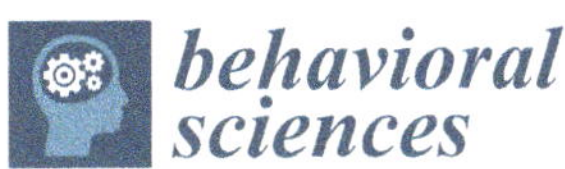
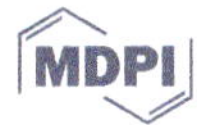

Review

Potential Benefits and Harms of Intermittent Energy Restriction and Intermittent Fasting Amongst Obese, Overweight and Normal Weight Subjects—A Narrative Review of Human and Animal Evidence

Michelle Harvie * and Anthony Howell

The Nightingale Centre, University Hospital of South Manchester NHS Foundation Trust, Southmoor Road, Manchester M23 9LT, UK; Tony.Howell@ics.manchester.ac.uk

* Correspondence: michelle.harvie@manchester.ac.uk; Tel.: +1-612-914-410

Academic Editors: Amanda Sainsbury and Felipe Luz
Received: 28 September 2016; Accepted: 13 December 2016; Published: 19 January 2017

Abstract: Intermittent energy restriction (IER) has become popular as a means of weight control amongst people who are overweight and obese, and is also undertaken by normal weight people hoping spells of marked energy restriction will optimise their health. This review summarises randomised comparisons of intermittent and isoenergetic continuous energy restriction for weight loss to manage overweight and obesity. It also summarises the potential beneficial or adverse effects of IER on body composition, adipose stores and metabolic effects from human studies, including studies amongst normal weight subjects and relevant animal experimentation. Six small short term (<6 month) studies amongst overweight or obese individuals indicate that intermittent energy restriction is equal to continuous restriction for weight loss, with one study reporting greater reductions in body fat, and two studies reporting greater reductions in HOMA insulin resistance in response to IER, with no obvious evidence of harm. Studies amongst normal weight subjects and different animal models highlight the potential beneficial and adverse effects of intermittent compared to continuous energy restriction on ectopic and visceral fat stores, adipocyte size, insulin resistance, and metabolic flexibility. The longer term benefits or harms of IER amongst people who are overweight or obese, and particularly amongst normal weight subjects, is not known and is a priority for further investigation.

Keywords: intermittent energy restriction; fasting; weight loss; weight gain

---

1. Introduction

Excess energy intake, weight gain and subsequent adiposity are consistently linked to illness, disability and mortality [1–3]. Randomised trials demonstrate that intentional weight loss reduces type 2 diabetes [4], all-cause mortality [5] and increases cognitive [6] and physical function [7]. The health benefits of weight loss and energy restriction in these human clinical trials are supported by a century of laboratory research in rodents, which has established that energy restriction (ER) prevents age-related disease including tumours, cardiovascular disease, diabetes and dementia; retards aging-related functional decline; and increases lifespan [8].

Most human and animal studies on weight loss have involved continuous energy restriction (CER) administered on a daily basis. More recently, interest has focussed on intermittent energy restriction (IER) defined as periods of energy restriction interspersed with normal energy intake.

IER is of potential interest to manage obesity and its metabolic sequelae and also for normal weight subjects hoping to optimise their health independent of weight loss for two main reasons: firstly, IER only requires the individual to focus on ER for defined days during the week which is potentially more achievable than the standard approach of CER which is associated with poor compliance [9]; and, secondly, many beneficial metabolic effects achieved with weight loss and energy restriction are related to the energy restriction per se and are attenuated when the individual is no longer in negative energy balance [10,11]. It is therefore possible that repeated spells of marked ER for short spells during the week could provide metabolic benefits to post obese individuals beyond the period of weight loss who are no longer in negative energy balance. IER may also provide metabolic benefits for normal weight subjects, although this requires further investigation.

The most studied IER approaches are either two consecutive days of ER per week ("two day") [12,13] or alternate days of ER (ADER) [14], typically with a restriction which is 60%–70% below estimated requirements, or a total fast on alternate days [15–18]. Confusingly, all three regimes have been called "intermittent fasting" in the literature. In this review we will use the term intermittent energy restriction (IER) to cover all of these approaches, "two day" for two consecutive days per week, alternate day energy restriction (ADER) when restriction is 60%–70% every other day and intermittent fasting (IF) when there is no energy intake on alternate days. It is important to distinguish IF from other IER regimens which allow food on restricted days as IF may evoke greater metabolic fluctuations (for example increased free fatty acids (FFA) and ketones) [19,20], induce stress in individuals [21] and may be associated with hyperphagia during non-restricted days [19].

The heightened scientific and lay interest in IER amongst overweight and normal weight subjects [22,23], indicates a need to summarise and evaluate the effectiveness and metabolic effects of IER compared with CER and assess the safety of IER. Recent IER reviews highlight the relative paucity of human data and concluded that IER is comparable to CER for weight loss with little evidence of a metabolic advantage [24,25]. However in most studies IER and CER were not matched for energy intake. In addition, reviewers did not consider the effects of IER amongst normal weight subjects or the important issue of potential harm of IER. This narrative review will examine how IER compares with CER in terms of weight loss, metabolic changes and safety.

2. Methods

A Medline search was undertaken from 1946 to October 2016 using the search terms "intermittent" or "alternate day" or "modified" or "fasting" or "diet" or "calorie" or "energy restriction" linking with "body weight", "body fat", "hepatic fat", "ectopic fat", "fat free mass (FFM)", "resting energy expenditure (REE)", "insulin resistance", "insulin sensitivity", "metabolic flexibility" (Table A1).

We include trials of IER with short periods of at least 50% energy restriction ($\leq$7 days) interspersed with days of normal eating ($\leq$10% energy restriction), but not studies of Ramadan, restriction for a few hours within the day (time restricted feeding) or studies with extended restricted periods, e.g., 2–5 weeks of dieting and not dieting which are testing different behavioural paradigms to weekly IER.

To compare adherence and weight loss success between IER and CER we include only randomised comparisons of IER and CER amongst free living individuals where the prescribed diets had been matched for overall energy intake. IER and IF are likely to have different effects on metabolic outcomes of interest, e.g., insulin resistance and REE during restricted and non–restricted phases. For this reason, the metabolic effects of IF and IER have only been reported from studies where authors have stated that measurements were undertaken on restricted or non-restricted days, which is critical to describe the overall metabolic effects of the IF and IER regimens.

3. Results

3.1. Is IER Associated with Greater Weight Control than CER?

3.1.1. Weight Loss amongst People with Overweight or Obesity

We identified 13 randomised comparisons of IER and CER [12–14,18,26–34]. Seven of the studies were excluded because energy intake was not equivalent between the IER and CER groups [18,28–32,34]. ADER is the most studied IER amongst humans [25], however most of these studies summarised in recent reviews [24,25] have either a no treatment comparison group or no comparison group and so were not included.

We present data on adherence and weight change with IER vs. CER for the remaining six studies [12–14,26,27,33]. These trials tested different IER regimens; three tested a two day IER [12,13,33], one a four day IER [27], one an alternating pattern of three to seven days of IER per week [26] and one study tested ADER [14]. Most of the IER regimens advised healthy eating on the non-restricted days, with the exception of Carter et al. [33] (Tables 1 and 2). The trials were relatively small with between 32 and 115 subjects randomised and between 25 and 88 completers within the trials. The trials were not powered to detect differences in body weight, and were relatively short duration (12–26 weeks). Drop out from the studies was between 0% and 40% and mainly comparable between the IER and CER groups, and to previous reports within CER studies [35]. Five of the studies reported an intention to treat analysis to account for these drop outs [12–14,27,33].

All of the selected studies demonstrate comparable reductions in body weight [12,14,26,27,33] between IER and CER. Four of the studies report equivalent reductions in body fat [12,26,27,33]; whilst one reported a greater loss of body fat with two different low carbohydrate IER regimens compared with CER over a four-month period [13]. The two IER regimens in this study allowed two consecutive days per week of either a low carbohydrate, low energy IER (70% ER, 2.7 MJ, 50 g carbohydrate/day) or a less restrictive low carbohydrate IER which allowed ad libitum protein and ad libitum monounsaturated fatty acids (MUFA, 55% ER, 4.78 MJ, 50 g carbohydrate/day). Both had 5 days of a healthy Mediterranean type diet, (45% energy from low glycaemic load carbohydrates, 30% fat; 15% MUFA, 8% polyunsaturated fatty acids and 7% saturated fatty acids). The IER regimens were compared to an isoenergetic 25% CER Mediterranean type diet. The differences in overall carbohydrate intake between the diet groups were modest (41% and 37% of energy for the two IER diets compared to 47% of energy for CER), which is unlikely to account for differences in adherence and reductions in adiposity between the diets [36].

Table 1. Randomised weight loss trials of intermittent energy restriction compared to isoenergetic continuous energy restriction in people who are obese or overweight.

Reference	IER Regimens	Study Population		Study Design			Primary End Point and Power of the Study
		N, Gender, Age	Baseline BMI (kg/m^2) Mean (SD) Range	Diet Groups (N)	Level of Support	Duration of Study	
Hill et al. 1989 [26]	3–7 day periods of alternating 70%, 60%, 45%, and 10% ER. Overall 40% CER	40 women (32 completers)	31 (3.0)	IER = 10 IER + exercise = 10 40% CER = 10 40% CER + exercise = 10	12 weekly group meetings. Menus provided.	12 weeks intervention and follow up 6 months after the weight loss programme	Weight loss No power calculation
Ash et al. 2003 [27]	4 consecutive days/week 50% ER (4.18 MJ liquid very low calorie diet 3 days/week, *ad lib* healthy eating) Overall 30% CER	51 men with Type 2 diabetes Age < 70 years	31.2 (3.4) 25–39.9	IER vs. 2 types of 30% CER IER = 14 30% CER = 20 (self-selected meals) 30% CER = 17 (pre-portioned meals)	Face to face visit the clinic dietitian and physician fortnightly and telephone contact with the dietitian on intervening weeks.	12 weeks	Weight loss and glycaemic control No power calculation
Varady et al. 2011 [14]	Alternate days of 75% ER (1.67–2.50 MJ/day) and AL low fat/American Heart Association diet: 30% kcal fat, 15% kcal protein, 55% kcal carbohydrate. Overall 25% CER	51 women and 9 men Age 35–65 years	32 (2.0) 25–39.9	IER = 15 (pre-portioned meals on fast days) 25% CER = 15 (pre-portioned meals) Exercise only =15 (180 minutes 70% max heart rate) Control = 15	No information	12 weeks	LDL and HDL particle size No power calculation
Harvie et al. 2011 [12]	2 consecutive days/week 70% ER (2.73 MJ/day, 50 g protein: 2 pints of milk, 1 portion of fruit and 4 portions of vegetables) 5 days ad libitum healthy eating. Overall 25% CER	107 premenopausal women Age 30–45 years	30.6 (5.1) 24–40	IER = 53 25% CER = 54	Fortnightly motivational phone calls and monthly clinical appointments with dietitian. Advised to maintain current levels of physical activity.	26 weeks	Insulin resistance 80% power to detect a 25% difference
Harvie et al. 2013 [13]	IECR: 2 consecutive days/week 70% ER (energy and carbohydrate restriction: 2.73 MJ/day, 70 g protein, 50 g carbohydrate) Overall 25% CER 2 days 60% ER. or IECR + PF: 2 consecutive days/week 50% ER (energy and carbohydrate restriction: ~4.18 MJ/day, 80 g protein, 50 g carbohydrate)	115 women aged 20–69 years	31 (5.0) 24–45	IECR = 37 IECR + PF = 38 25% CER = 40 2 days/week IECR vs. IECR + PF 1 days/week vs. isoenergetic CER diet	Fortnightly motivational phone calls and monthly clinical appointments with dietitian. Advised to achieve 5 × 45 min of moderate intensity physical activity per week—but achieved minimal changes in the three groups	13 weeks weight loss phase. 4 weeks weight maintenance phase.	Insulin resistance 80% power to detect a 20% difference
Carter et al. 2016 [33]	IECR 2 days per week 1.67–2.5 MJ/day (70%–85% restriction) and habitual eating for 5 days	63 30 men 33 women Type 2 diabetes Age > 18 Mean (SD) age 61 (7.5)	35 (4.8)	IECR = 31 + exercise (2000 steps) CER = 32 5.0–6.5 MJ (35%–45%) + exercise (2000 steps)	Asked to record dietary intake throughout the 12-week study. Fortnightly appointments with dietitian	12 weeks	HbA1c No power calculation

Mean (SD); IER, intermittent energy restriction; CER, continuous energy restriction; IECR, intermittent energy and carbohydrate restriction; IECR + PF, intermittent energy and carbohydrate restriction and ad libitum protein and MUFA.

Table 2. Adherence, weight loss and changes in metabolic markers in randomised trials of intermittent energy restriction compared to isoenergetic continuous energy restriction in people who are obese or overweight.

Reference	Dropout % of Subjects	Dietary Adherence Methodology	Final Analysis	Outcomes		
				Weight change Mean (SD) % Weight Loss	Change in Body Fat and fat Free Mass (FFM) Method of Assessment	Metabolic Effects
Hill et al. 1989 [26]	12 weeks/6 months after intervention IER = 40%/60% IER + exercise = 0%/0% 40% CER = 20%/70% 40% CER + exercise = 20%/40% Combined IER + IER + exercise = 20%/30% Combined CER + CER + exercise = 20%/55%	12 week diet records Average daily intake IER = 4.97 (0.59) MJ IER + exercise = 4.58 (2.92) MJ 40% CER = 5.46 (1.49) MJ 40% CER + exercise = 4.59 (0.30) MJ $p > 0.05$	Completers analysis	12 week data Combined IER/CER diet only groups Weight −6.5 (0.9) kg (−7.6%) Combined IER/CER + exercise −8.6 (0.9) kg (−8.8%)	Body density from underwater weighing IER = CER Fat loss (kg): IER 6.0 (0.8) CER 6.1 (0.6) $p > 0.05$ Loss of FFM: Combined all groups 47.6 (1.1) to 46.0 (1.0) $p < 0.05$	Equal reductions in blood pressure and triglycerides with IER vs. CER. No change in insulin with IER or CER ($p > 0.05$) Reduced total cholesterol IER −14% vs. CER −6% ($p < 0.05$)
Ash et al. 2003 [27]	IER = 0% 30% CER (self-selected meals) = 0% 30% CER (pre-portioned meals) = 0%	24 hour recalls All groups mean (SD) reduction in average daily energy intake −2.36 (2.78) MJ ~30% energy restriction	Completers as no drop outs	IER = CER Combined IER/CER group 6.5 (6%)	DEXA IER = CER % Body fat loss: IER −2.0 (1.1)% CER (self-selected meals) −0.9 (1.4)% CER (pre-portioned meals) −2.6 (1.6) % ($p = 0.41$) FFM: no data	Reduced HbA1c and triglycerides IER = CER $p > 0.05$
Varady et al. 2011 [14]	IER = 13% 25% CER = 20% Exercise = 20% Control = 20%	No data	BOCF	IER −5.2 ± 1.1% CER −5.0 ± 1.4% Exercise −5.1 ± 0.9% Control −0.2 ± 0.4%	No data	Increase in LDL particle size IER = CER $p > 0.05$
Harvie et al. 2011 [12]	IER = 20% 25% CER = 13% 9% of potential recruits did not tolerate the 2 day trial of the restricted days of IER and did not enter the study Drop out due to problems adhering to the diet: IER = 5%, CER = 5%. At the end of the trial, 31 of IER (58%) and 46 of CER (85%) subjects planned to continue the diet allocated at randomization.	IER 7 day food diaries at baseline, 1, 3 and 6 months Potential restricted days completed 0–6 months: mean (95% CI) 66 (55%–77%) Overall average daily reduction in energy intake: mean (95% CI) 12 weeks IER −2.40 (−2.94 to −1.87) MJ (~30% restriction) CER −1.65 (−2.11 to −1.18) (~21% restriction), $p = 0.04$ 26 weeks IER −2.40 (−2.94 to −1.87) (~30% restriction) CER −1.73 (−2.13 to −1.37) MJ (~21% restriction), $p = 0.04$	LOCF	IER = CER 12 weeks IER −6.3 (4.5)% CER −5.0 (3.6)% $p = 0.11$ 24 weeks IER −7.8 (5.9%) CER −6.6 (5.0%) $p = 0.26$	Bioelectrical impedance IER = CER 12 weeks % Body fat loss: IER −2.4 (2.3)% CER −2.0 (2.1)%, p= 0.42 Body fat mass: IER −3.8 (2.9) kg CER −3.3 (3.0) kg, $p = 0.43$ 24 weeks % Body fat loss: IER −3.4 (3.2%) CER −2.8 (2.7) %, $p = 0.35$ Body fat mass: IER −5.0 (4.4) kg CER −4.4 (3.9) kg, $p = 0.34$ 21% of weight lost as FFM in IER and CER $p = 0.99$	Reduction in HOMA insulin resistance IER > CER at 12 and 24 weeks. Mean difference (95% CI) 12 weeks: −17 (−33.2 to −0.2), p = 0.046. 24 weeks: −23% (−38 to −8.6)%, p = 0.001. Reduced total LDL cholesterol, triglycerides and blood pressure IER = CER $p > 0.05$

Table 2. *Cont.*

Reference	Dropout % of Subjects	Dietary Adherence Methodology	Final Analysis	Outcomes		
				Weight change Mean (SD) % Weight Loss	Change in Body Fat and fat Free Mass (FFM) Method of Assessment	Metabolic Effects
Harvie et al. 2013 [13]	IECR = 11% IECR + PF = 26% 25% CER = 33% Drop out due to problems adhering to the diet: IECR 0% IECR + PF 5% CER 5%	7 day food diaries at baseline, 1, 3 and 4 months Potential restricted days 0–4 months mean (95% CI): IECR 76 (67%–81%) IECR + PF 74 (64%–84%) Overall average daily reduction in intake median, %: 12 weeks IECR = −2.97 MJ, −36% IECR + PF = −2.3 MJ, −29% DER = −2.63 MJ, −33% $p = 0.046$ 16 weeks IECR = −2.38 MJ, 32% IECR + PF = −2.06 MJ, 26% DER = −2.16 MJ, 25% $p = 0.765$	LOCF	No difference in % weight loss between groups at 12 weeks IECR −6.2 (4.6) IECR + PF −5.7 (3.9) CER −4.3 (4.6). % weight change during 1 month of weight loss maintenance: IECR −0.49 (1.7) IECR + PF −0.34 (0.9) CER −0.13 (0.88) $p = 0.431$ % weight lost as FFM median (95%CI): IECR 36.0 (26.4 to 41.3) IECR + PF 20.4 (13.2 to 27.2) DER 29.3 (25 to 38.1) $p = 0.048$	Bioelectrical impedance reduction in body fat mass at 12 weeks IER > CER, $p = 0.019$ Body fat mass: IECR −3.7 (3.7) kg IECR + PF −3.7 (2.2) kg CER −2.0 (3.3) kg No difference during 1 month of weight loss maintenance: Reduction in body fat/kg IECR −0.58 (1.2) IECR + PF −0.31 (0.7) CER + 0.26 (0.90) $p = 0.313$	Reduction in HOMA insulin resistance IECR > CER. Mean (95% CI) change at 12 weeks: −0.2 (−0.19 to 0.66) unit; $p = 0.02$ After 4 weeks of weight loss maintenance: IECR −0.06 (0.51) IECR + PF + 0.03 (0.6) CER −0.25 (0.53) Unit, $p = 0.084$ Reduced total LDL cholesterol, triglycerides and blood pressure IECR = IECR + PF = CER
Carter et al. 2016 [33]	IECR 16% CER 22%	No data	ITT	IECR −6.2 (3.6)% CER −5.6 (4.4)% $p = 0.6$	DEXA IER 3.8.(2.7)% CER −4.0 (3.2)% $p = 0.8$	HbA1C IER −0.6 (1)% CER −0.5 (0.8)

Mean (SD); IECR + PF, intermittent energy and carbohydrate restriction and ad libitum protein and MUFA; BOCF, baseline observation carried forward; LOCF, last observation carried forward; HOMA, Homeostasis Model Assessment; LDL, low-density lipoprotein; DEXA, dual energy x ray absorptiometry.

3.1.2. Adherence to IER and CER amongst People with Overweight or Obesity

Adherence to diets within trials is notoriously difficult to assess due to missing dietary records and well documented underreporting amongst overweight subjects [37]. This notwithstanding, dietary records in four of the studies [12,13,26,27] provided some information of the relative adherence and overall energy intake of IER vs. CER which was broadly comparable between the two groups.

Two of the studies of a two-day IER explored weekly adherence to the ER days and also intake on intervening non-restricted days to assess whether there is any evidence of energy compensation on these days [12,13]. The first study used a simple IER with two consecutive restricted days of 2.73 MJ, from milk, fruit and vegetables. An intention to treat analysis assuming women who left the study or who did not complete food records were non-adherent reported that mean (95% CI) 66% (55%–77%) of the potential IER days were completed. The low carbohydrate IER tested in the second study [13], allowed a larger range of foods than the previously tested regimen and appeared to have a greater adherence; mean (95% CI) potential IER days completed for the low carbohydrate, low energy IER and the less restrictive IER were respectively 76% (67%–81%) and 74% (64%–84%).

Neither of the IER tested were associated with compensatory hyperphagia on the non-dieting days. These trials have instead reported an important "carry over effect" of reduced energy intake by ~20% on non-restricted days (Figure 1). Energy intake on the non-restricted days of the IER regimen was similar to the planned 25% restriction of the CER regimen [12,13]. Food records amongst the CER group in this study showed that 55% were achieving their daily 25% and an overall 25% CER. Thus the greater loss of fat reported with the two day low carbohydrate IER diets compared to CER in the 2013 study appears to be linked to better dietary adherence with IER vs. CER, partly linked to good adherence to the two restricted days each week and the spontaneous restriction of energy intake on non-restricted days [13].

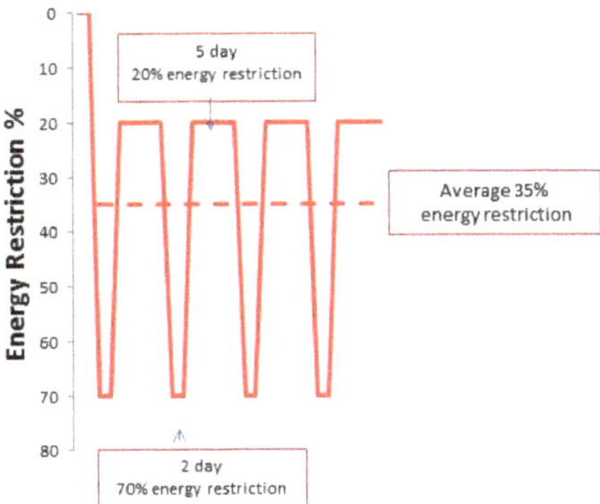

Figure 1. Degree of dietary energy restriction with IER in Manchester studies. The IER cohort undertook a 70% energy restriction on two consecutive days per week and additionally undertook an unplanned carry-over energy restriction to an average of 20% below their baseline intake on the remaining five days of the week (*solid line*). The restricted days and the unplanned carry-over energy restriction resulted in an equivalent overall 35% energy restriction over the trial period (*dashed line*).

Energy intake was not presented in the RCT of ADER compared to CER [14], however previous reports of ADER have similarly found a small carry over effect with a 5% reduction in energy on the non-restricted days of the regimen [38]. A number of studies were testing combined IER/CER and exercise interventions [13,26,33] and reported exercise to be feasible alongside both IER and CER diets, but there are no reported interactions between diet allocation and levels of activity and weight loss.

3.1.3. Maintaining Weight Loss amongst People with Overweight or Obesity

Dietary approaches must demonstrate the ability to maintain weight loss. Estimates of successful weight loss maintenance with CER (defined as >10% weight loss maintained at ≥12 months), vary between 20% and 50% depending on the level of support provided at later time points [9,39]. There are few data on weight loss maintenance using IER. One month of a weight maintenance IER (one day of ER and six days of an ad libitum Mediterranean type diet per week) successfully maintained reductions in weight and of insulin resistance which had been achieved with three months of a weight loss IER (two days of ER and five days of an ad libitum Mediterranean type diet) in the 2013 IER trial described above [13]. However, one month is too short a period to draw any conclusions about the longer term efficacy of IER. They had previously reported that after six months of dieting, 58% of the IER group compared to 85% of CER subjects planned to continue the diet allocated at randomisation [12]. Unpublished data from this trial show, by 12 months, 33% of the initial IER randomisation group were still undertaking one or two days of IER each week. An intention to treat analysis based on last observation carried forward showed no difference in the percentage of women in the IER and CER groups losing 5%–10% of body weight (25% vs. 30%) or losing 10% or more at 12 months (19% vs. 19%, $\chi^2 = 0.370$, $p = 0.83$) (Harvie et al. unpublished).

In summary, randomised trials to date have found IER to be equivalent to CER for weight loss in six studies [12–14,26,27,33] and superior to CER for reducing body fat in one study [13]. All studies were relatively small and in the author's estimations only powered to show absolute differences of 4%–5% between the groups. Larger studies would be required to investigate if there are smaller differences in weight loss between IER and CER regimens (2%–3% weight loss differences), which would still be clinically meaningful. Studies were mainly conducted amongst women and included motivated groups of subjects who had answered adverts [14,26,27], or were recruited from a clinic for women at increased risk of breast cancer [12,13]. Interventions have been short term at ≤26 weeks, and tested under highly supervised conditions with high levels of dietetic support and sometimes meal provision [14,27]. Larger, longer term, real world weight loss trials are required to inform how IER performs longer term in a variety of settings in comparison to the standard approach of CER.

3.2. Prevention of Weight Gain amongst Normal Weight Subjects

There are currently no randomised data to compare the relative efficacy of IER vs. CER to prevent adult weight gain amongst normal weight subjects. Two studies have tested the metabolic effects of IER amongst groups of normal and overweight subjects (BMI 20–30 Kg/m^2). These studies have been designed to assess short term metabolic effects, mainly for two to three weeks and involved highly controlled situations in which participants were instructed to increase dietary intake on non–restricted days to ensure they did not have an overall energy deficit [15,40]. The studies report sustained hunger with IF [15,40], and difficulties maintaining daily living activities during restricted days of an ADER regimen [41]. This suggests limited compliance and efficacy of these specific regimens amongst cohorts of normal and overweight subjects. However, other patterns of IER, e.g., one restricted day per week, may be better tolerated and warrant study.

4. Metabolic Effects of IER vs. CER

4.1. Adipose Stores and Adipocyte Size

4.1.1. Human Studies

Reductions in adiposity, specifically visceral and ectopic (i.e., hepatic/abdominal and intramuscular) fat stores are a therapeutic target of ER. Hepatic and visceral fat stores rapidly mobilise with marked ER as they are thought to be more sensitive to the lipolytic effects of catecholamines during negative energy balance than subcutaneous fat [41]. Marked CER (>50% ER) is related to rapid decreases in hepatic fat in people with obesity [42,43]. Lim et al. [43] reported a 30% reduction in hepatic fat after seven days of a 60%–70% CER in subjects with type 2 diabetes (nine men and two women), which normalised hepatic insulin sensitivity. There are currently no human data concerning the long term or chronic effects of IER on hepatic, intra-abdominal and intramyocellular triglyceride stores. Reports of significant reductions in hepatic fat stores (−29%) after two days of ER and carbohydrate restriction in men and women with obesity [42], suggest reductions could occur during the repeated spells of restriction with IF/IER each week. Such reductions may account for the reported improvements in homeostatic model assessment (HOMA) insulin resistance, i.e., hepatic insulin resistance with IER described below [12,13], (see Section 4.4) but require further study.

In contrast, short term fasting studies raise the possibility of harm with IER amongst normal weight subjects. Periods of IER each week will induce lipolysis and fluxes in FFAs. The 1–2 days of IF/IER each week will lead to large fluxes in FFA which are typically three-fold greater than those seen after a normal overnight fast [44], and will be larger with IF rather than IER [19]. These fluxes can lead to skeletal muscle insulin resistance. Single bouts of total fasts (24–48 h) in non-obese subjects have been associated with modest increases in hepatic and intramyocellular triglyceride content which are not seen after the normal 12 h overnight fast. Specifically a single spell of fasting of between 24–48 h leads to modest increases in intramyocellular triglycerides (2.4%–3.6%) but not hepatic fat in non-obese premenopausal women, mainly in the second 24 h period of fasting [45], whilst men have modest increases in hepatic fat (0.42%–0.74%) within the first 24 h of fasting, but do not accumulate intramyocellular triglycerides [45,46]. The clinical significance of the modest changes in hepatic triglycerides in men [46], and intramyocellular triglycerides in women [45] in these short term studies is not known. Some [45,47] but not all [48] studies have associated increased intramyocellular triglycerides with reduced insulin sensitivity upon refeeding amongst women. Possible mechanisms for increased hepatic fat with fasting in men include reduced apolipoprotein B-100 production and hepatic lipid export, and/or impaired mitochondrial function and fat oxidation resulting from increased oxidative stress, with diversion of fatty acids for esterification [49]. The effects of repeated IER each week on hepatic and intramyocellular triglyceride stores and whole body insulin sensitivity needs to be assessed in longer term studies and also amongst people who are overweight or obese.

4.1.2. Animal Studies

Studies in rodents report mixed effects of IER vs. CER on hepatic and visceral fat stores. One month of alternate days of either fasting or a 75% or 85% energy restriction without an overall energy restriction in female C57BL/6J mice did not change weight or total amounts of body fat, but led to redistribution of fat from visceral (−40%) to subcutaneous stores (+65%) [50]. A similar investigation amongst male C57BL/6J mice did not find that alternate days of fasting or ER had effects on total or visceral fat stores. However, in this study, alternate days of a 50% ER and ad libitum feeding reduced fat cell size in the inguinal (subcutaneous) fat pads by 50% and in epididymal (visceral) fat pads by 35% [51], despite there being no overall energy restriction. Marked reductions in fat cell size are thought to reduce risk of inflammation and metabolic diseases [52].

However in other animal models (four week old male Sprague Dawley rats and LDL-receptor knockout mice) IF regimens reduced energy intake and weight but increased visceral fat, fat cell size and had adverse effects on insulin sensitivity compared to heavier ad libitum fed animals [53,54]. The variable effects of IER vs. CER on fat stores in different animal models means extrapolating findings from specific animal models to the human situation is problematic. The adverse effects of IF in these studies may be because IF animals adopt a gorging pattern of eating which in turn can shift normal night time grazing to a pattern of overfeeding during daylight hours. This disturbance of circadian rhythms may lead to the reported accumulation of abdominal and hepatic fat and adverse metabolic effects [55]. The adverse effects of fasting and ER seen in these rodent studies are important to consider, but may not be an issue for humans. In contrast to rodent studies, people who are overweight or obese undertaking IER appear to reduce intake on the non-restricted days [12,13,38] and do not display compensatory overfeeding (see Section 3.1). The effects of IER and CER on circadian rhythm is important, however this has not been studied.

4.2. Fat Free Mass

Human Studies

Weight loss and weight maintenance diets should reduce body fat stores and, as far as possible, preserve FFM to maintain physical function and attenuate declines in resting REE and help to prevent weight gain. CER is known to reduce FFM in addition to body fat. Typically 10%–60% of weight reduction using CER is FFM, depending on initial body fat, the degree of energy restriction, extent of exercise and protein intake [56]. Proponents of IER and IF diets claim they may preserve FFM more than CER from cross study comparisons of IER and CER interventions which may have allowed our Palaeolithic hunter gatherer ancestors to survive spells of food shortage [57]. However the concern is that spells of severe restriction with IER and IF (i.e., fasting or intakes of <2.0 MJ/day) could lead to greater losses of FFM than the modest daily energy restriction with CER. There are, however, few data to inform this question, as the modest sized IER trials undertaken are unlikely to be powered sufficiently to demonstrate difference in FFM loss [58]. Weight loss trials amongst people who are overweight or obese suggest losses of FFM with IER and CER are equivalent within the bounds of small numbers and are dependent on the overall protein content of the IER and CER diet rather than the pattern of energy restriction [59]. The first IER trial reported an equivalent loss of weight as FFM between IER and CER (both 20% of weight loss) when both diets provided 0.9 g protein/kg body weight [12]. Likewise the 2013 trial reported equal losses of FFM (both 30% of weight loss) with a standard protein IER (1.0 g protein/kg body weight) compared to a standard protein CER (1.0 g protein/kg body weight) [13]. There was however a greater preservation of FFM (20% of weight loss) with a high protein IER (1.2 g protein/kg weight) compared to the standard protein CER (30% with 1.0 g protein/kg body weight ($p < 0.05$) [13]. Likewise Hill et al. [26] reported 27% of weight loss from FFM with IER and CER which both provided 0.7 g protein/kg body weight. Studies of ADER reported the proportion of weight lost as FFM as low as 10% in women with obesity [60] and as high as 30% amongst non-obese subjects [61]. Subsequent studies show that exercise helps to retain FFM amongst subjects undergoing IER [26] and ADER [62] which is well documented with CER [63].

One study assessed muscle protein turnover before and after 14 days of alternate day fasting in normal weight healthy men [17]. This study reported lowered mechanistic target of rapamycin (mTOR) phosphorylation in muscle which was thought to reflect decreased muscle protein synthesis and a failure to reduce muscle proteolysis. These changes could lead to a reduced muscle mass, thus suggesting that long term alternate day fasting could lead to reduced muscle mass in normal weight subjects [17].

4.3. Resting Energy Expenditure

Human Studies

Resting energy expenditure accounts for 60% to 75% of the total daily energy requirement in an individual, thus it is important in determining overall energy balance and whether an individual is weight stable or gaining or losing weight. REE is known to be reduced during CER in association with reduced FFM and fat mass [64], as well as to reduced circulating leptin and thyroid hormones and sympathetic nerve activity [65]. Total energy expenditure may be reduced 10% within two-weeks of starting 25% CER [65].

There are few data on the effects of IER on REE. REE could be acutely decreased during the short restricted periods each week, which could normalise during the normal eating days of the week. However, an increase in REE of ~5% is seen during the first days of starvation [66], perhaps as a result to the increased energy cost of fatty acid recycling, glucose storage, gluconeoegenesis, increased sympathetic nervous activity and catecholamine concentrations [67]. Studies to date have assessed REE after non-restricted days of IER and have mostly shown reductions in REE amongst subjects who are overweight or obese [26,28,68] and overweight or a normal weight [15,17]. One exception is a recent trial of ADF amongst 26 subjects with obesity, where REE decreased with CER but not IER [18]. Most studies suggest IER evokes the same adaptive response as CER at least on non-restricted days. Future studies should assess the effects of IER on REE during restricted days to assess the overall impact of IER on metabolic rate.

4.4. Peripheral and Hepatic Insulin Resistance

4.4.1. Human Studies

Insulin acts on skeletal muscle to increase glucose uptake and inhibit protein catabolism, on adipose tissue to increase glucose uptake, lipogenesis, lipoprotein lipase and uptake of triglycerides, and on the liver to reduce lipolysis, gluconeogenesis and increases glycogen synthesis. Obesity is associated with both peripheral and hepatic insulin resistance where normal or elevated insulin levels have an attenuated biological response in these tissues [69]. Studies in obese, overweight and normal weight subjects have assessed the effects of IER on whole body, peripheral and hepatic insulin sensitivity using a variety of methods, with variable results.

We assessed HOMA insulin resistance, a measure of hepatic insulin sensitivity, in two RCTS of a two-day IER versus CER amongst subjects who are overweight or obese. As indicated above, the first trial compared IER (two consecutive days of 70% ER per week) to an isoenergetic CER (25% ER Mediterranean type diet seven days per week) amongst 105 healthy women [12]. The IER led to greater reductions in HOMA compared to CER when measured on the morning after five normal eating days. The mean (95% CI) % change in HOMA over six months IER was −24 (−35 to −13)% and CER was −4 (−20 to +12)%, (p = 0.001). We also measured HOMA on the morning after the two energy restricted days, which showed an additional 25% reduction compared with CER at this time. These differences in insulin sensitivity occurred despite comparable reductions in body fat between the groups (IER −4.5 vs. CER −3.6 kg, p = 0.34).

The follow up study tested two low carbohydrate IER regimens which allowed two consecutive days per week of either a low carbohydrate, low energy IER (70% ER, 2.7 MJ, 50 g carbohydrate per day) or a less restrictive low carbohydrate IER which allowed ad libitum protein and MUFA (55% ER, 4.18 MJ, 50 g carbohydrate per day). These regimens led to equivalent reductions in body fat which were both greater than CER as described above (see Section 3.1) [13]. However, reductions in serum insulin and HOMA insulin resistance measured after non-restricted days were significantly lower than CER only with the lower energy IER (p = 0.02), but not the less restrictive IER regimen (p = 0.21). The reasons for the apparent greater improvement in insulin resistance with more restrictive IER is independent of changes in body fat and may be specifically linked to the more marked energy restriction on restricted days (70% vs. 55%). A recent small trial amongst 26 subjects with obesity reported successful weight loss with IF, −8.8 (0.9)% or a 16% CER, −6.2 (0.9)%. However, neither group experienced changes in insulin resistance assessed using an insulin-augmented frequently sampled intravenous glucose tolerance test measured after a non-restricted day [18].

There are few data of the effects of IER vs. CER on glucose control amongst overweight and obese individuals with type 2 diabetes Ash et al. (2003) reported that a four day IER over 12 weeks led to equivalent reductions in percentage body fat (see Section 3.1) and in HbA1c compared with isoenergetic CER although this small study may have been underpowered to show significant differences [27]. Carter reported equivalent reductions in HbA1c in individuals with Type 2 diabetes with 12 weeks of IER or CER which had been achieved with greater (albeit non-significant) reductions in insulin medications within the IER group [33]. Williams et al. [57] assessed the effect of enhancing a standard 25% CER diet with periods of 75% ER (either five days per week every five weeks or one day per week for 15 weeks). Predictably, additional periods of ER increased weight loss. The five days per week intervention resulted in the greatest normalisation of HbA1c, independent of weight loss, suggesting a potential specific insulin-sensitising effect of this pattern of IER added to CER [30]

Three studies assessed the effects of two to three weeks of IF (alternating 20–24 h periods of a total fast interspersed with 24–28 h periods of hyperphagia (175%–200% of estimated energy requirements) [16–18]. They were designed to ensure there was no overall energy deficit or weight loss, and results have varied between the studies. Halberg et al. [16] assessed the effects of two weeks of IF (a total fast for 20 h from 22.00 and ending at 18.00 the following day) in eight overweight young men. Improvements in insulin mediated whole body glucose uptake and insulin induced inhibition of adipose tissue lipolysis assessed using a euglycaemic hyperinsulinaemic clamp were seen when measured after two normal feeding days, which the authors suggested may be related to higher adiponectin concentrations seen during the 20 h fast [16]. Soeters et al. [17] tested an identical two week IF intervention in normal weight men in a cross over design. However IF was not associated with changes in peripheral glucose uptake or hepatic insulin sensitivity assessed with a hyperinsulinaemic clamp, or lipid or protein metabolism. Heilbronn et al. [47] assessed the effects of three weeks of IF (alternating 24 h total fast and 24 h ad libitum feeding) amongst 16 overweight men and women. Glucose uptake during a test meal was assessed at baseline after a 12 h fast and after three weeks of IF on the morning after a fasting day, i.e., after a 36-h fast. Men had a significant reduction in insulin response and improved glucose uptake and insulin sensitivity, whilst women had impaired glucose uptake and apparent skeletal muscle insulin resistance. This observation is likely to be related to greater fluxes of FFA during this 36-hour fast amongst fasting women [70], which most likely reflects a normal physiological adaptation to fasting rather than a cause for concern. Reduced glucose uptake in skeletal muscle limits the competition between skeletal muscle and the central nervous system and other glucose obligate tissues for circulating glucose in situations with low glucose availability, which reduces gluconeogenesis and has protein sparing effects in turn has protein sparing effects [71]. The short term studies of IF outlined above report mixed results on peripheral and hepatic insulin sensitivity and raise the possibility of different responses to IF according to gender. Further studies are required using robust measures of insulin sensitivity.

4.4.2. Animal Studies

Variable effects of IF regimens on insulin sensitivity have also been reported in animal studies [72–74]. Higashida et al. [74] tested whether energy restriction with IF could prevent the development of muscle insulin resistance induced by a high fat diet. Young male Wistar rats were given a high fat diet for four weeks and then allocated to a continued high fat diet (n = 12) or an IF with alternate days of fasting and an ad libitum high fat diet for six weeks (n = 12). These animals were compared with a group who had been fed a 36% CER chow diet for the 10 week study (n = 12). The IF and CER rats had a reduced weight (IF −27%, CER −14%), and reduced intra-abdominal body fat (IF −39%, CER −50%) compared to the high fat diet fed animals. IF failed to improve insulin stimulated glucose uptake in muscles (measured after a feed day) despite their lower adiposity. Both IF and ad libitum fed animals had reductions in muscle GLUT–4 proteins compared to CER (−30% and −42%). However IF animals had increased serum concentrations of adiponectin (+92%) and reduced HOMA insulin resistance (−49%) compared to the high fat fed animals indicating improved hepatic insulin sensitivity with IF [74]. Thus, in this animal model, IF had a favourable effect on hepatic, but not muscle insulin resistance compared with CER.

The apparent greater reductions in HOMA insulin resistance with a two day IER compared with CER in premenopausal women who are overweight or obese [12,13], and in some relevant animal models [74] raises the possibility that IER may improve hepatic insulin sensitivity. However, IER did not appear to evoke greater improvements in insulin sensitivity than CER in three other human comparator trials [18,27,33].

IF has been shown to have variable effects on peripheral and hepatic insulin stimulated uptake of glucose in non-obese subjects. The health implications of repeated short term increases in FFA and increases in peripheral insulin resistance with IF and IER each week are not known and need further investigation. This may be particularly important for groups which experience the largest fluxes of FFA, i.e., normal weight individuals and women [75].

5. Metabolic Flexibility

Periods of energy restriction or prolonged exercise switch liver, skeletal muscle and cardiac tissues to fat oxidation, and the catabolism of amino acids, whilst the post prandial state favours glucose uptake and oxidation. The reciprocal regulation of fat and glucose oxidation is controlled systematically by insulin and glucagon, and in response to changes in cellular levels of metabolites such as fatty acids, pyruvate, citrate and malonyl CoA which regulate mitochondrial enzymes. Energy metabolism is considered to be optimal when the body can readily switch between oxidising glucose or fat in response to nutrient availability and physiological stress [76]. This is considered to maintain metabolic health and the optimal cellular functioning. The switch in energy metabolism is known as metabolic flexibility. Metabolic inflexibility is seen in overfed individuals who do not easily switch between fat and glucose oxidation. There is simultaneous oxidation of fat, glucose and amino acids all of which increase oxidative stress, diacylglycerols, ceramides, and acylation of mitochondrial proteins, which in turn results in perturbations of mitochondrial function. Metabolic inflexibility is thought to be the root cause of insulin resistance [76].

Distinct periods of ER interspersed with normal energy intake each week may be akin to hunter-gatherer lifestyles and may promote maintenance of metabolic flexibility compared to standard daily diets, especially since IER contains longer periods of ER than our usual overnight fast. A recent study in rats of ADF supports this notion. Male Wistar rats were subjected to 48 days of IF (eight repeated cycles of three days of fasting and three days refeeding) or an isoenergetic 20% CER. The IF mice showed up regulation of genes for both lipid storage (PPARγ 2 and *Fsp27*) and fat oxidation (MCPT1) reflecting good metabolic flexibility with increased fat oxidation during fasting days and lipogenesis on non-restricted days of IF. These changes were not induced with an isoenergetic 20% CER [77].

In humans, six months of a 25% CER has been shown to improve metabolic flexibility, as evidenced by increased shift in fasting-to-postprandial concentrations of acyl carnitine (important for transfer of fatty acids into the mitochondrion prior to oxidation) [78]. There are currently no data of the effects of IER on metabolic flexibility in humans.

5.1. Is IER Safe?

There are theoretical concerns that IER could promote erratic eating patterns, binging, and low mood. A recent systematic review of 15 clinical trials concluded that marked CER (>60%) reduced binge eating behaviour amongst overweight or obese individuals with pre-treatment binge eating disorder, and did not appear to trigger binge eating in those without previous binge eating disorder [79].

Hoddy et al. [68] reported reductions in depression and binge eating and improved body image perception after eight weeks of following ADER. In contrast, four weeks of IER (four consecutive days of a 70% ER and three days of ad libitum eating) amongst nine normal weight young women, classified as unrestrained eaters, resulted in increased feelings of hunger, worse mood, heightened irritability, difficulties concentrating, increased fatigue, eating-related thoughts, fear of loss of control and over eating during non-restricted days [80]. We have reported comparable reductions in profile of mood state scores for tension, depression, anger, fatigue and confusion, an increase in vigour and an overall decline in total mood disturbance with a two day IER and CER [12,13]. Thus existing data show IER can improve eating behaviours and mood amongst subjects with overweight and obesity, but may have the potential for harm amongst normal weight individuals with unrestrained eating styles.

Another frequent concern is whether the spells of marked energy restriction with IER could perturb the hypothalamic-pituitary-gonadal axis in women and alter the frequency and length of menstrual cycles. Such effects are likely to be related to the starting weight of the individual, overall energy balance and the number of consecutive restricted days with IER. The 2011 IER study amongst obese and overweight women reported a longer average menstrual cycle length in women following IER for six months (two consecutive days of 70% ER per week) compared to 25% CER group (29.7 $\pm$ 3.8 days vs. 27.4 $\pm$ 2.7 days, $p < 0.005$) [12]. A study amongst normal weight, sedentary, normal cycling women found that three consecutive days of a total fast during the mid-follicular phase affected luteinising hormone dynamics, but were insufficient to perturb follicle development, or menstrual cycle length [81]. The effect of IER on the reproductive axis amongst obese, overweight and normal weight subjects requires further study, especially regimens which include longer periods of energy restriction.

IER does not appear to limit an individuals' ability to exercise. A 12 week combined ADER and exercise trial amongst subjects with obesity reported equal attendance to a supervised exercise programme (40 min of 75% max heart rate on three days per week) on both restricted and non-restricted days of ADER [62]. Similarly Carter et al. [33] reported a comparable increase in daily average step count in the IER and CER groups and Hill et al. [26] reported comparable and good adherence to a moderate intensity walking programme (five 20–50 min sessions of brisk walking 60%–70% max heart rate per week) amongst dieters undertaking IER and CER [26].

The majority of studied IER regimens have recommended healthy eating and not feasting on non-restricted days. Feasting on non-restricted days of IER may have adverse effects on health, despite weight loss. For example, a high fat ADER (45% fat) produced equivalent weight loss to a low fat ADER; 5.4 (1.5) kg vs. −4.2 (0.6) kg [82]. However, despite weight loss in this study, the high fat ADER group had decreased brachial artery flow mediated dilation which could increase risk of atherosclerosis and hypertension.

Thus, limited data to date suggest that IER is not associated with disordered or binge eating, perturbation of the hypothalamic-pituitary-gonadal axis, and does not limit the ability to exercise amongst in individuals who are overweight or obese. However the safety longer term and amongst normal weight individuals is not known.

5.2. Is There an Optimal IER Regimen?

The optimal duration, frequency and severity of ER needs to strike a pragmatic balance of being achievable, whilst also delivering supposed beneficial metabolic effects. There are numerous potential permutations of IER and IF which could be studied. IER is likely to be preferable to IF regimens amongst humans, as it is likely to have greater compliance and lower stress and cortisol responses [21]. IER regimens may need to provide some energy and protein intake on restricted days (i.e., 2.5 MJ and 50 g protein) to maintain nitrogen balance and FFM, which does not seem to be achieved with spells of total fasting [83]. IER evokes smaller fluctuations in FFAs and ketones than IF [19,20]. The latter is linked to short term impaired glucose tolerance during the resumption of normal feeding. The longer term implications of short term impairments in glucose tolerance with repeated IF each week is not known.

The timing of energy intake during the restricted days of IER does not appear to be important for compliance and weight loss. Hoddy et al. [84] reported equal reductions in weight with a 75% ADER with either one meal at lunch or dinner or three small meals throughout the day.

6. Conclusions

This review highlights a lack of high quality data to inform adherence and benefits or harms of IER vs. CER. Research findings and gaps in the evidence comparing IER to CER for weight control and metabolic health are summarised in Table 3. The few randomised comparisons of IER vs. CER amongst overweight and obese subjects report equivalent weight loss, with one trial of a two day low carbohydrate IER reporting greater reductions in body fat compared to CER [13]. These studies were not powered to detect a difference in loss of weight or fat, thus study finding are suggestive but not conclusive of no difference between IER and CER. No studies to date have tested whether IER can prevent weight gain amongst normal weight subjects, however IER regimens based on alternate days of total fasting or marked energy restriction (70% restriction) have not been well tolerated amongst normal and overweight populations (BMI 20–30 kg/m^2) [15,40].

This review highlights numerous gaps in knowledge of the effects of IER vs. CER on ectopic and visceral fat stores, adipocyte size, FFM, insulin resistance, REE and metabolic flexibility, particularly amongst normal weight subjects. In the absence of these data, we have drawn on findings of short term studies and highlighted some potential beneficial or adverse effects. The variable and sometimes adverse effects of IER on fat stores and metabolism in some rodent models reported in this review are a concern. However, this may relate in part to shifts in night and day eating patterns and circadian rhythm [55], which may not translate to the human situation.

Future IER research requires two types of randomised comparison trials. Firstly, longer term RCTs of IER and CER (>6 months) to show whether IER is sustainable long term and has long term benefits or yet undiscovered harmful effects on weight, body composition, and metabolic health compared to CER. Secondly, detailed metabolic proof of principle studies in controlled conditions to assess the effects of IER and matched isoenergetic CER on FFM, hepatic and intramuscular fat stores, insulin sensitivity and metabolic flexibility using robust methodology such as DXA, MRI and insulin clamps. These studies need to assess the metabolic effects of IER during restricted and feed phases of the diet to fully characterise its biological effects amongst people of any weight.

Well documented differences in metabolic responses to periods of fasting and marked energy restriction between pre-menopausal women (i.e., increased ketones and free fatty acids) compared to men and post-menopausal women suggest possible different metabolic responses, and perhaps better tolerance to IER within certain populations [85]. Future IER studies should include males, older subjects, individuals with morbid obesity or type 2 diabetes, as well as normal weight subjects. There is also a need to explore optimum patterns of restriction, e.g., two days per week, alternate days, five days per month [86] or other permutations and the best mode of restriction on the restricted and intervening days (e.g., low carbohydrate, low protein).

The popularity of IER within the general public coupled with the gaps in the evidence we have identified indicate that IER deserves further rigorous study. We do not know conclusively whether long term IER is a safe effective method of weight control for subjects who are overweight or obese or whether IER may confer health benefits to people of any weight independent of weight loss. High quality research comparing long term outcomes of IER and CER are required to ascertain any true benefits or detrimental effects which IER may have for controlling weight and improving metabolic health in the population.

Table 3. Summary of research findings and gaps in research comparing intermittent energy restriction/intermittent fasting to CER for weight control and metabolic health.

Outcome	Effects in People Who Are Obese or Overweight	Effects in People Who Are Normal Weights	Effects in Rodent Studies
Weight loss/prevention of weight gain	IER = CER for weight loss in six studies which were not powered to detect differences in weight. The study finding are suggestive but not conclusive of no difference between IER and CER weight [12–14,26,27,33]	No long term data	N/A
Proportion of body fat stored as visceral and subcutaneous fat	No data	No data	Mixed results: Reduced visceral and increased subcutaneous fat in female C57BL/6J mice [50]. No change in male C57BL/6J mice [51]. Increased visceral and decreased subcutaneous fat in 4 week old male Sprague Dawley rats [53] and LDL-receptor knockout mice [54].
Fat cell size	No data	No data	Reduced in male C57BL/6J mice [51]
Hepatic fat	No data	Modest increase after a single 24 h fast in men not women [46]	Mixed results: Deposition in IER > CER [53,54] IER = CER [87].
Intra myocellular triglycerides	No data	Modest increase after a single 48 hour fast in women but not men [45]	No data
Insulin sensitivity	Mixed results IER > CER (HOMA) [12,13] Reduced HbA1c IER = CER $p > 0.05$ [27,33]	Mixed results IER > CER [16] IER = CER [17]	Mixed results IER > CER total body and hepatic insulin sensitivity [73]. IER < CER peripheral insulin sensitivity [74] IER > CER hepatic insulin sensitivity [74]
Fat free mass	IER = CER [12,26]	No data	No data
Resting energy expenditure	IER = CER [26,28] IER > CER [18]	No comparison data	No data
Metabolic flexibility	No data	No data	IER > CER [77].

IER, intermittent energy restriction; CER, continuous energy restriction; LDL, low-density lipoprotein; N/A, not applicable.

Acknowledgments: We thank Mary Pegington and Helen Ruane for proof reading and Kath Sellers for formatting the manuscript.

Author Contributions: Michelle Harvie and Tony Howell conceived and designed the review; Michelle Harvie wrote the review, and Tony Howell edited the manuscript.

Conflicts of Interest: The authors declare no conflict of interest. Michelle Harvie and Anthony Howell have written three self-help books for the public to follow intermittent diets. All author proceeds are paid directly to the charity Prevent Breast Cancer Limited (formally known as Genesis Breast Cancer Prevention Appeal Ltd., Registered Charity Number: 1109839) to fund breast cancer research.

Abbreviations

ER	energy restriction
CER	continuous energy restriction
IER	Intermittent energy restriction
ADER	alternate day energy restriction
IF	Intermittent fasting
FFA	free fatty acids
FFM	fat free mass
REE	resting energy expenditure
MUFA	monounsaturated fatty acid
HOMA	homeostatic model assessment

Appendix A

Table A1. Search strategy.

#	Searches	Results
1	((intermittent or "alternate day" or modified) adj1 (fasting or diet or "energy restriction" or "calor* restriction")).mp. [mp=title, abstract, original title, name of substance word, subject heading word, keyword heading word, protocol supplementary concept word, rare disease, supplementary concept word, unique identifier]	854
2	(body adj1 (fat or weight)).mp. [mp=title, abstract, original title, name of substance word, subject heading word, keyword heading word, protocol supplementary concept word, rare disease supplementary concept word, unique identifier]	308923
3	(fat adj1 (liver or hepatic)).mp. [mp=title, abstract, original title, name of substance word, subject heading word, keyword heading word, protocol supplementary concept word, rare disease supplementary concept word, unique identifier]	2661
4	"ectopic fat".mp.	445
5	("fat free mass" or "muscle mass").mp. [mp=title, abstract, original title, name of substance word, subject heading word, keyword heading word, protocol supplementary concept word, rare disease supplementary concept word, unique identifier]	15776
6	"resting energy expenditure".mp.	2708
7	Insulin/ or insulin.mp.	340396
8	"metabolic flexibility".mp.	371
9	body weight/ or exp body weight changes/ or exp overweight/	365308
10	exp Adipose Tissue/	82804
11	Insulin/ or Insulin Resistance/	199942
12	exp Calorimetry, Indirect/ or exp Basal Metabolism/ or exp Energy Metabolism/ or exp Energy Intake/	361348
13	2 or 3 or 4 or 5 or 6 or 7 or 8 or 9 or 10 or 11 or 12	1115315
14	1 and 13	424

References

1. Whitlock, G.; Lewington, S.; Sherliker, P.; Clarke, R.; Emberson, J.; Halsey, J.; Qizilbash, N.; Collins, R.; Peto, R. Body-mass index and cause-specific mortality in 900,000 adults: Collaborative analyses of 57 prospective studies. *Lancet* **2009**, *373*, 1083–1096. [PubMed]
2. Sun, Q.; Townsend, M.K.; Okereke, O.I.; Franco, O.H.; Hu, F.B.; Grodstein, F. Adiposity and weight change in mid-life in relation to healthy survival after age 70 in women: Prospective cohort study. *BMJ* **2009**, *339*, b3796. [CrossRef] [PubMed]
3. Forouzanfar, M.H.; Alexander, L.; Anderson, H.R.; Bachman, V.F.; Biryukov, S.; Brauer, M.; Burnett, R.; Casey, D.; Coates, M.M.; Cohen, A.; et al. Global, regional, and national comparative risk assessment of 79 behavioural, environmental and occupational, and metabolic risks or clusters of risks in 188 countries, 1990–2013: A systematic analysis for the Global Burden of Disease Study 2013. *Lancet* **2015**, *386*, 2287–2323. [CrossRef]
4. Knowler, W.C.; Fowler, S.E.; Hamman, R.F.; Christophi, C.A.; Hoffman, H.J.; Brenneman, A.T.; Brown-Friday, J.O.; Goldberg, R.; Venditti, E.; Nathan, D.M. 10-year follow-up of diabetes incidence and weight loss in the diabetes prevention program outcomes study. *Lancet* **2009**, *374*, 1677–1686. [PubMed]
5. Kritchevsky, S.B.; Beavers, K.M.; Miller, M.E.; Shea, M.K.; Houston, D.K.; Kitzman, D.W.; Nicklas, B.J. Intentional weight loss and all-cause mortality: A meta-analysis of randomized clinical trials. *PLoS ONE* **2015**, *10*, e0121993. [CrossRef] [PubMed]
6. Veronese, N.; Facchini, S.; Stubbs, B.; Luchini, C.; Solmi, M.; Manzato, E.; Sergi, G.; Maggi, S.; Cosco, T.; Fontana, L. Weight loss is associated with improvements in cognitive function among overweight and obese people: A systematic review and meta-analysis. *Neurosci. Biobehav. Rev.* **2016**, *72*, 87–94. [CrossRef] [PubMed]
7. Christensen, R.; Bartels, E.M.; Astrup, A.; Bliddal, H. Effect of weight reduction in obese patients diagnosed with knee osteoarthritis: A systematic review and meta-analysis. *Ann. Rheum. Dis.* **2007**, *66*, 433–439. [CrossRef] [PubMed]
8. Chung, K.W.; Kim, D.H.; Park, M.H.; Choi, Y.J.; Kim, N.D.; Lee, J.; Yu, B.P.; Chung, H.Y. Recent advances in calorie restriction research on aging. *Exp. Gerontol.* **2013**, *48*, 1049–1053. [CrossRef] [PubMed]
9. Anastasiou, C.A.; Karfopoulou, E.; Yannakoulia, M. Weight regaining: From statistics and behaviors to physiology and metabolism. *Metabolism* **2015**, *64*, 1395–1407. [CrossRef] [PubMed]
10. Wing, R.R.; Blair, E.H.; Bononi, P.; Marcus, M.D.; Watanabe, R.; Bergman, R.N. Caloric restriction per se is a significant factor in improvements in glycemic control and insulin sensitivity during weight loss in obese NIDDM patients. *Diabetes Care* **1994**, *17*, 30–36. [CrossRef] [PubMed]
11. Henry, R.R.; Scheaffer, L.; Olefsky, J.M. Glycemic effects of intensive caloric restriction and isocaloric refeeding in noninsulin-dependent diabetes mellitus. *J. Clin. Endocrinol. Metab.* **1985**, *61*, 917–925. [CrossRef] [PubMed]
12. Harvie, M.N.; Pegington, M.; Mattson, M.P.; Frystyk, J.; Dillon, B.; Evans, G.; Cuzick, J.; Jebb, S.A.; Martin, B.; Cutler, R.G.; et al. The effects of intermittent or continuous energy restriction on weight loss and metabolic disease risk markers: A randomized trial in young overweight women. *Int. J. Obes.* **2011**, *35*, 714–727. [CrossRef] [PubMed]
13. Harvie, M.; Wright, C.; Pegington, M.; McMullan, D.; Mitchell, E.; Martin, B.; Cutler, R.G.; Evans, G.; Whiteside, S.; Maudsley, S.; et al. The effect of intermittent energy and carbohydrate restriction v. daily energy restriction on weight loss and metabolic disease risk markers in overweight women. *Br. J. Nutr.* **2013**, *110*, 1534–1547. [CrossRef] [PubMed]
14. Varady, K.A.; Bhutani, S.; Klempel, M.C.; Kroeger, C.M. Comparison of effects of diet versus exercise weight loss regimens on LDL and HDL particle size in obese adults. *Lipids Health Dis.* **2011**, *10*, 119. [CrossRef] [PubMed]
15. Heilbronn, L.K.; Smith, S.R.; Martin, C.K.; Anton, S.D.; Ravussin, E. Alternate-day fasting in nonobese subjects: Effects on body weight, body composition, and energy metabolism. *Am. J. Clin. Nutr.* **2005**, *81*, 69–73. [PubMed]
16. Halberg, N.; Henriksen, M.; Soderhamn, N.; Stallknecht, B.; Ploug, T.; Schjerling, P.; Dela, F. Effect of intermittent fasting and refeeding on insulin action in healthy men. *J. Appl. Physiol.* **2005**, *99*, 2128–2136. [CrossRef] [PubMed]

17. Soeters, M.R.; Lammers, N.M.; Dubbelhuis, P.F.; Ackermans, M.; Jonkers-Schuitema, C.F.; Fliers, E.; Sauerwein, H.P.; Aerts, J.M.; Serlie, M.J. Intermittent fasting does not affect whole-body glucose, lipid, or protein metabolism. *Am. J. Clin. Nutr.* **2009**, *90*, 1244–1251. [CrossRef] [PubMed]
18. Catenacci, V.A.; Pan, Z.; Ostendorf, D.; Brannon, S.; Gozansky, W.S.; Mattson, M.P.; Martin, B.; MacLean, P.S.; Melanson, E.L.; Troy, D.W. A randomized pilot study comparing zero-calorie alternate-day fasting to daily caloric restriction in adults with obesity. *Obesity* **2016**, *24*, 1874–1883. [CrossRef] [PubMed]
19. Antoni, R.; Johnston, K.L.; Collins, A.L.; Robertson, M.D. Investigation into the acute effects of total and partial energy restriction on postprandial metabolism among overweight/obese participants. *Br. J. Nutr.* **2016**, *115*, 951–959. [CrossRef] [PubMed]
20. Anderson, J.W.; Herman, R.H. Effect of fasting, caloric restriction, and refeeding on glucose tolerance of normal men. *Am. J. Clin. Nutr.* **1972**, *25*, 41–52. [PubMed]
21. Nakamura, Y.; Walker, B.R.; Ikuta, T. Systematic review and meta-analysis reveals acutely elevated plasma cortisol following fasting but not less severe calorie restriction. *Stress* **2015**, *19*, 1–21. [CrossRef] [PubMed]
22. NHS Choices. News Analysis: Does the 5:2 Fast Diet Work? *NHS Choices*. 1 May 2013. Available online: http://www.nhs.uk/news/2013/01January/Pages/Does-the-5--2-intermittent-fasting-diet-work.aspx (accessed on 8 December 2016).
23. Young, E. Deprive yourself: The real benefits of fasting. *New Scientist*. 12 November 2012. Available online: https://www.newscientist.com/article/mg21628912--400-deprive-yourself-the-real-benefits-of-fasting/ (accessed on 8 December 2016).
24. Davis, C.S.; Clarke, R.E.; Coulter, S.N.; Rounsefell, K.N.; Walker, R.E.; Rauch, C.E.; Huggins, C.E.; Ryan, L. Intermittent energy restriction and weight loss: A systematic review. *Eur. J. Clin. Nutr.* **2016**, *70*, 292–299. [CrossRef] [PubMed]
25. Seimon, R.V.; Roekenes, J.A.; Zibellini, J.; Zhu, B.; Gibson, A.A.; Hills, A.P.; Wood, R.E.; King, N.A.; Byrne, N.M.; Sainsbury, A. Do intermittent diets provide physiological benefits over continuous diets for weight loss? A systematic review of clinical trials. *Mol. Cell Endocrinol.* **2015**, *418*, 153–172. [CrossRef] [PubMed]
26. Hill, J.O.; Schlundt, D.G.; Sbrocco, T.; Sharp, T.; Pope-Cordle, J.; Stetson, B.; Kaler, M.; Heim, C. Evaluation of an alternating-calorie diet with and without exercise in the treatment of obesity. *Am. J. Clin. Nutr.* **1989**, *50*, 248–254. [PubMed]
27. Ash, S.; Reeves, M.M.; Yeo, S.; Morrison, G.; Carey, D.; Capra, S. Effect of intensive dietetic interventions on weight and glycaemic control in overweight men with Type II diabetes: A randomised trial. *Int. J. Obes. Relat. Metab. Disord.* **2003**, *27*, 797–802. [CrossRef] [PubMed]
28. de Groot, L.C.; van Es, A.J.; van Raaij, J.M.; Vogt, J.E.; Hautvast, J.G. Adaptation of energy metabolism of overweight women to alternating and continuous low energy intake. *Am. J. Clin. Nutr.* **1989**, *50*, 1314–1323. [PubMed]
29. Keogh, J.B.; Pedersen, E.; Petersen, K.S.; Clifton, P.M. Effects of intermittent compared to continuous energy restriction on short-term weight loss and long-term weight loss maintenance. *Clin. Obes.* **2014**, *4*, 150–156. [CrossRef] [PubMed]
30. Williams, K.V.; Mullen, M.L.; Kelley, D.E.; Wing, R.R. The effect of short periods of caloric restriction on weight loss and glycemic control in type 2 diabetes. *Diabetes Care* **1998**, *21*, 2–8. [CrossRef] [PubMed]
31. Wing, R.R.; Jeffery, R.W. Prescribed "breaks" as a means to disrupt weight control efforts. *Obes. Res.* **2003**, *11*, 287–291. [CrossRef] [PubMed]
32. Wing, R.R.; Blair, E.; Marcus, M.; Epstein, L.H.; Harvey, J. Year-long weight loss treatment for obese patients with type II diabetes: Does including an intermittent very-low-calorie diet improve outcome? *Am. J. Med.* **1994**, *97*, 354–362. [CrossRef]
33. Carter, S.; Clifton, P.M.; Keogh, J.B. The effects of intermittent compared to continuous energy restriction on glycaemic control in type 2 diabetes; a pragmatic pilot trial. *Diabetes Res. Clin. Pract.* **2016**, *122*, 106–112. [CrossRef] [PubMed]
34. Zuo, L.; He, F.; Tinsley, G.M.; Pannell, B.K.; Ward, E.; Arciero, P.J. Comparison of high-protein, intermittent fasting low-calorie diet and heart healthy diet for vascular health of the obese. *Front. Physiol.* **2016**, *7*, 350. [CrossRef] [PubMed]
35. Moroshko, I.; Brennan, L.; O'Brien, P. Predictors of dropout in weight loss interventions: A systematic review of the literature. *Obes. Rev.* **2011**, *12*, 912–934. [CrossRef] [PubMed]

36. Sacks, F.M.; Bray, G.A.; Carey, V.J.; Smith, S.R.; Ryan, D.H.; Anton, S.D.; McManus, K.; Champagne, C.M.; Bishop, L.M.; Laranjo, N.; et al. Comparison of weight-loss diets with different compositions of fat, protein, and carbohydrates. *N. Engl. J. Med.* **2009**, *360*, 859–873. [CrossRef] [PubMed]
37. Hill, R.J.; Davies, P.S. The validity of self-reported energy intake as determined using the doubly labelled water technique. *Br. J. Nutr.* **2001**, *85*, 415–430. [CrossRef] [PubMed]
38. Klempel, M.C.; Bhutani, S.; Fitzgibbon, M.; Freels, S.; Varady, K.A. Dietary and physical activity adaptations to alternate day modified fasting: Implications for optimal weight loss. *Nutr. J.* **2010**, *9*, 35. [CrossRef] [PubMed]
39. Wing, R.R.; Phelan, S. Long-term weight loss maintenance. *Am. J. Clin. Nutr.* **2005**, *82*, 222S–225S. [PubMed]
40. Wegman, M.P.; Guo, M.; Bennion, D.M.; Shankar, M.N.; Chrzanowski, S.M.; Goldberg, L.A.; Xu, J.; Williams, T.A.; Lu, X.; Hsu, S.I.; et al. Practicality of intermittent fasting in humans and its effect on oxidative stress and genes related to aging and metabolism. *Rejuvenation Res.* **2014**, *18*, 162–172. [CrossRef] [PubMed]
41. Taylor, R. Banting Memorial lecture 2012: Reversing the twin cycles of type 2 diabetes. *Diabet. Med.* **2013**, *30*, 267–275. [CrossRef] [PubMed]
42. Kirk, E.; Reeds, D.N.; Finck, B.N.; Mayurranjan, S.M.; Patterson, B.W.; Klein, S. Dietary fat and carbohydrates differentially alter insulin sensitivity during caloric restriction. *Gastroenterology* **2009**, *136*, 1552–1560. [CrossRef] [PubMed]
43. Lim, E.L.; Hollingsworth, K.G.; Aribisala, B.S.; Chen, M.J.; Mathers, J.C.; Taylor, R. Reversal of type 2 diabetes: Normalisation of beta cell function in association with decreased pancreas and liver triacylglycerol. *Diabetologia* **2011**, *54*, 2506–2514. [CrossRef] [PubMed]
44. Salgin, B.; Marcovecchio, M.L.; Humphreys, S.M.; Hill, N.; Chassin, L.J.; Lunn, D.J.; Hovorka, R.; Dunger, D.B. Effects of prolonged fasting and sustained lipolysis on insulin secretion and insulin sensitivity in normal subjects. *Am. J. Physiol. Endocrinol. Metab.* **2009**, *296*, E454–E461. [CrossRef] [PubMed]
45. Browning, J.D.; Baxter, J.; Satapati, S.; Burgess, S.C. The effect of short-term fasting on liver and skeletal muscle lipid, glucose, and energy metabolism in healthy women and men. *J. Lipid. Res.* **2012**, *53*, 577–586. [CrossRef] [PubMed]
46. Moller, L.; Stodkilde-Jorgensen, H.; Jensen, F.T.; Jorgensen, J.O. Fasting in healthy subjects is associated with intrahepatic accumulation of lipids as assessed by 1H-magnetic resonance spectroscopy. *Clin. Sci.* **2008**, *114*, 547–552. [CrossRef] [PubMed]
47. Heilbronn, L.K.; Civitarese, A.E.; Bogacka, I.; Smith, S.R.; Hulver, M.; Ravussin, E. Glucose tolerance and skeletal muscle gene expression in response to alternate day fasting. *Obes. Res.* **2005**, *13*, 574–581. [CrossRef] [PubMed]
48. Soeters, M.R.; Sauerwein, H.P.; Groener, J.E.; Aerts, J.M.; Ackermans, M.T.; Glatz, J.F.; Fliers, E.; Serlie, M.J. Gender-related differences in the metabolic response to fasting. *J. Clin. Endocrinol. Metab.* **2007**, *92*, 3646–3652. [CrossRef] [PubMed]
49. Gan, S.K.; Watts, G.F. Is adipose tissue lipolysis always an adaptive response to starvation?: Implications for non-alcoholic fatty liver disease. *Clin. Sci.* **2008**, *114*, 543–545. [CrossRef] [PubMed]
50. Varady, K.A.; Allister, C.A.; Roohk, D.J.; Hellerstein, M.K. Improvements in body fat distribution and circulating adiponectin by alternate-day fasting versus calorie restriction. *J. Nutr. Biochem.* **2010**, *21*, 188–195. [CrossRef] [PubMed]
51. Varady, K.A.; Roohk, D.J.; Loe, Y.C.; McEvoy-Hein, B.K.; Hellerstein, M.K. Effects of modified alternate-day fasting regimens on adipocyte size, triglyceride metabolism, and plasma adiponectin levels in mice. *J. Lipid Res.* **2007**, *48*, 2212–2219. [CrossRef] [PubMed]
52. Goossens, G.H. The role of adipose tissue dysfunction in the pathogenesis of obesity-related insulin resistance. *Physiol. Behav.* **2008**, *94*, 206–218. [CrossRef] [PubMed]
53. Cerqueira, F.M.; da Cunha, F.M.; Caldeira da Silva, C.C.; Chausse, B.; Romano, R.L.; Garcia, C.C.; Colepicolo, P.; Medeiros, M.H.; Kowaltowski, A.J. Long-term intermittent feeding, but not caloric restriction, leads to redox imbalance, insulin receptor nitration, and glucose intolerance. *Free Radic. Biol. Med.* **2011**, *51*, 1454–1460. [CrossRef] [PubMed]

54. Dorighello, G.G.; Rovani, J.C.; Luhman, C.J.; Paim, B.A.; Raposo, H.F.; Vercesi, A.E.; Oliveira, H.C. Food restriction by intermittent fasting induces diabetes and obesity and aggravates spontaneous atherosclerosis development in hypercholesterolaemic mice. *Br. J. Nutr.* **2014**, *111*, 979–986. [CrossRef] [PubMed]
55. Kliewer, K.L.; Ke, J.Y.; Lee, H.Y.; Stout, M.B.; Cole, R.M.; Samuel, V.T.; Shulman, G.I.; Belury, M.A. Short-term food restriction followed by controlled refeeding promotes gorging behavior, enhances fat deposition, and diminishes insulin sensitivity in mice. *J. Nutr. Biochem.* **2015**, *26*, 721–728. [CrossRef] [PubMed]
56. Chaston, T.B.; Dixon, J.B.; O'Brien, P.E. Changes in fat-free mass during significant weight loss: A systematic review. *Int. J. Obes.* **2007**, *31*, 743–750. [CrossRef] [PubMed]
57. Varady, K.A. Intermittent versus daily calorie restriction: Which diet regimen is more effective for weight loss? *Obes. Rev.* **2011**, *12*, 593–601. [CrossRef] [PubMed]
58. Heymsfield, S.B.; Gonzalez, M.C.; Shen, W.; Redman, L.; Thomas, D. Weight loss composition is one-fourth fat-free mass: A critical review and critique of this widely cited rule. *Obes. Rev.* **2014**, *15*, 310–321. [CrossRef] [PubMed]
59. Soenen, S.; Martens, E.A.; Hochstenbach-Waelen, A.; Lemmens, S.G.; Westerterp-Plantenga, M.S. Normal protein intake is required for body weight loss and weight maintenance, and elevated protein intake for additional preservation of resting energy expenditure and fat free mass. *J. Nutr.* **2013**, *143*, 591–596. [CrossRef] [PubMed]
60. Varady, K.A.; Bhutani, S.; Church, E.C.; Klempel, M.C. Short-term modified alternate-day fasting: A novel dietary strategy for weight loss and cardioprotection in obese adults. *Am. J. Clin. Nutr.* **2009**, *90*, 1138–1143. [CrossRef] [PubMed]
61. Varady, K.A.; Bhutani, S.; Klempel, M.C.; Kroeger, C.M.; Trepanowski, J.F.; Haus, J.M.; Hoddy, K.K.; Calvo, Y. Alternate day fasting for weight loss in normal weight and overweight subjects: A randomized controlled trial. *Nutr. J.* **2013**, *12*, 146. [CrossRef] [PubMed]
62. Bhutani, S.; Klempel, M.C.; Kroeger, C.M.; Trepanowski, J.F.; Varady, K.A. Alternate day fasting and endurance exercise combine to reduce body weight and favorably alter plasma lipids in obese humans. *Obesity* **2013**, *21*, 1370–1379. [CrossRef] [PubMed]
63. Weinheimer, E.M.; Sands, L.P.; Campbell, W.W. A systematic review of the separate and combined effects of energy restriction and exercise on fat-free mass in middle-aged and older adults: Implications for sarcopenic obesity. *Nutr. Rev.* **2010**, *68*, 375–388. [CrossRef] [PubMed]
64. Schwartz, A.; Kuk, J.L.; Lamothe, G.; Doucet, E. Greater than predicted decrease in resting energy expenditure and weight loss: Results from a systematic review. *Obesity* **2012**, *20*, 2307–2310. [CrossRef] [PubMed]
65. Rosenbaum, M.; Leibel, R.L. Adaptive thermogenesis in humans. *Int. J. Obes.* **2010**, *34*, S47–S55. [CrossRef] [PubMed]
66. Siervo, M.; Faber, P.; Lara, J.; Gibney, E.R.; Milne, E.; Ritz, P.; Lobley, G.E.; Elia, M.; Stubbs, R.J.; Johnstone, A.M. Imposed rate and extent of weight loss in obese men and adaptive changes in resting and total energy expenditure. *Metabolism* **2015**, *64*, 896–904. [CrossRef] [PubMed]
67. Soeters, M.R.; Soeters, P.B.; Schooneman, M.G.; Houten, S.M.; Romijn, J.A. Adaptive reciprocity of lipid and glucose metabolism in human short-term starvation. *Am. J. Physiol. Endocrinol. Metab.* **2012**, *303*, E1397–E1407. [CrossRef] [PubMed]
68. Hoddy, K.K.; Kroeger, C.M.; Trepanowski, J.F.; Barnosky, A.R.; Bhutani, S.; Varady, K.A. Safety of alternate day fasting and effect on disordered eating behaviors. *Nutr. J.* **2015**, *14*, 1–3. [CrossRef] [PubMed]
69. Wilcox, G. Insulin and insulin resistance. *Clin. Biochem. Rev.* **2005**, *26*, 19–39. [PubMed]
70. Hedrington, M.S.; Davis, S.N. Sexual dimorphism in glucose and lipid metabolism during fasting, hypoglycemia, and exercise. *Front. Endocrinol.* **2015**, *6*, 61. [CrossRef] [PubMed]
71. Gormsen, L.C.; Gjedsted, J.; Gjedde, S.; Norrelund, H.; Christiansen, J.S.; Schmitz, O.; Jorgensen, J.O.; Moller, N. Dose-response effects of free fatty acids on amino acid metabolism and ureagenesis. *Acta Physiol.* **2008**, *192*, 369–379. [CrossRef] [PubMed]
72. Anson, R.M.; Guo, Z.; de Cabo, R.; Iyun, T.; Rios, M.; Hagepanos, A.; Ingram, D.K.; Lane, M.A.; Mattson, M.P. Intermittent fasting dissociates beneficial effects of dietary restriction on glucose metabolism and neuronal resistance to injury from calorie intake. *Proc. Natl. Acad. Sci. USA* **2003**, *100*, 6216–6220. [CrossRef] [PubMed]

73. Belkacemi, L.; Selselet-Attou, G.; Hupkens, E.; Nguidjoe, E.; Louchami, K.; Sener, A.; Malaisse, W.J. Intermittent fasting modulation of the diabetic syndrome in streptozotocin-injected rats. *Int. J. Endocrinol.* **2012**, *2012*, 962012. [CrossRef] [PubMed]
74. Higashida, K.; Fujimoto, E.; Higuchi, M.; Terada, S. Effects of alternate-day fasting on high-fat diet-induced insulin resistance in rat skeletal muscle. *Life Sci.* **2013**, *93*, 208–213. [CrossRef] [PubMed]
75. Bloom, W.L.; Azar, G.; Clark, J.; MacKay, J.H. Comparison of metabolic changes in fasting obese and lean patients. *Ann. N. Y. Acad. Sci.* **1965**, *131*, 623–631. [CrossRef] [PubMed]
76. Muoio, D.M. Metabolic inflexibility: When mitochondrial indecision leads to metabolic gridlock. *Cell* **2014**, *159*, 1253–1262. [CrossRef] [PubMed]
77. Karbowska, J.; Kochan, Z. Intermittent fasting up-regulates Fsp27/Cidec gene expression in white adipose tissue. *Nutrition* **2012**, *28*, 294–299. [CrossRef] [PubMed]
78. Huffman, K.M.; Redman, L.M.; Landerman, L.R.; Pieper, C.F.; Stevens, R.D.; Muehlbauer, M.J.; Wenner, B.R.; Bain, J.R.; Kraus, V.B.; Newgard, C.B.; et al. Caloric restriction alters the metabolic response to a mixed-meal: Results from a randomized, controlled trial. *PLoS ONE* **2012**, *7*, e28190. [CrossRef] [PubMed]
79. Da Luz, F.Q.; Hay, P.; Gibson, A.A.; Touyz, S.W.; Swinbourne, J.M.; Roekenes, J.A.; Sainsbury, A. Does severe dietary energy restriction increase binge eating in overweight or obese individuals? A systematic review. *Obes. Rev.* **2015**, *16*, 652–665. [CrossRef] [PubMed]
80. Laessle, R.G.; Platte, P.; Schweiger, U.; Pirke, K.M. Biological and psychological correlates of intermittent dieting behavior in young women. A model for bulimia nervosa. *Physiol. Behav.* **1996**, *60*, 1–5. [CrossRef]
81. Olson, B.R.; Cartledge, T.; Sebring, N.; Defensor, R.; Nieman, L. Short-term fasting affects luteinizing hormone secretory dynamics but not reproductive function in normal-weight sedentary women. *J. Clin. Endocrinol. Metab.* **1995**, *80*, 1187–1193. [PubMed]
82. Varady, K.A.; Bhutani, S.; Klempel, M.C.; Phillips, S.A. Improvements in vascular health by a low-fat diet, but not a high-fat diet, are mediated by changes in adipocyte biology. *Nutr. J.* **2011**, *10*, 8. [CrossRef] [PubMed]
83. Birkenhager, J.C.; Haak, A.; Ackers, J.G. Changes in body composition during treatment of obesity by intermittent starvation. *Metabolism* **1968**, *17*, 391–399. [CrossRef]
84. Hoddy, K.K.; Kroeger, C.M.; Trepanowski, J.F.; Barnosky, A.; Bhutani, S.; Varady, K.A. Meal timing during alternate day fasting: Impact on body weight and cardiovascular disease risk in obese adults. *Obesity* **2014**, *22*, 2524–2531. [CrossRef] [PubMed]
85. Morrow, P.G.; Marshall, W.P.; Kim, H.J.; Kalkhoff, R.K. Metabolic response to starvation. II. Effects of sex steroid administration to pre- and postmenopausal women. *Metabolism* **1981**, *30*, 274–278. [CrossRef]
86. Brandhorst, S.; Choi, I.Y.; Wei, M.; Cheng, C.W.; Sedrakyan, S.; Navarrete, G.; Dubeau, L.; Yap, L.P.; Park, R.; Vinciguerra, M.; et al. A periodic diet that mimics fasting promotes multi-system regeneration, enhanced cognitive performance, and healthspan. *Cell Metab.* **2015**, *22*, 86–99. [CrossRef] [PubMed]
87. Rusli, F.; Boekschoten, M.V.; Zubia, A.A.; Lute, C.; Muller, M.; Steegenga, W.T. A weekly alternating diet between caloric restriction and medium fat protects the liver from fatty liver development in middle-aged C57BL/6J mice. *Mol. Nutr. Food Res.* **2015**, *59*, 533–543. [CrossRef] [PubMed]

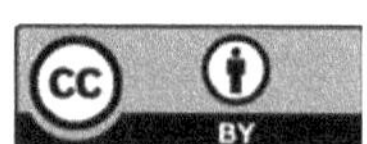

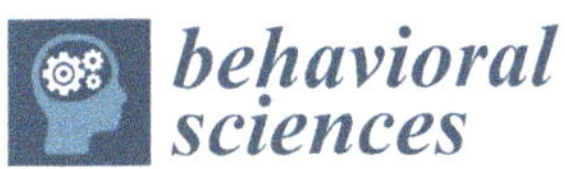
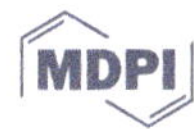

Review

Strategies to Improve Adherence to Dietary Weight Loss Interventions in Research and Real-World Settings

Alice A. Gibson * and Amanda Sainsbury

The Boden Institute of Obesity, Nutrition, Exercise & Eating Disorders, Sydney Medical School, Charles Perkins Centre, The University of Sydney, Camperdown, NSW 2006, Australia; amanda.salis@sydney.edu.au
* Correspondence: alice.gibson@sydney.edu.au; Tel.: +61-02-8627-1920

Received: 16 June 2017; Accepted: 7 July 2017; Published: 11 July 2017

Abstract: Dietary interventions are the cornerstone of obesity treatment. The optimal dietary approach to weight loss is a hotly debated topic among health professionals and the lay public alike. An emerging body of evidence suggests that a higher level of adherence to a diet, regardless of the type of diet, is an important factor in weight loss success over the short and long term. Key strategies to improve adherence include designing dietary weight loss interventions (such as ketogenic diets) that help to control the increased drive to eat that accompanies weight loss, tailoring dietary interventions to a person's dietary preferences (and nutritional requirements), and promoting self-monitoring of food intake. The aim of this paper is to examine these strategies, which can be used to improve adherence and thereby increase the success of dietary weight loss interventions.

Keywords: adherence; obesity; diet-reducing; appetite

---

1. Introduction

The obesity epidemic is one of the greatest public health challenges globally. In Australia, obesity has affected every facet of our population, with almost two thirds (63.4%) of adults now considered overweight or obese [1]. Obesity places an enormous burden on society, costing an estimated $8.6 billion dollars annually in Australia alone [2]. Clinicians are at the forefront of the obesity epidemic, often with limited time and resources. In order for clinicians to tackle the obesity epidemic, they need evidenced-based treatments that are practical, affordable and feasible to implement in real word settings.

The core principle of any obesity treatment is that it must shift the balance between energy intake and energy expenditure. Diet-induced weight loss, or 'dieting' as it is usually referred to, is the most common approach to weight loss. For a person dieting to lose weight, the energy balance principle dictates that they must restrict their energy intake to below their total energy expenditure in order to induce an energy deficit. However, there are many ways to achieve energy restriction due to the complex interplay of human metabolism, eating behaviours and the food supply, and this has contributed to the seemingly endless array of dieting books, products and programs available. The optimal dietary approach to weight loss is thus a hotly debated topic among health professionals and the lay public alike.

While the debate about the optimal weight loss diet continues, an emerging body of evidence suggests that higher levels of adherence to a diet, regardless of the type of diet, is an important factor in weight loss success [3–6]. There are numerous factors that may influence an individual's level of adherence to a dietary intervention, and clinicians will likely need to utilise a range of strategies to promote adherence. This paper will first narratively review the evidence supporting adherence as a key factor in weight loss success. It will then narratively review three key strategies that can be used to improve adherence and thereby increase the success of dietary weight loss interventions. These three strategies to be reviewed here are designing dietary weight loss interventions that help to control the increased drive to eat that accompanies weight loss, tailoring weight loss interventions to a person's dietary preferences (and nutritional requirements), and promoting self-monitoring of food intake. Although not the only strategies that can be utilised in practice to promote dietary adherence, we selected these specific strategies because they are practical, feasible, and applicable in both research and real-world settings, in diverse clinical populations.

2. Adherence is the Key to Weight Loss Success

A diverse body of research supports the idea that dietary adherence—the degree to which an individual 'sticks' to a diet—is a more important factor in weight loss success that the 'type' of diet an individual is prescribed. Dansinger et al. [3] reported a strong curvilinear association ($r = 0.60$; $p < 0.01$) between self-reported dietary adherence (on a scale of 1 to 10) and weight loss after following one of four popular weight loss diets (Atkins, Zone, Ornish or Weight Watchers), with no association between diet type and weight loss [3]. The Atkins, Zone, Ornish and Weight Watchers diets represent fairly wide extremes in macronutrient distribution. The Atkins diet is very low in carbohydrate (<20 g per day initially); the Zone diet aims to maintain a macronutrient balance with 40-30-30 per cent of energy coming from carbohydrate, protein and fat, respectively; the Ornish diet is a very low-fat (<10% of energy) vegetarian diet; and Weight Watches uses a 'points' food exchange system to reduce energy intake [3]. Similarly, results from the A TO Z weight loss study found that dietary adherence score (calculated by comparing self-reported food intake with the dietary goals of the respective diets) was significantly correlated with weight loss at 12-months within each of the three diets tested in that study (Atkins, Zone and Ornish) [4]. Therefore, in these two studies, it was the level of adherence to a diet, not which type of diet an individual followed, that predicted weight loss success. As the diets tested in these two studies are quite contrasting in their macronutrient distributions, it would suggest that in order to increase the success of weight loss diets, more emphasis should be placed on strategies for increasing adherence, rather than on the macronutrient composition of the diet *per se*.

Adherence has also been shown to be an important predictor of longer-term weight loss success in studies where individuals are all prescribed the same diet. Corral et al. [5] quantified dietary adherence based on metabolised energy intake, which was calculated using doubly labelled water to measure energy expenditure, coupled with dual-energy X-ray absorptiometry to measure change in body energy stores before and after a low energy diet (LED; $\geq$3350 kJ/day or $\geq$800 kcal/day). All food was provided to participants, and the composition of the LED was 20–23% of energy from fat, 20–23% of energy from protein, and 56–59% of energy from carbohydrate [5]. People in the highest tertile of adherers were found to consume an average of 2692 $\pm$ 309 kJ/day (644 $\pm$ 74 kcal/day), in contrast to those in the lowest tertile of adherers, who consumed an average of 6575 $\pm$ 138 kJ/day (1573 $\pm$ 33 kcal/day) [5]. Consequently, high adherers were more successful, losing weight at twice the rate as low adherers (126.5 $\pm$ 7.7 g/day versus 56.9 + 2.7 g/day; $p < 0.001$) [5]. Further, adherence during the weight loss phase predicted weight maintenance at two years, with the high adherers regaining only 50% of the weight that was lost, compared with 99% regain for the low adherers [5]. Thus, identifying poor adherence during the early phases of a weight loss diet might be an important indicator of poorer long-term outcomes. Poor dietary adherence has also recently been shown, through the use of mathematical models predicting energy intake, to be the primary reason for the less than expected weight loss associated with energy-restricted diets [7–10]. The mathematical models are based on the energy balance principle, which calculates average energy intake over a given period of time by deducting changes in energy stores from measures of energy expenditure. As the models take into account the concomitant reduction in energy expenditure with weight loss, it has been shown that it is fluctuating energy intake (i.e., poor dietary adherence) that is the primary driver of the weight loss plateau that typically occurs around 6-months into a diet [7]. Taken together, the studies highlighted above suggest that whether individuals are given the same diet or different diets, and whether adherence to the diet is determined through self-report, gold standard procedures or mathematical modelling, adherence is strongly associated with weight loss success over the short and long term.

Adherence is surprisingly high with very low energy diets (VLED). VLEDs involve severely restricting energy intake to ≤3350 kJ/day (≤800 kcal/day), which results in substantial and rapid initial weight loss [11]. VLEDs are the most intensive dietary intervention for obesity and the single most effective dietary intervention [12]. The rapid weight loss of VLEDs is very motivating for people and may be one reason they are associated with high adherence. A recent study showed that a person commencing a VLED has an ~80% chance of losing ≥12.5% of their initial body weight, compared to only ~50% for people commencing a diet involving moderate energy restriction [13]. Further, rapid initial weight loss has been shown to be predictive of long term success in maintaining a lower body weight [14–17]. The use of VLEDs to induce rapid weight loss, in contrast to many of the other weight loss products on the market, is backed by decades of medical research, and VLEDs have been in clinical use for almost 40 years [18,19]. The National Health and Medical Research Council (NHMRC) of Australia and the Dietitians Association of Australia (DAA) clinical practice guidelines for the treatment of overweight and obesity in adults suggest that VLEDs are useful as an intensive medical therapy option and are effective for supporting weight loss in adults with a BMI > 30 kg/m^2, or with a BMI > 27 kg/m^2 and obesity-related comorbidities, taking into account the individual situation and when used under medical supervision [20,21]. However, a 2008 survey of Australian dietitians revealed that only 1.5% of respondents reported prescribing a rapid weight loss program to their clients [22]. This is in line with an earlier survey of Australian dietitians, conducted in 2002, in which only 3.2% of respondents reported using a VLED to manage overweight and obesity in their clients [23]. Thus, despite the efficacy of and medical research behind VLEDs, they appear to be underutilised by clinicians, and should be explored further as a means of improving adherence to a weight loss program.

In summary, adherence to a dietary weight loss intervention is strongly associated with weight loss success over the short and long term [3–7,9]. This review will now examine three key strategies to improve adherence to dietary weight loss interventions. These are: designing diets to help reduce the weight loss-induced drive to eat, tailoring the diet to match dietary preferences (whilst meeting nutritional requirements), and promoting self-monitoring of food intake.

3. Strategies to Improve Adherence

3.1. Reducing the Drive to Eat with Diets that Induce Ketosis

Adherence to dietary weight loss interventions could be improved by strategies that help to control the physical drive to eat that occurs during energy restriction. An increase in the drive to eat in response to energy restriction and weight loss is one of a range of compensatory responses that collectively oppose ongoing weight loss and promote weight regain [24]. An increase in the drive to eat may contribute to the high rate of attrition in weight loss attempts and the inability of most individuals to maintain weight loss [25–28]. Indeed, the degree of hunger experienced by individuals with overweight or obesity in response to an energy restricted diet has been shown to be a predictor of subsequent weight regain [29], presumably due to increased food intake. However, not all studies have shown an association between changes in hunger and weight regain [30]. The compensatory increase in the drive to eat during weight loss is likely induced by multiple pathways, including alterations in expression of hypothalamic regulators of energy balance [31], as well as adaptive changes in gut function, which alter the concentration of appetite-regulating hormones such as ghrelin [30,32,33], cholecystokinin [30,34,35] and peptide YY [30,34,36]. Thus, designing dietary strategies that 'block' the compensatory increase in the drive to eat associated with energy-restricted diets represents a key target to improve adherence.

One dietary strategy that is frequently reported to suppress the drive to eat is diets that induce ketosis. Ketosis is a coordinated metabolic response to a low carbohydrate intake, resulting in an increased circulating concentration of ketones bodies or 'ketones' (β-hydroxybutyrte, aceotoacetate and acetone) that are produced by the liver from β-oxidation of free fatty acids. Suppression in the drive to eat associated with ketosis is thought to be a key factor in the efficacy of VLEDs, by allowing individuals to adhere to a severe restriction of energy intake and lose weight rapidly, without a compensatory increase in hunger [18,19,37–40]. Indeed, our recent systematic review and meta-analysis showed that individuals are indeed slightly, but significantly, less hungry and exhibit significantly greater fullness/satiety when adhering to a VLED, than when they are in energy balance before the diet [41]. Another type of diet that induces ketosis is ketogenic low carbohydrate diets (KLCDs), which severely restrict dietary carbohydrate intake but allow ad libitum consumption of protein and fat. However, although both KLCDs and VLEDs induce ketosis, KLCDs can result in several-fold higher circulating levels of ketones compared to VLEDs, as KLCDs limit carbohydrate intake to less than 20 g/day, while VLEDs typically provide at least 50–60 g/day [42,43]. The reason why KLCDs induce weight loss is attributed to suppression of the drive to eat, resulting in a spontaneous decrease in energy intake [42,44–46]. In keeping with this, our review also found that individuals adhering to KLCDs report feeling significantly less hungry and report feeling a significantly reduced desire to eat compared with baseline measures; albeit due to inclusion of only three KLCDs in the review the evidence should be considered carefully [41]. As the absolute changes shown in the meta-analysis may be considered small, and for some aspects of appetite were not significant, the clinical relevance of these findings to improve adherence is in the clear lack of an *increase* in the drive the eat, particularly for the VLEDs. Thus, the compensatory increase in the drive to eat that typically occurs during energy restriction [24–28] appears to be 'blocked' by VLEDs or KLCDs, aiding adherence to the energy restriction required for weight loss via VLEDs or KLCDs. For further discussion of the evidence for possible reasons underpinning the hunger suppressing effects of ketosis and ketogenic diets, see our recent review [41].

Determining whether ketosis per se is involved in the mechanism of hunger suppression during ketogenic diets, and if so, what level of ketosis is needed to result in a suppressed drive to eat, could lead to the development of novel weight management strategies. After all, VLEDs are only intended for short term use [47], and KLCDs, while efficacious in inducing weight loss in the short term, cannot be adhered to in the long term for most individuals [48]. Further, in order for a person to remain in ketosis, they must sustain a severely restricted carbohydrate intake, which involves the elimination, or extremely limited intake, of whole food groups that are beneficial to health (e.g., wholegrains, legumes, fruits, dairy and starchy vegetables). However, if ketosis were found to be involved in the mechanism underlying a suppressed drive to eat, ketosis could potentially be mimicked via the administration of synthetic ketones, thereby aiding adherence via increased hunger control while allowing consumption of a diet that is more aligned with healthy eating guidelines. Alternatively, if the level of ketosis needed for suppressing the drive to eat was found to be low, a diet less restrictive in carbohydrate could be followed, which might be easier for individuals to adhere to and is also more nutritionally sound. In our systematic review and meta-analysis, it was not possible to determine whether ketosis had a dose-dependent effect on the drive to eat, as differences in ketosis levels between the studies were insufficient for performance of a meaningful meta-regression analysis (all studies in the review reported an average circulating ketone level of about 0.5 mM). Elucidating what level of ketosis is required to suppress the drive to eat in response to energy restriction would have important implications for clinical practice. For example, it could allow for the design of KLCDs that are more aligned with dietary guidelines through the inclusion of some healthful carbohydrate containing foods. In turn, the diet would be more adaptable to a person's usual diet, and therefore more likely to be adhered to in the long term [6,49].

In contrast to inducing ketosis via a carbohydrate restricted diet, a novel approach to weight management could be to mimic ketosis through exogenous administration of synthetic ketones. Synthetic ketones administered orally as part of a meal replacement diet have recently been shown to be safe and well tolerated in humans [50]. Although synthetic ketones were developed as an alternative means of mimicking ketosis for the purposes of treating neurological conditions, such as refractory epilepsy, Parkinsons Disease and Alzheimer's Disease [51,52], artificially mimicking ketosis could potentially allow individuals to reap the benefits of hunger suppression, while adhering to a diet with a more flexible—and thus sustainable and health-promoting—macronutrient distribution. Further investigation would be required to test this possibility.

In summary, while it appears that ketogenic diets do suppress a compensatory increase in the drive to eat in response to energy restriction and weight loss, and that ketosis provides a plausible mechanism underlying the effect, it is not clear what level of ketosis needs to be reached for this effect to occur. Future research should investigate the minimum level of ketosis required to achieve a suppression in the drive to eat, and the level of carbohydrate intake and/or dosage of synthetic ketones required to achieve this, as a potential means of promoting long term adherence to energy restricted diets via increased control of the drive to eat.

3.2. Tailoring Diets to Dietary Preferences (Whilst Meeting Nutritional Requirements)

While controlling the drive to eat may be a key target for improving adherence to dietary weight loss interventions, physical hunger is not the only reason people eat (or drink) (see [53] for further discussion of non-hunger-related factors affecting adherence). Level of adherence may also be influenced by how different a dietary intervention is from a person's usual diet. Indeed, one study which used a Mediterranean diet intervention found that adherence to the Mediterranean diet at one and four years follow-up (as assessed by a score of $\geq$7 in the Mediterranean dietary score) was associated with how similar their usual diet was to the Mediterranean diet at baseline [49]. Another study showed that adherence to one of four diets that were high or average in protein, or high or low in fat (2 $\times$ 2 factorial design), was better in those who were randomly assigned to a diet which reflected the macronutrient profile of their baseline diet [6]. Therefore, adherence to a dietary intervention is likely influenced by how 'different' the dietary intervention is from an individual's usual diet. This is probably why individuals have difficulty adhering to severely carbohydrate-restricted diets over the long term [6,48], as carbohydrates are a major contributor to energy in most people's diets [54]. In summary, a dietary intervention that is flexible and can be individualised and adapted according to a person's dietary preferences may lead to better adherence to dietary prescriptions.

As well as individualisation according to a person's usual diet and dietary preferences, dietary weight loss interventions should take into account a person's nutritional requirements and be nutritionally sound. Notably, protein is a nutrient that is particularly important during weight loss for promoting satiety (which may also improve adherence by controlling the drive to eat), as well as helping to prevent loss of fat-free mass [55–58]. However, there are currently no practical resources (or information in clinical practice guidelines) on how to tailor dietary interventions that allow dietary preferences to be taken into account while also achieving adequate protein intake for individuals with varying requirements. Further, in published studies of dietary weight loss interventions in which protein intake has been individualised to requirements, there is limited information about how the diet was designed and how the diet is typically provided to the participants, be it as specially formulated meal replacements [59,60], or pre-prepared meals [42,61,62]. The diets used in these research studies, while important for establishing efficacy, are difficult to directly translate into clinical practice in real world settings, where individuals purchase commercial meal replacement products or are responsible for purchasing and preparing their own food. In summary, there is a need for practical clinical guidance on how to design dietary interventions that can be tailored to individual dietary preferences and dietary requirements (particularly protein) to improve adherence, that are also applicable in real world settings.

To demonstrate how to achieve a flexible and individualised diet according to a person's dietary preferences and nutritional requirements on a practical level, we recently published a modelling study which outlines the design process and underlying rationale for the dietary interventions of a clinical trial of fast versus slow weight loss (The TEMPO Diet Trial, ACTRN: 12612000651886) [63]. For the slow weight loss arm of the TEMPO diet trial, that paper demonstrated the feasibility of designing a food-based, moderately energy-restricted diet that can be individualized to a person's dietary preferences, while still aligning with the Australian Dietary Guidelines and containing adequate protein for women of various sizes. Although the TEMPO Diet Trial is more of an efficacy study than an effectiveness study, due to being conducted in a research setting with a narrowly defined population, it was designed to maximize clinical utility by drawing on existing resources and clinical practice guidelines [20,64]. By demonstrating how to operationalize the Australian Dietary Guidelines for weight loss, this paper provides clinicians with a practical, affordable and feasible intervention that can be adapted and implemented into research or real-world settings.

Taking into account nutritional requirements is particularly important with VLEDs, as they involve the use of specially formulated meal replacement products that replace all usual food intake (except low energy vegetables or broth). The nutritional formulation and cost of meal replacement products used for VLEDs can vary widely, as demonstrated by our recent survey of products available in Australia (several of which are available internationally) [65]. However, as we have shown in our recent papers [63,65], it is possible to tailor VLEDs to suit individuals' nutrient requirements based on age- and sex-appropriate dietary recommendations [66]. While this does not make the VLED closer to a person's usual diet, because a VLED is very unlike a person's usual diet due to the use of meal replacement products, it does make the diet closer to a person's nutritional requirements. Tailoring to meet individual protein requirements may be particularly important for promoting adherence by helping to control the drive to eat [55–58]. Tailoring VLEDs to meet nutritional requirements may also help to reduce complications. Although modern VLEDs are accepted as being safe, there are several potential complications associated with VLEDs. These side effects include, but are not limited to, lethargy, light headedness or dizziness, constipation, menstrual irregularities, gastrointestinal upsets, cold intolerance, dry skin and gallstones [67]. The majority of side effects are generally considered insufficient in magnitude or duration to warrant stopping the diet, and usually resolve upon the reintroduction of food. However, VLEDs should ideally be commenced in consultation with an appropriately qualified health care practitioner, particularly for people with weight-related comorbidities such as diabetes. Ensuring that VLEDs contain adequate fat and fibre levels may help to promote adherence by reducing the risk of complications such as gallstones and constipation—the risk of which is higher with VLEDs than with LEDs [68].

3.3. *Self-Monitoring of Food Intake*

Another potential target for improving adherence to a dietary intervention is recording of food intake. Keeping a food record, or 'food diary', is common in research and real-world settings for promoting and measuring adherence to dietary interventions, particularly for weight management [69–71]. In a systematic review of self-monitoring in weight management, all 15 studies that focused on dietary self-monitoring (in the form of a paper or electronic food diary) found significant associations between the frequency or consistency of self-monitoring of diet and weight loss [71]. Further, self-monitoring via recording of food intake has been shown to be a strong predictor of dietary change, as well as being a strong predictor of maintenance of dietary change over the long term [72]. However, food records can be subject to large errors, particularly with estimation of portion sizes [73]. A key aspect of any dietary intervention is providing dietary guidance on what and how much (i.e., portion size) to eat. Portion size estimation is difficult, but particularly when individuals are away from home and without access to scales or other portion size estimation aids (such as household measuring cups and spoons). A number of strategies have been developed to help individuals estimate portion sizes more accurately, including using comparison to common objects (such as tennis balls, mobile phones, matchstick boxes) as well as using the hands. For example, 'a fist', 'thumb tip' and 'fingertip' are used to estimate one cup, one tablespoon and one teaspoon, respectively. Although the accuracy of these estimation methods may be challenging in a research setting, efforts are currently underway to address this [74]. However, in a real world setting the value of a person self-monitoring their food intake is more so on increasing a person's awareness of their food intake, rather than accuracy of portion size estimation. This is reflected in the review mentioned above which found associations with the frequency and/or consistency of reporting and weight loss, not necessary the degree of accuracy. In summary, to promote adherence to dietary interventions, clinicians should encourage individuals to self-monitor their food intake.

4. Conclusions

Adherence is an important key to weight loss success, and there are a number of strategies that can be used to improve adherence that are applicable in research or real-world settings. An increased drive to eat is a major contributor to unsuccessful weight loss attempts, and thus it is a key target in improving adherence. Diets which induce ketosis (such as VLEDs or KLCDs) may help to control the increased drive to eat associated with weight loss, but further research is needed on the level of carbohydrate restriction that is required to achieve this. Ensuring that a diet contains adequate protein may also help to prevent an increase in the drive to eat. In addition, a dietary intervention that is tailored to a person's dietary preferences (whilst still aligning with nutritional recommendations), may also improve adherence. For this reason, government-based dietary guidelines are a very useful tool to use when tailoring a dietary intervention, as they are intended as population approach that are designed to be adapted to different dietary, cultural and cost preferences. Encouraging individuals to self-monitor their food intake has also been shown to improve the success of weight loss attempts and maintaining dietary changes overtime.

As alluded to in our Introduction, strategies that can be used to increase adherence are not limited to those discussed herein. There are numerous other strategies that have the potential influence an individual's level of adherence to a dietary intervention, and clinicians will likely need to utilise a range of strategies, both dietary and behavioural. For instance, increased dietary fibre intake may help to control the drive to eat [75]. However, further evidence for the effect over the long term, and during weight loss and maintenance in individuals with overweight or obesity is required. As well as dietary factors, other behavioural strategies in addition to self-monitoring, such as meal planning [76] may also help to promote adherence and increase the success of weight loss. Given the emerging body of evidence suggesting that higher levels of adherence to a diet, regardless of the type of diet, is an important factor in weight loss success, research efforts should be focused on increasing the evidence based for strategies to improve adherence.

Acknowledgments: This work was supported by the Australian Government: Department of Education & Training via an Australian Postgraduate Award to A.A.G., and via the National Health and Medical Research Council (NHMRC) of Australia via a Project Grant and Senior Research Fellowship to A.S.

Author Contributions: A.A.G. conceived the idea for the review and wrote the manuscript. A.S. provided supervision and mentoring in the form of discussions about the content and ordering of the review, as well as key ideas on areas of literature to include.

Conflicts of Interest: A.A.G. has received payment for oral presentations from the Pharmacy Guild of Australia and Nestlé Health Sciences. A.S. has received payment from Eli Lilly, the Pharmacy Guild of Australia, Novo Nordisk, the Dietitians Association of Australia, Shoalhaven Family Medical Centres and the Pharmaceutical Society of Australia for seminar presentation at conferences, and has served on the Nestlé Health Science Optifast® VLCD™ Advisory Board since 2016. She is also the author of The Don't Go Hungry Diet (Bantam, Australia and New Zealand, 2007) and Don't Go Hungry for Life (Bantam, Australia and New Zealand, 2011).

References

1. Australian Bureau of Statistics. 4364.0.55.001—National Health Survey: First Results, 2014–2015. Available online: http://www.abs.gov.au/ausstats/abs@.nsf/Lookup/by%20Subject/4364.0.55.001~2014--15~Main%20Features~Overweight%20and%20obesity~22 (accessed on 28 June 2016).
2. Obesity Australia. *No Time to Weight 2, Obesity: Its Impact on Australia and a Case for Action*; Obesity Australia: Sydney, Australia, 2015.

3. Dansinger, M.L.; Gleason, J.A.; Griffith, J.L.; Selker, H.P.; Schaefer, E.J. Comparison of the Atkins, Ornish, Weight Watchers, and Zone diets for weight loss and heart disease risk reduction: A randomized trial. *JAMA* **2005**, *293*, 43–53. [CrossRef] [PubMed]
4. Alhassan, S.; Kim, S.; Bersamin, A.; King, A.C.; Gardner, C.D. Dietary adherence and weight loss success among overweight women: Results from the A TO Z weight loss study. *Int. J. Obes.* **2008**, *32*, 985–991. [CrossRef] [PubMed]
5. Corral, P.D.; Bryan, D.R.; Garvey, W.T.; Gower, B.A.; Hunter, G.R. Dietary Adherence During Weight Loss Predicts Weight Regain. *Obesity* **2011**, *19*, 1177–1181. [CrossRef] [PubMed]
6. Sacks, F.M.; Bray, G.A.; Carey, V.J.; Smith, S.R.; Ryan, D.H.; Anton, S.D.; McManus, K.; Champagne, C.M.; Bishop, L.M.; Laranjo, N.; et al. Comparison of Weight-Loss Diets with Different Compositions of Fat, Protein, and Carbohydrates. *N. Engl. J. Med.* **2009**, *360*, 859–873. [CrossRef] [PubMed]
7. Thomas, D.M.; Martin, C.K.; Redman, L.M.; Heymsfield, S.B.; Lettieri, S.; Levine, J.A.; Bouchard, C.; Schoeller, D.A. Effect of dietary adherence on the body weight plateau: A mathematical model incorporating intermittent compliance with energy intake prescription. *Am. J. Clin. Nutr.* **2014**. [CrossRef] [PubMed]
8. Hall, K.D. Predicting metabolic adaptation, body weight change, and energy intake in humans. *Am. J. Physiol.* **2010**, *298*, E449–E466. [CrossRef] [PubMed]
9. Hall, K.D.; Sacks, G.; Chandramohan, D.; Chow, C.C.; Wang, Y.C.; Gortmaker, S.L.; Swinburn, B.A. Quantification of the effect of energy imbalance on bodyweight. *Lancet* **2011**, *378*, 826–837. [CrossRef]
10. Heymsfield, S.B.; Harp, J.B.; Reitman, M.L.; Beetsch, J.W.; Schoeller, D.A.; Erondu, N.; Pietrobelli, A. Why do obese patients not lose more weight when treated with low-calorie diets? A mechanistic perspective. *Am. J. Clin. Nutr.* **2007**, *85*, 346–354. [PubMed]
11. Mustajoki, P.; Pekkarinen, T. Very low energy diets in the treatment of obesity. *Obes. Rev.* **2001**, *2*, 61–72. [CrossRef] [PubMed]
12. Anderson, J.W.; Konz, E.C.; Frederich, R.C.; Wood, C.L. Long-term weight-loss maintenance: A meta-analysis of US studies. *Am. J. Clin. Nutr.* **2001**, *74*, 579–584. [PubMed]
13. Purcell, K.; Sumithran, P.; Prendergast, L.A.; Bouniu, C.J.; Delbridge, E.; Proietto, J. The effect of rate of weight loss on long-term weight management: A randomised controlled trial. *Lancet Diabetes Endocrinol.* **2014**, *2*, 954–962. [CrossRef]
14. Astrup, A.; Rossner, S. Lessons from obesity management programmes: Greater initial weight loss improves long-term maintenance. *Obes. Rev.* **2000**, *1*, 17–19. [CrossRef] [PubMed]
15. Nackers, L.M.; Ross, K.M.; Perri, M.G. The association between rate of initial weight loss and long-term success in obesity treatment: Does slow and steady win the race? *Int. J. Behav. Med.* **2010**, *17*, 161–167. [CrossRef] [PubMed]
16. Unick, J.L.; Hogan, P.E.; Neiberg, R.H.; Cheskin, L.J.; Dutton, G.R.; Evans-Hudnall, G.; Jeffery, R.; Kitabchi, A.E.; Nelson, J.A.; Pi-Sunyer, F.X.; et al. Evaluation of early weight loss thresholds for identifying nonresponders to an intensive lifestyle intervention. *Obesity* **2014**, *22*, 1608–1616. [CrossRef] [PubMed]
17. Unick, J.L.; Neiberg, R.H.; Hogan, P.E.; Cheskin, L.J.; Dutton, G.R.; Jeffery, R.; Nelson, J.A.; Pi-Sunyer, X.; West, D.S.; Wing, R.R.; et al. Weight change in the first 2 months of a lifestyle intervention predicts weight changes 8 years later. *Obesity* **2015**, *23*, 1353–1356. [CrossRef] [PubMed]
18. Howard, A.N. The historical development, efficacy and safety of very-low-calorie diets. *Int. J. Obes.* **1981**, *5*, 195–208. [PubMed]
19. Howard, A.N. The historical development of very low calorie diets. *Int. J. Obes.* **1989**, *13* (Suppl. 2), 1–9. [PubMed]
20. National Health and Medical Research Council. *Clinical Practice Guidelines for the Management of Overweight and Obesity in Adults, Adolescents and Children in Australia*; National Health and Medical Research Council: Melbourne, Australia, 2013.
21. Dietitians Association of Australia. *DAA Best Practice Guildeines for the Treatment of Overweight and Obesity in Adults*; Dietitians Association of Australia: Deakin, ACT, Australia, 2012.
22. Purcell, K. The rate of weight loss does not influence long term weight maintenance. Ph.D. Thesis, The University of Melbourne, Melbourne, Australia, 2014.
23. Collins, C. Survey of dietetic management of overweight and obesity and comparison with best practice criteria. *Nutr. Diet.* **2003**, *60*, 177–184.

24. Maclean, P.S.; Bergouignan, A.; Cornier, M.A.; Jackman, M.R. Biology's response to dieting: The impetus for weight regain. *Am. J. Physiol.* **2011**, *301*, R581–R600. [CrossRef] [PubMed]
25. Doucet, E.; St-Pierre, S.; Alméras, N.; Tremblay, A. Relation between appetite ratings before and after a standard meal and estimates of daily energy intake in obese and reduced obese individuals. *Appetite* **2003**, *40*, 137–143. [CrossRef]
26. Westerterp-Plantenga, M.S.; Saris, W.H.; Hukshorn, C.J.; Campfield, L.A. Effects of weekly administration of pegylated recombinant human OB protein on appetite profile and energy metabolism in obese men. *Am. J. Clin. Nutr.* **2001**, *74*, 426–434. [PubMed]
27. Drapeau, V.; King, N.; Hetherington, M.; Doucet, E.; Blundell, J.; Tremblay, A. Appetite sensations and satiety quotient: Predictors of energy intake and weight loss. *Appetite* **2007**, *48*, 159–166. [CrossRef] [PubMed]
28. Gilbert, J.-A.; Drapeau, V.; Astrup, A.; Tremblay, A. Relationship between diet-induced changes in body fat and appetite sensations in women. *Appetite* **2009**, *52*, 809–812. [CrossRef] [PubMed]
29. Pasman, W.J.; Saris, W.H.; Westerterp-Plantenga, M.S. Predictors of weight maintenance. *Obes. Res.* **1999**, *7*, 43–50. [CrossRef] [PubMed]
30. Sumithran, P.; Prendergast, L.A.; Delbridge, E.; Purcell, K.; Shulkes, A.; Kriketos, A.; Proietto, J. Long-term persistence of hormonal adaptations to weight loss. *N. Engl. J. Med.* **2011**, *365*, 1597–1604. [CrossRef] [PubMed]
31. Sainsbury, A.; Zhang, L. Role of the arcuate nucleus of the hypothalamus in regulation of body weight during energy deficit. *Mol. Cell. Endocrinol.* **2010**, *316*, 109–119. [CrossRef] [PubMed]
32. Olszanecka-Glinianowicz, M.; Zahorska-Markiewicz, B.; Kocelak, P.; Janowska, J.; Semik-Grabarczyk, E. The effect of weight reduction on plasma concentrations of ghrelin and insulin-like growth factor 1 in obese women. *Endokrynol. Pol.* **2008**, *59*, 301–304. [PubMed]
33. Cummings, D.E.; Weigle, D.S.; Frayo, R.S.; Breen, P.A.; Ma, M.K.; Dellinger, E.P.; Purnell, J.Q. Plasma ghrelin levels after diet-induced weight loss or gastric bypass surgery. *N. Engl. J. Med.* **2002**, *346*, 1623–1630. [CrossRef] [PubMed]
34. Sumithran, P.; Proietto, J. The defence of body weight: A physiological basis for weight regain after weight loss. *Clin. Sci.* **2013**, *124*, 231–241. [CrossRef] [PubMed]
35. Chearskul, S.; Delbridge, E.; Shulkes, A.; Proietto, J.; Kriketos, A. Effect of weight loss and ketosis on postprandial cholecystokinin and free fatty acid concentrations. *Am. J. Clin. Nutr.* **2008**, *87*, 1238–1246. [PubMed]
36. Pfluger, P.T.; Kampe, J.; Castaneda, T.R.; Vahl, T.; D'Alessio, D.A.; Kruthaupt, T.; Benoit, S.C.; Cuntz, U.; Rochlitz, H.J.; Moehlig, M.; et al. Effect of human body weight changes on circulating levels of peptide YY and peptide YY3–36. *J. Clin. Endocrinol. Metab.* **2007**, *92*, 583–588. [CrossRef] [PubMed]
37. Lappalainen, R.; Sjoden, P.O.; Hursti, T.; Vesa, V. Hunger/craving responses and reactivity to food stimuli during fasting and dieting. *Int. J. Obes.* **1990**, *14*, 679–688. [PubMed]
38. Lieverse, R.J.; van Seters, A.P.; Jansen, J.B.; Lamers, C.B. Relationship between hunger and plasma cholecystokinin during weight reduction with a very low calorie diet. *Int. J. Obes. Relat. Metab. Disord.* **1993**, *17*, 177–179. [PubMed]
39. Hoie, L.H.; Bruusgaard, D. Compliance, clinical effects, and factors predicting weight reduction during a very low calorie diet regime. *Scand. J. Prim. Health Care* **1995**, *13*, 13–20. [CrossRef] [PubMed]
40. Rosen, J.C.; Gross, J.; Loew, D.; Sims, E.A. Mood and appetite during minimal-carbohydrate and carbohydrate-supplemented hypocaloric diets. *Am. J. Clin. Nutr.* **1985**, *42*, 371–379. [PubMed]
41. Gibson, A.A.; Seimon, R.V.; Lee, C.M.; Ayre, J.; Franklin, J.; Markovic, T.P.; Caterson, I.D.; Sainsbury, A. Do ketogenic diets really suppress appetite? A systematic review and meta-analysis. *Obes. Rev.* **2015**, *16*, 64–76. [CrossRef] [PubMed]
42. Johnstone, A.M.; Horgan, G.W.; Murison, S.D.; Bremner, D.M.; Lobley, G.E. Effects of a high-protein ketogenic diet on hunger, appetite, and weight loss in obese men feeding ad libitum. *Am. J. Clin. Nutr.* **2008**, *87*, 44–55. [PubMed]
43. Sumithran, P.; Prendergast, L.A.; Delbridge, E.; Purcell, K.; Shulkes, A.; Kriketos, A.; Proietto, J. Ketosis and appetite-mediating nutrients and hormones after weight loss. *Eur. J. Clin. Nutr.* **2013**. [CrossRef] [PubMed]

44. Yancy, W.S., Jr.; Olsen, M.K.; Guyton, J.R.; Bakst, R.P.; Westman, E.C. A low-carbohydrate, ketogenic diet versus a low-fat diet to treat obesity and hyperlipidemia: A randomized, controlled trial. *Ann. Intern. Med.* **2004**, *140*, 769–777. [CrossRef] [PubMed]
45. Brehm, B.J.; Seeley, R.J.; Daniels, S.R.; D'Alessio, D.A. A randomized trial comparing a very low carbohydrate diet and a calorie-restricted low fat diet on body weight and cardiovascular risk factors in healthy women. *J. Clin. Endocrinol. Metab.* **2003**, *88*, 1617–1623. [CrossRef] [PubMed]
46. Boden, G.; Sargrad, K.; Homko, C.; Mozzoli, M.; Stein, T.P. Effect of a low-carbohydrate diet on appetite, blood glucose levels, and insulin resistance in obese patients with type 2 diabetes. *Ann. Intern. Med.* **2005**, *142*, 403–411. [CrossRef] [PubMed]
47. Delbridge, E.; Proietto, J. State of the science: VLED (Very Low Energy Diet) for obesity. *Asia Pac. J. Clin. Nutr.* **2006**, *15*, 49–54. [PubMed]
48. Foster, G.D.; Wyatt, H.R.; Hill, J.O.; McGuckin, B.G.; Brill, C.; Mohammed, B.S.; Szapary, P.O.; Rader, D.J.; Edman, J.S.; Klein, S. A randomized trial of a low-carbohydrate diet for obesity. *N. Engl. J. Med.* **2003**, *348*, 2082–2090. [CrossRef] [PubMed]
49. Beunza, J.J.; Toledo, E.; Hu, F.B. Adherence to the Mediterranean diet, long-term weight change, and incident overweight or obesity: The Seguimiento Universidad de Navarra (SUN) cohort. *Am. J. Clin. Nutr.* **2010**, *92*. [CrossRef] [PubMed]
50. Clarke, K.; Tchabanenko, K.; Pawlosky, R.; Carter, E.; Todd King, M.; Musa-Veloso, K.; Ho, M.; Roberts, A.; Robertson, J.; Vanitallie, T.B.; et al. Kinetics, safety and tolerability of (R)-3-hydroxybutyl (R)-3-hydroxybutyrate in healthy adult subjects. *Regul. Toxicol. Pharmacol.* **2012**, *63*, 401–408. [CrossRef] [PubMed]
51. Hashim, S.A.; VanItallie, T.B. Ketone body therapy: From the ketogenic diet to the oral administration of ketone ester. *J. Lipid Res.* **2014**, *55*, 1818–1826. [CrossRef] [PubMed]
52. Newport, M.T.; VanItallie, T.B.; Kashiwaya, Y.; King, M.T.; Veech, R.L. A new way to produce hyperketonemia: Use of ketone ester in a case of Alzheimer's disease. *Alzheimer's Dement.* **2015**, *11*, 99–103. [CrossRef] [PubMed]
53. Gibson, A.; Franklin, J.; Sim, K.; Partridge, S.; Caterson, I. Obesity: Making it less weighty. *Endocrinol. Today* **2014**, *2*, 8–15.
54. Australian Bureau of Statistics. 4364.0.55.007—Australian Health Survey: Nutrition First Results—Foods and Nutrients, 2011–2012: Table 1 Mean daily energy and nutrient intake. Available online: http://www.abs.gov.au/AUSSTATS/abs@.nsf/DetailsPage/4364.0.55.0072011--12?OpenDocument (accessed on 1 November 2015).
55. Westerterp-Plantenga, M.S.; Lemmens, S.G.; Westerterp, K.R. Dietary protein—Its role in satiety, energetics, weight loss and health. *Br. J. Nutr.* **2012**, *108* (Suppl. 2), S105–S112. [CrossRef] [PubMed]
56. Westerterp-Plantenga, M.S.; Luscombe-Marsh, N.; Lejeune, M.P.G.M.; Diepvens, K.; Nieuwenhuizen, A.; Engelen, M.P.K.J.; Deutz, N.E.P.; Azzout-Marniche, D.; Tome, D.; Westerterp, K.R. Dietary protein, metabolism, and body-weight regulation: Dose-response effects. *Int. J. Obes.* **2006**, *30*, S16–S23. [CrossRef]
57. Westerterp-Plantenga, M.S.; Nieuwenhuizen, A.; Tome, D.; Soenen, S.; Westerterp, K.R. Dietary protein, weight loss, and weight maintenance. *Annu. Rev. Nutr.* **2009**, *29*, 21–41. [CrossRef] [PubMed]
58. Leidy, H.J.; Clifton, P.M.; Astrup, A.; Wycherley, T.P.; Westerterp-Plantenga, M.S.; Luscombe-Marsh, N.D.; Woods, S.C.; Mattes, R.D. The role of protein in weight loss and maintenance. *Am. J. Clin. Nutr.* **2015**, *101*, 1320S–1329S. [CrossRef] [PubMed]
59. Soenen, S.; Hochstenbach-Waelen, A.; Westerterp-Plantenga, M.S. Efficacy of alpha-lactalbumin and milk protein on weight loss and body composition during energy restriction. *Obesity* **2011**, *19*, 370–379. [CrossRef] [PubMed]
60. Soenen, S.; Martens, E.A.P.; Hochstenbach-Waelen, A.; Lemmens, S.G.T.; Westerterp-Plantenga, M.S. Normal Protein Intake Is Required for Body Weight Loss and Weight Maintenance, and Elevated Protein Intake for Additional Preservation of Resting Energy Expenditure and Fat Free Mass. *J. Nutr.* **2013**, *143*, 591–596. [CrossRef] [PubMed]
61. Weigle, D.S.; Breen, P.A.; Matthys, C.C.; Callahan, H.S.; Meeuws, K.E.; Burden, V.R.; Purnell, J.Q. A high-protein diet induces sustained reductions in appetite, ad libitum caloric intake, and body weight despite compensatory changes in diurnal plasma leptin and ghrelin concentrations. *Am. J. Clin. Nutr.* **2005**, *82*, 41–48. [PubMed]

62. Leidy, H.J.; Carnell, N.S.; Mattes, R.D.; Campbell, W.W. Higher Protein Intake Preserves Lean Mass and Satiety with Weight Loss in Pre-obese and Obese Women. *Obesity* **2007**, *15*, 421–429. [CrossRef] [PubMed]
63. Gibson, A.A.; Seimon, R.V.; Franklin, J.; Markovic, T.P.; Byrne, N.M.; Manson, E.; Caterson, I.D.; Sainsbury, A. Fast versus slow weight loss: Development process and rationale behind the dietary interventions for the TEMPO Diet Trial. *Obes. Sci. Prac.* **2016**, *2*, 162–173. [CrossRef] [PubMed]
64. Australian Government National Health and Medical Research Council. Healthy Eating for Adults. Available online: http://www.eatforhealth.gov.au/sites/default/files/files/the_guidelines/n55g_adult_brochure.pdf (accessed on 30 January 2017).
65. Gibson, A.A.; Franklin, J.; Pattinson, A.L.; Cheng, Z.G.Y.; Samman, S.; Markovic, T.P.; Sainsbury, A. Comparison of Very Low Energy Diet Products Available in Australia and How to Tailor Them to Optimise Protein Content for Younger and Older Adult Men and Women. *Healthcare* **2016**, *4*, 71. [CrossRef] [PubMed]
66. Australian Government Department of Health and Ageing. *Nutrient Reference Values For Australia and New Zealand*; National Health and Medical Research Council: Canberra, Australia, 2006.
67. Franklin, J.; Sweeting, A.; Gibson, A.; Caterson, I. Adjunctive therapies for obesity: VLEDs, pharmacotherapy and bariatric surgery. *Endocrinol. Today* **2014**, *3*, 32–37.
68. Johansson, K.; Sundstrom, J.; Marcus, C.; Hemmingsson, E.; Neovius, M. Risk of symptomatic gallstones and cholecystectomy after a very-low-calorie diet or low-calorie diet in a commercial weight loss program: 1-year matched cohort study. *Int. J. Obes.* **2014**, *38*, 279–284. [CrossRef] [PubMed]
69. Carter, M.C.; Burley, V.J.; Nykjaer, C.; Cade, J.E. Adherence to a smartphone application for weight loss compared to website and paper diary: Pilot randomized controlled trial. *J. Med. Internet Res.* **2013**, *15*, e32. [CrossRef] [PubMed]
70. Carter, M.C.; Burley, V.J.; Nykjaer, C.; Cade, J.E. My Meal Mate (MMM): Validation of the diet measures captured on a smartphone application to facilitate weight loss. *Br. J. Nutr.* **2013**, *109*, 539–546. [CrossRef] [PubMed]
71. Burke, L.E.; Wang, J.; Sevick, M.A. Self-Monitoring in Weight Loss: A Systematic Review of the Literature. *J. Am. Diet. Assoc.* **2011**, *111*, 92–102. [CrossRef] [PubMed]
72. Tinker, L.F.; Rosal, M.C.; Young, A.F.; Perri, M.G.; Patterson, R.E.; Van Horn, L.; Assaf, A.R.; Bowen, D.J.; Ockene, J.; Hays, J.; et al. Predictors of Dietary Change and Maintenance in the Women's Health Initiative Dietary Modification Trial. *J. Am. Diet. Assoc.* **2007**, *107*, 1155–1165. [CrossRef] [PubMed]
73. Young, L.R.; Nestle, M.S. Portion sizes in dietary assessment: Issues and policy implications. *Nutr. Rev.* **1995**, *53*, 149–158. [CrossRef] [PubMed]
74. Gibson, A.A.; Hsu, M.S.H.; Rangan, A.M.; Seimon, R.V.; Lee, C.M.Y.; Das, A.; Finch, C.H.; Sainsbury, A. Accuracy of hands v. household measures as portion size estimation aids. *J. Nutr. Sci.* **2016**, *5*, e29. [CrossRef] [PubMed]
75. Clark, M.J.; Slavin, J.L. The effect of fiber on satiety and food intake: A systematic review. *J. Am. Coll. Nutr.* **2013**, *32*, 200–211. [CrossRef] [PubMed]
76. Ducrot, P.; Méjean, C.; Aroumougame, V.; Ibanez, G.; Allès, B.; Kesse-Guyot, E.; Hercberg, S.; Péneau, S. Meal planning is associated with food variety, diet quality and body weight status in a large sample of French adults. *Int. J. Behav. Nutr. Phys. Act.* **2017**, *14*, 12. [CrossRef] [PubMed]

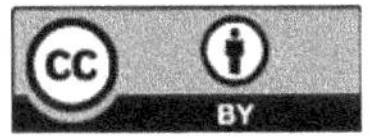

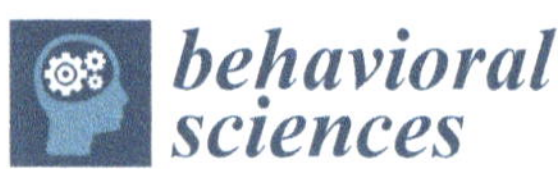

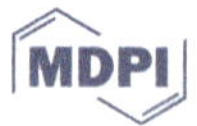

Article

Investigating Philosophies Underpinning Dietetic Private Practice

Claudia Harper [1,*] and Judith Maher [2]

1 The Boden Institute of Obesity, Nutrition, Exercise and Eating Disorders, Sydney Medical School, The University of Sydney, Level 2, Charles Perkins Centre, John Hopkins Drive, Camperdown, NSW 2006, Australia

2 Faculty of Science, Health, Education and Engineering, University of the Sunshine Coast, 90 Sippy Downs Dr, Sippy Downs, QLD 4556, Australia; jmaher@usc.edu.au

* Correspondence: claudia.harper@sydney.edu.au

Academic Editors: Amanda Sainsbury and Felipe Luz
Received: 23 November 2016; Accepted: 21 February 2017; Published: 1 March 2017

Abstract: There is limited theory or knowledge regarding dietitians' practice philosophies and how these philosophies are generated and incorporated into their professional practices. For the purposes of this study, a conceptual framework will explain and define the 'philosophies' as three different types of knowledge; episteme, techne, and phronesis. This study aimed to develop an explanatory theory of how dietitians in private practice source, utilise, and integrate practice philosophies. A grounded theory qualitative methodology was used to inform the sampling strategy, data collection, and analytical processes. Semi-structured interviews with dietitians in private practice were undertaken and data were collected and analysed concurrently. The results show that dietitians form collaborative relationships with their clients, in order to nurture change over time. They use intrinsic and intertwined forms of episteme, techne, and phronesis, which allow them to respond both practically and sensitively to their clients' needs. The learning and integration of these forms of knowledge are situated in their own practice experience. Dietitians adapt through experience, feedback, and reflection. This study highlights that private practice offers a unique context in which dietitians deal with complex issues, by utilising and adapting their philosophies.

Keywords: grounded theory; health care professionals; diet therapy; knowledge utilization; philosophy; relationships; patient-provider; theory development

---

1. Introduction

The profession of dietetics, consistent with medicine, nursing, and other allied health care providers, is firmly based in 'Evidence-Based Practice' (EBP). Sackett et al., the forefather of EBP, stated that EBP is the "conscientious, explicit and judicious use of current best evidence in making decisions about the care of individual patients" [1] (p. 71). The rationale behind EBP, which originated in the medical field, was to increase patient safety and to ensure that the best known intervention was being employed [1]. Health practitioners and their auditors feel confident that, when using EBP guidelines, the applied therapy is based on sound theory and evidence. In Australia, the accrediting professional body/organisation for Dietitians, the Dietitians Association of Australia (DAA), explicitly requires that EBP is used [2,3].

The DAA and the International Confederation of Dietetic Associations (ICDA) states that dietitians need to utilize EBP in conjunction with both the "dietitians' expertise and judgment, and the clients' or communities' unique values and circumstances to guide decision-making in dietetics" [2,4]. This is particularly true for dietitians in private practice; an area of practice which has been poorly researched, despite the rapidly growing numbers in this sector in recent years [5]. In addition, although encouraging a practice that integrates clinical judgment and patient values with EBP, accreditation requirements for dietetic university programs heavily emphasize a biomedical reductionist model of practice [6]. Despite these codes of practice, there is no description of the level of expertise needed to effectively carry out this practice and there is little knowledge of whether or how dietitians should do this in practice [2,4].

Nutrition and food behavior is a complex area with many competing influences, posing challenges to the formulation and application of applicable EBP. Such influences include, but are not limited to: 'taste and food preferences, weight concerns, physiology, time and convenience, environment, abundance of foods, economics, media/marketing, perceived product safety, culture, and attitudes/beliefs' [7].

While there are no questions about whether or not EBP works under the conditions that the research was pursued, there is a realization that these conditions are rarely reproduced in individual circumstances [8]. Additionally, evidence based on a single intervention is not congruent in a clinical setting, where a range of treatment approaches are often required [8]. Other health modalities have also noted that EBP constrains practice to quantifiable aspects and that there are areas within the patient-practitioner relationship that have been overlooked.

Perspectives and studies on exerting change in nutrition behavior have been primarily generated in the public health sector and, as such, possible problems and solutions have also largely been discussed in this context. On a public health scale, EBP has failed to exert meaningful change in the health behavior of targeted populations [9]. Buchanan suggests this could be due to social science attempting to apply a natural science perspective to the complexity of human behavior [9]. In effect, natural or biomedical science cannot adequately study, explain, or address phenomena in which the subjects have volition to choose their own actions [9]. Others call for more social research to explore the areas that are poorly understood when it comes to applying successful interventions within the social and environmental contexts of nutrition and health behavior [10,11].

Schubert et al. and Buchanan suggest that the analytical approach to nutrition science fails to recognize diet and nutritional disease as a complex set of processes outside of predictable scientific models [9,10]. Further, research is greatly removed from the human level, where dietitians interact with their clients and their dietary practices within the consultation process [10]. Studies that have explored nutrition and dietetic consultation practices generally focus on dietitians working in the hospital or community health arenas, and on singular aspects of practice. Some of these aspects include verbal and non-verbal communication skills [12], trust in communication between dietitians and clients [13], patients' experiences of dietetic consultations [14], dietitians use of EBP [15–17], and dietitians' opinions of client-centered nutrition counselling. Most studies investigate what dietary interventions are needed to effect nutritional change; however, less attention is paid to counselling approaches in dietetic consultation [14]. To date, no studies have explored the knowledge types in relation to nutrition and dietetic practices.

Proponents within medicine and nursing have noted gaps in research where EBP has failed to address important areas of practice that exist on the human level, in consultation with the patient [18–21]. They have proposed a practice framework which incorporates three philosophies that arguably underpin the skillsets and behaviors of practitioners whom are able to practice in a holistic way, working to address the particular needs of the patient [18–24]. These philosophies encompass reflective practice and clinical judgement, as well as skills that are not easily identifiable in a quantitative way [18,22,24,25]. These philosophies; episteme, techne, and phronesis, are identified as types of knowledge and originate from Aristotle's Nicomachean Ethics [26].

Practitioners who possess the knowledge types episteme and techne are said to be competent practitioners. However, those practitioners who possess phronesis, in addition to episteme and techne, utilize knowledge and skillsets that show expert characteristics [25,27–29]. It has been shown within nursing, that practitioners exhibiting the use of these three concepts, are better able to respond contextually and appropriately to their patients [30,31]. Others have noted that practice and research which incorporates phronesis with episteme and techne, may help bridge the gap between theory and practice, and encompass knowledge and skills that are not effectively conceived within a biomedical science paradigm [18,21,23,29].

Episteme, translated to epistemology, refers to 'the branch of philosophy which investigates the origin, nature, method and limits of human knowledge' [32]. In essence, episteme encompasses what is seen as true scientific knowledge based on evidence, which is the basis of dietetic practice. The term epistemology has come to be understood as scientific knowledge which is universal, invariable, and context independent. The most highly respected form of scientific knowledge in healthcare comes from randomly controlled clinical trials, in which theories are tested and found to be true or untrue.

Techne denotes production, namely art, workmanship, or skill (the 'know how'). It describes the endeavor of using technical rationality to produce a certain outcome [28]. Technical rationality describes a practice of systematically performing a set of discrete tasks, in order to produce a generic product [28]. This ensures that the practice is efficient, standardized, and 'practitioner proof' [28]. In this way, it can be replicated and controlled, and lends itself to practice criteria that are easily assessed and accounted for [28]. This aligns with clinical reasoning in medicine, in that, decisions made objectively whilst remaining neutral and which are based on the strongest evidence, should produce results free from conflict; with respect to multiple values and interests [28]. By utilizing both episteme and techne in practice, evidential knowledge is combined with a good technique. However, relying on technique alone may be inappropriate within complex contemporary situations [29]. Expert judgement in contextual situations requires practical judgement, and phronesis helps fill the gaps that good technique alone cannot address [21,29].

Phronesis is most often translated as 'practical wisdom' or prudence, and denotes the ability or character trait of being able to use one's collective knowledge in a different way, in order to produce the most optimal outcome of a specific situation [32]. A phronetic practitioner is able to draw on their knowledge, recognize what is needed in that situation, and deal with it effectively [28]. This ability requires a high level of perception and flexibility, in combination with an understanding of which epistemic and technical knowledge to apply for the best outcome [28]. Benner et al. state that phronesis is necessary to evaluate and integrate evidence and techne [18]. Phronetic action is not easily formulated as it requires creative insight and the ability to actuate knowledge with appropriateness to the situation [18,28]. Phronesis is concerned with the highest good in a situation and requires moral deliberation [33]. Phronesis is dependent on experiential learning, is changeable, and develops in practical endeavors [18,33]. It is also described as being ethical and reflective in practice, and develops through interactions with others [29,34].

Based on the above, our aim was to investigate which forms of knowledge dietitians use, and how these are developed and incorporated within the practices of dietitians in private practice. We are using Gustavsson's description of knowledge to guide us: "Knowledge is not merely theoretical, it is also practical, it is about what we know, what we do and how we act" [35].

In this text, we alternate between the use of the terms, patient and client, as well as, participant and dietitian.

2. Method

Constructivist grounded theory, developed by Charmaz, was used to explore what types of knowledge dietitians use in private practice in Australia [36]. How these knowledge philosophies are acquired, developed, and integrated into practice, was also investigated. Consistent with Blumer and Charmaz, sensitizing concepts were used to shape the research topic and guide the questions [36,37]. We used Aristotle's philosophical concepts of knowledge to provide us with a starting point for our investigation. These three types of knowledge, stemming from Aristotle's intellectual virtues, are: episteme, techne, and phronesis [38]. Our awareness of these knowledge philosophies assisted our discernment between diverse types of knowledge, despite their acquisition and use being simultaneous and interconnected.

It is important to note, however, that these concepts were not used to force the data into preconceived perspectives. According to Charmaz, researchers using constructivist grounded theory construct theories through interactions, perspectives, and practices [36]. Charmaz explicitly states that theories formulated by researchers using constructive methodology, are an interpretive description of the phenomena under study [36]. This study was approved by the University of the Sunshine Coast Human Ethics Committee.

2.1. Recruitment and Sampling

Accredited Practicing Dietitians (APD) in private practice, registered with the Dietitians Association of Australia (DAA), were identified via the DAA website. The DAA is the regulatory body for dietitians in Australia. It is a requirement that practicing dietitians register with the DAA, in order to gain APD status. Dietitians may then be listed on their website and searched for by the public. It is assured that all dietitians listed as an APD on the DAA website hold the credentials to practice as a dietitian.

Invitation emails were sent to 89 dietitians listed as APDs on the DAA website, inviting them to take part in the study. The first round of dietitians were chosen randomly and, as analysis progressed, the recruitment of dietitians became more specified, with the aim of testing emerging concepts within broader sample characteristics. To add robustness to our categories, once we had noted similar concepts within less experienced dietitians, more experienced dietitians were targeted, in order to expand our sample. For example, when a theme of dietitians experiencing a 'fast learning curve' and then a levelling out of this learning, emerged in dietitians with less than five years of experience, dietitians with more than 20 years experience were asked whether they remembered a similar process. As a result, an additional theme of 'lifelong learning' emerged in those dietitians with more experience.

Eleven dietitians, registered as APDs at the time of this study, agreed to participate in the study. This represents a 12% response rate. The length of time that had been spent working as a dietitian in private practice spanned between seven months and 30 years. All but one dietitian was self-employed. Two dietitians included in the sample were male. The dietitians in this study were a mixture of generalist and specialist dietitians, and two dietitians held double degrees, with the additional degree being held in another allied health modality. One dietitian held a Diabetes Educator status.

2.2. Data Collection and Analysis

Data were collected via semi structured interviews with dietitians, who responded affirmatively to invitation emails. A pilot interview was conducted prior to the commencement of data collection. The pilot interview indicated that the interview format was appropriate for gathering rich data associated with our subject matter. One-on-one, in depth, semi structured interviews were conducted in person (eight interviews), or on the telephone (three interviews). Telephone interviews were conducted to gain access to dietitians who were not close enough to interview in person. This also helped broaden the sample. The interviews were recorded with a recording device and a recording service was used to record the phone interviews. All interviews were transcribed by the researcher verbatim. This process allowed the researcher to become more familiar with the data.

In the interview, participants were asked to describe an interesting or recent case which they had worked on. The purpose of this was to explore a case that the participants could recollect in more detail. Subsequent questions allowed an exploration of the participant's thoughts, decisions, and reasoning, before, during, and after the case. At times, the interview process became reflective, due to the participant needing to reflect on why they chose to do things in a certain way, or how they arrived at the decisions that they had made. As data collection and analysis proceeded, and emerging concepts became apparent, additional questions were asked, in order to develop the categories more fully. For example, when data analysis indicated that being a self-employed business owner significantly contributed to the subject matter, this area was explored in more detail in subsequent interviews.

Observations and perceptions made during the interview were recorded as field notes at a convenient time and were used to provide further context on the emerging categories. During transcription and throughout analysis, further thoughts surrounding the data were recorded as memos and used to add depth to the analytical process [36].

Consistent with grounded theory, data analysis occurred concurrently with data collection [36]. In the initial open coding phase, preliminary codes were ascribed to words, lines, or incidents within the data. The data were preliminarily open-coded in Microsoft WordPerfect10 (Microsoft, Washington, DC, USA). We then used NVivo10 qualitative software (QSR International Pty Ltd, Melbourne, Australia) to store and group the data. Codes were crosschecked across the data set, to ensure the accuracy of the emerging concepts. Codes that appeared frequently or seemed significant across the data, were focused into categories.

Theoretical coding, according to Charmaz, conceptualizes possible relationships between the categories that were developed during the previous analytical stage [36]. For instance, the category 'applying evidence contextually and collaboratively' subsumed a number of codes that described strategies and information which dietitians used to determine appropriate therapies in practice. One other category, 'non prescriptive', encompassed various approaches to nutrition therapy favored by the dietitians. These categories were then encompassed within the conceptual category, 'collaborative therapy', as a way in which dietitians make decisions on nutrition therapy. Other major categories, 'nurturing change' and 'evolution and adaptation', also subsumed various processes and strategies.

Because our area of interest was the types of knowledge that dietitians use, the contextual information detected during this study, along with observational memos, were used to create a model of the knowledge philosophies that underpin the key strategies and skills which dietitians used in this study. This model of private practice also described the contexts and processes within which dietitians acquired, developed, and integrated these knowledge philosophies into practice skills.

3. Results

In the presentation of our results, we will first describe the overview of our theoretical model of private practice, summarized in Figure 1. This model of private practice was generated from the data, as themes which were common across the data set became apparent, and were elevated and organized into concepts and overarching categories.

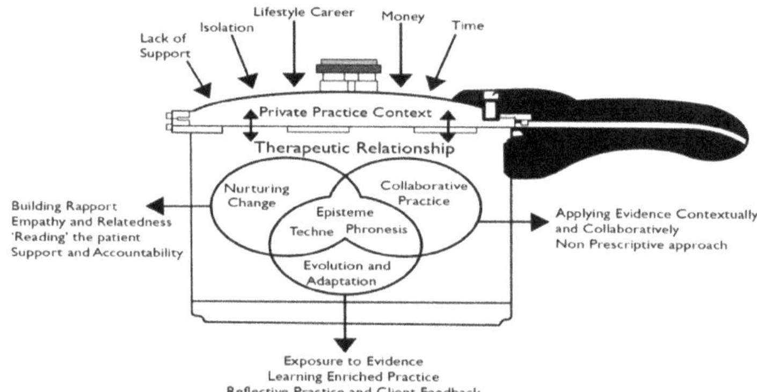

Figure 1. Philosophies Underpinning Dietetic Private Practice.

We will then, in turn, explain each component of the model, beginning with describing the unique context of private practice. We will describe the therapeutic relationships and the individual key strategies and processes that dietitians utilize to foster these in private practice. Finally, we will elucidate the knowledge philosophies underpinning these processes and show how these philosophies are integrated within processes that allow dietitians to adapt and evolve their practices.

3.1. Overview

As depicted in Figure 1, private practice is a complex and pressured environment within which dietitians adapt and evolve their practices. The unique context of private practice (described below) compels dietitians to modify their practices and foster mutually beneficial therapeutic relationships with their patients.

Synergistically, the therapeutic relationships themselves provide a context in which dietitians hone the skills and strategies needed within their practices. The key strategies used by dietitians with their patients: 'nurturing change' and 'collaborative practice', are continuously being refined using the third strategy of 'evolution and adaptation'. Underpinning and intertwined within these strategies, the three intellectual virtues: episteme, techne, and phronesis, were evident. These knowledge types remain at the center of this model. This is due to their presence being fundamental to the way in which dietitians adapt and evolve their strategies, in relation to the therapeutic relationships that are cultivated in the context of private practice. We will consider these concepts separately, explaining each of them in turn. Firstly, we will set the scene in the context of private practice.

3.2. Private Practice Context

Private practice dietetics appears to be a unique context within which dietitians acquire skills and use knowledge specific to that setting. It presents as a complex and pressured environment, within which dietitians adapt and evolve their practices. Private practitioners experience concerns over money and time, a lack of support, isolation, and enmeshment of their work and personal life. The private practitioners in this study acknowledged the challenging aspects of working in a private practice, which involved many hours of unpaid work, running a business, and doing the necessary paperwork that goes along with being both a dietitian, and being a business owner. Unpaid time was spent on business endeavors, preparing and updating education material, reading, keeping up to date, and professional development. Positive aspects of working in private practice included the freedom to choose which areas of interest they would focus their practice on and being one's own boss. These positive aspects were more prevalent among more established dietitians. The dietitians in this study indicated that running a business was more suitable for their perceived personalities.

Dietitians in this study spoke of the necessity of entering private practice due to the lack of work for dietitians. The more established dietitians expressed concerns that new graduates are entering private practice with no support or experience, and who are accepting an income well below what they should, thus creating a negative impression of the dietetic profession as a whole. Dietitians expressed that there was a lack of education on the complex aspects of private practice. These aspects included the wide array of conditions encountered, business acumen, people skills needed for dealing with frequently emotional patients, and the psychological aspects of feeling emotionally drained or experiencing death in long term patients with whom close therapeutic relationships have been established.

A sense of isolation from peers was experienced by the dietitians that worked alone. Some spoke of being comfortable with this isolation and had no desire to change. Others had sought out opportunities to connect with other dietitians, to varying degrees. Competition with other local dietitians, in some cases, was expressed as paradoxical to making connections.

The participants expressed the desire to deliver the best service that they could, and were continuously adapting their practice and knowledge base in an effort to better serve their client base. On account of this, dietitians spoke of the all-encompassing nature of being a dietitian in private practice. When they weren't actively working in their practice, they were learning, reading, and thinking about nutrition and business. In effect, this created a career which could be described as a 'lifestyle career', as it was often difficult to 'turn off', even when outside of the practice. The high exposure which nutrition, food, and cooking has within society through various outlets, also added to this feeling. Those that also lived in the community which they worked in described the balancing act of seeing clients both professionally and in a more casual setting, and being conscious of the relationship which they had with their clients. Overall, private practice provided a rich context in which dietitians worked and in which they learned the skills which are needed to be successful.

3.3. *Therapeutic Relationship*

The therapeutic relationship is the foundation of the practitioner-patient alliance. Research suggests that this relationship has two parts: building a relationship and facilitating positive action [39]. A successful therapeutic relationship requires the practitioner to build a good rapport, show empathy, and gain the trust of their client [39]. Braude states that within the intersubjective space between the practitioner and patient, elements exist that are beyond the cognitions of the practitioner and patient [20]. Despite being beyond cognition, these nonverbal, tacit clues that exist within the context of the therapeutic relationship, provide valuable information to the practitioner, which they draw upon to appropriately respond to their patient [20].

Dietitians in private practice recognized the importance of developing a therapeutic relationship as the foundation of their practice. They have developed strategies that directly relate to fostering a mutually satisfying therapeutic relationship with their clients. The motivations for dietitians in private practice to foster these relationships are multi-faceted. The participants in this study described the importance of the therapeutic relationship for facilitating change and positive outcomes for their clients. Furthermore, they noted that positive outcomes were more likely in clients who received ongoing support through follow-up consultations over time. Follow-up consultations and the resultant positive outcomes were mediated by the therapeutic relationships that dietitians fostered from the outset of contact. Additionally, dietitians in this study were aware that building these relationships were crucial to their professional reputation with both doctors and patients, and that, in turn, they had a direct effect on their income. In this way, the therapeutic relationship was vital to both the client's wellbeing and the practitioner's livelihood.

3.4. *Collaborative Therapy*

Collaborative therapy refers to the key strategy that dietitians in this study used to formulate their education focus and nutrition interventions with their clients. Using a non-prescriptive approach, and applying evidence both contextually and collaboratively, are ways in which the dietitians in this study worked collaboratively with their clients. These processes were the most commonly described approaches across the data set and they are elucidated below.

3.4.1. Evidence Applied Contextually and Collaboratively

Dietitians in this study described working with their patients to design therapies that were informed by EBP, but that were, more importantly, collaboratively formulated with the patient. The clients' social contexts were often barriers to implementing strict EBPs and necessitated a flexible approach. One dietitian showed awareness of the clinical guidelines for a low salt diet, but access to suitable foods and the clients' lifestyle prohibited recommending a diet which was strictly based on clinical guidelines:

> 'It wasn't a clinical low salt diet, it's quite difficult to access that sort of food here unless you're going to cook absolutely everything from scratch which wasn't quite realistic for her. We also discussed how to, you know, eat out, get take away in a sensible manner. She had become quite reliant on take away for small periods of time there, she had her children, came back home and was doing lots of events of the evening, so she needed to do that sort of thing so it was about, so if you need to do take away how can we do that well?' (Dietitian 7)

The primary goal of the dietitians was to ascertain the client's abilities, requirements, and wishes, and to collaborate with their client in order to tailor a suitable intervention protocol. Facilitating client autonomy within this collaborative process, where possible and practical, was seen by dietitians as a necessary part of gaining trust, enhancing a rapport, and increasing compliance with their clients. They described the approach of telling a client what they had to do as having the potential of alienating the client and getting them off side. One dietitian described a client who arrived with a diet plan that she wanted to follow, and which had previously allowed her to successfully lose weight. The dietitian chose to facilitate this to show support for the client and encourage follow-up visits. Over time, taking into consideration her previous failures, the dietitian hoped to work with the client to make her diet more easily sustainable over the long term:

> '(She) had specifically come to me because she said she wanted some accountability and just a little bit of support along the way so, in many ways I was guided by what she wanted to do. . . given her previous failures, that we would have to look at something that I think would be a bit more sustainable for her. But in the first appointment I decided to let her run with what she wanted to start with because I wanted to show, demonstrate to her that I was, you know, being supportive of what she wanted to do.' (Dietitian 8)

Evidence applied contextually and collaboratively as episteme and techne. Episteme as a knowledge type underpinning practice is evident in the use of evidence-based guidelines for nutrition interventions and counselling techniques. Techne, as a knowledge type, is present when dietitians have the technical acumen to use this knowledge and apply it appropriately to suit their clients' needs. In this way, episteme and techne underpin the DAA competency standards which state that, for dietitians to be competent, they must be able to use client care in collaboration with clients.

3.4.2. Non Prescriptive

The dietitians in this study most often used a non-prescriptive diet approach during intervention. Increasing awareness whilst eating and educating to increase nourishment within an often imperfect diet, was seen as more desirable than promoting prescriptive diets. Some others spoke of supplying a diet plan to their clients, when they felt that the client preferred that approach. One participant described how being non-prescriptive worked well for her clients:

> 'It's not prescriptive; it's them figuring it out for themselves. That's how I work anyway and it works really well.' (Dietitian 3)

Non-prescriptive as episteme and techne. Using a non-prescriptive diet for clients would be underpinned by episteme and techne, in the use of evidence which signifies that changes are needed in the diet and using the techniques to apply changes in a non-prescriptive way.

3.5. *Nurturing Change*

Nurturing change refers to the key strategy that the dietitians in this study used to foster an environment in which their clients felt heard and supported. The processes that constitute 'nurturing change' are, 'building rapport', 'empathy and relatedness', 'reading the patient', and 'support and accountability'. These relational and interpersonal skills were the most commonly described processes across the data set. They are individually considered below.

3.5.1. Building Rapport and Relationships

The dietitians in this study were conscious of establishing a good relationship with their clients. They were aware that, prior to any education or intervention being delivered or being successful, they need to establish a relationship in which the client feels comfortable and feels as though they are engaged in the consultation process. The techniques that they use to build a rapport and relationships vary, according to the dietitian and the client.

The dietitians reported changing their approach, depending on the type of client that they had. They use a range of techniques to show the client that they are interested, respectful, and willing to listen. In doing so, they were more confident that the client would be more engaged with them and more likely to return to see them. Repeat visits were seen as much more conducive to successful outcomes for the client, as well as being advantageous for the business. One dietitian spoke of the importance of engaging the client and making them comfortable, in order to be able to help them:

> 'I know if I can't engage that patient that I'm not going to be able to help them so it's of primary importance to make sure you are on that level with the patient and they're happy with you, you know, if they're not happy with you, or comfortable with me I'm not going to be able to help them so I need to kind of establish that right from the beginning.' (Dietitian 6)

Another dietitian described being aware that more than one consultation is usually needed to help a client achieve positive outcomes, and that facilitating follow-up visits hinged on establishing a rapport and connection, right from the first consult:

> 'Generally I try and establish a really good rapport and connection with the person because I know that if I can establish that rapport then I know that I can keep them coming back and I know that I can help them, whereas if we can't establish that connection, so that's what I sort of try to establish in that first consult.' (Dietitian 9)

Building rapport and relationships as episteme and techne. Although not stated explicitly in the competency standards, building a rapport with clients is a fundamental element of counselling models and is implied in dietetic counselling practice. In this way, episteme and techne are evident as knowledge types underpinning the techniques used to a build rapport and relationships when counselling clients.

3.5.2. Empathy and Relatedness

All participants described the amount of emotionality that they encounter in consultations with their clients. Some dietitians felt this emotionality was due to the more personal and unregimented atmosphere of the private practice consultation process. This atmosphere was contrasted with consults in hospital wards by dietitians who had experience in both areas. Depression is often encountered and crying was encountered on a very regular basis by all dietitians in this study. Dietitians in this study felt that being respectful and empathetic during these encounters was crucial. Often, dietitians described crying as flattering and showing trust, and also as cathartic, moving the consultation in a more beneficial direction. All dietitians reported that when the emotionality became counterproductive to moving forward, they would encourage clients to seek professional help. The dietitians in this study recognized the importance of understanding the client from their perspective and being able to relate to their circumstances. The older dietitians also described scenarios in which having personal experience helped them relate to their client's situation. The younger dietitians revealed how they had grown more comfortable with clients' emotions over time. Anger was also encountered, although to a much lesser extent, and was usually dealt with by listening to the clients' concerns and reassuring them that they are there to help. A dietitian describes becoming comfortable with dealing with crying patients over time:

> 'I go through many boxes of tissues in a week, but it's a tough situation and I remember when I first had my client cry on me, I didn't know what to do, I didn't know what to say but I think through experience you get to know it's part of the whole process—it's part of that process of change because it's a realization.' (Dietitian 2)

An older dietitian described being able to relate to different life stages of her clients, after having the same experiences:

> 'I think that it allows you to relate to people at that stage, so when I had young children I could relate to how tired and busy young mums are, when I had teenage daughters I could relate to, you know, so the mother drags the teenage daughter in sits her in the chair and says 'she eats terribly, fix her diet' you know, so you can relate to fact that the child is sitting there going, 'yeah mum I don't want to be here' so yeah.' (Dietitian 4)

Empathy and relatedness as phronesis. Being empathic is a necessary element of being a skillful counsellor [40]. Svenaus (2003) draws a direct comparison between empathy and phronesis, and suggests that empathy is a fundamental component of being a phronetic practitioner who seeks the good for his patient in each situation [41]. In this way, phronesis underpins the practice of being empathetic in the context of this situation.

3.5.3. 'Reading' the Patient

The dietitians in this study frequently alluded to 'picking up' signals from their clients which helped them decide how to proceed within the consultation. They used a variety of ways to describe this process. These included, 'gut feel', 'intuition', 'reading the person', 'instinct', 'clever questioning', and 'tone'. These non-verbal cues or the tone of the conversation, despite being hard for the dietitians to describe, played a significant role in how the dietitians chose to proceed and respond throughout the consultation. During the interviews, the dietitians could recall how the patient was feeling and described asking direct questions, if they weren't sure.

Most dietitians described this as a natural ability that they had, but which they honed over time:

> 'Yeah, I guess I think I naturally can read people pretty well that sort of one area I can adapt the way I speak with people, so yeah that instinct as well—it kind of gets better as you go.' (Dietitian 2)

Most dietitians described using this perceptive ability to help them make clinical decisions:

> 'I think you've really just got to tailor everything to the individual and that's all on gut feel. I don't know that's the way I operate anyway—it's—it is a bit gut feel.' (Dietitian 1)

Reading the patient and phronesis. Braude suggests that perception connects cognition and consciousness, and that it is important for clinical reasoning [20]. He suggests that these perceptions are present within the therapeutic relationship and contends that, when perception and intuition are combined with the explicit, phronesis is a fitting concept to apply to clinical decisions [20]. Phronesis, then, underpins the practice of using tacit clues which are implicit within the consultation process, to assist in being responsive to the patients' needs.

3.5.4. Support and Accountability

Dietitians who saw clients regularly over a period of time, reported that their roles moved more towards providing support and accountability, rather than nutritional advice or changes. These consultations became less structured than the first consultations. This dynamic was the most successful in helping their clients change nutritional and lifestyle habits. Slow, long term incremental changes were seen as being more successful in the long run, and repeat visits gave these dietitians the freedom to more successfully support clients and make necessary changes:

> 'For review consultations, subsequent consultations, probably a lot more of my energy would be focused on motivational interviewing, health coaching and supportive counselling, that sort of thing. So it's gradual changes occurring but I think they're coming about from her having that accountability of coming in and seeing me every week and that's her decision.' (Dietitian 10)

3.6. Evolution and Adaptation

Acquisition, development, and integration encompass how dietitians are exposed to knowledge, how they seek it out, and how they learn and integrate information and strategies in their practice.

3.6.1. Exposure

In line with the concept of dietetics in private practice being a lifestyle career, dietitians are constantly exposed to nutritional information from the media, social media, supermarkets, newspapers, and magazines, as well as their own clients. They report that, in addition to these sources, they also seek out information on Google Scholar and access online resources provided through dietetic professional organizations, in particular, Practice Based Evidence in Nutrition (PEN). The DAA website provides registered dietitians with online forum style 'interest groups', in which dietitians can discuss various topics relating to nutrition and dietetics. Most of the participants in this study found that these forums were an interesting and valuable source of information, and also participated in these groups. Mentors were also described as being useful and valuable sources of information, with some dietitians continuing to choose mentoring options long after the DAA stipulation of one year. In cases where opportunities to speak to other dietitians were taken or sought out, these contacts were described as very helpful. Professional development is a necessity for all accredited dietitians, and dietitians in private practice most often sought learning opportunities in areas that taught motivational interviewing or other courses that concentrated on the psychological aspects of dietetic counselling, rather than the nutritional aspects. One dietitian described how social media and the interest groups provided a constant stream of information:

> 'I like loads of different nutrition and dietetic sorts of pages, and it's probably the quickest and easiest way along with email to [get information]. I've always got social media or my emails up there where the interest group stuff is coming through all the time so, yeah so they probably are the two quickest and easiest ways that I'm sort of updating things all the time.' (Dietitian 5)

All dietitians used PEN and google scholar as sources of evidence:

> '(The) first port of call would probably be PEN, so the data base associated with the DAA and then I'd probably just go google scholar somewhere like that and start looking up papers.' (Dietitian 11)

Exposure as episteme and techne. Episteme and techne, as knowledge types, underpin having a knowledge base of evidential information and the technique to search for and discern relevant sources of evidence and information, and integrate them into practice.

3.6.2. Learning Enriched in Practice

The development of sound nutrition and practice philosophies occurred most quickly and thoroughly within the context of the consultation process, with secondary input coming from exposure to other information sources. New graduates entering private practice reported a steep learning curve which levelled out in a matter of months with increased exposure to the consultation process, although all dietitians reported continuous learning and improvement over their career span. Dietitians described that building these skills occurred over time with experience, but that they were also building on pre-existing skills and knowledge that they felt they naturally possessed. All dietitians reported constantly adapting their practice and approach, in relation to the perceived needs of their clients. Over time, this process becomes embedded in practice and becomes intrinsic within the dietitian, permitting them become continuously responsive to the changing environment of private practice. One participant described how, through experience, existing skills improve:

> 'I think just through experience, I think you know as an initial dietitian you know you can do everything that an experienced dietitian can do just about but you can't, you can't

> convert that into that kind of people skill connection. You can have people skills but through experience you get to know what people respond to, and I think that's where it's definitely built from. I'd like to think that my people skills are really good and have always been really good but you still can't put that into a consultation situation until you've been able to do it many times I think.' (Dietitian 7)

Learning enriched in practice as phronesis. Phronesis requires experiential learning across time, as is evident in our participants, where knowledge is honed, corrected, or rejected [18]. Phronesis is a knowledge type that is essentially changeable and particular to situations. Therefore, it requires experiential learning, during which it can be improved, corrected, and responsive to real events [18].

3.6.3. Reflective Practice and Client Feedback

Practice philosophies are integrated through the process of reflective practice and client feedback. Reflective practice was carried out via mentoring, and through thinking about their performance and what they needed to change. One dietitian set a specific time each week to reflect on where her gaps in knowledge were and how she could improve them. All the dietitians spoke in a reflective manner during the interviews and they were self-aware in knowing their strengths and weaknesses. They described their character traits and their personality types, and how these fitted with private practice and consultations with clients. The participants also reflected on circumstances with patients, both inside and outside of consultations. They thought about and described how they felt about them, how they thought the patient felt, and at times, how they might do things differently, if a similar circumstance happened in future.

Client feedback was provided in the forms of both physical biomarkers and the observation that clients who are happy with the service they are receiving will return for follow-up visits, and that these repeat clients had better success rates. Physical biomarkers were seen as a secondary source of success to any psychological aspects that had changed positively in the client over time and which helped to ensure the continued compliance of any implemented healthy lifestyle changes. One participant described how reflecting on practice culminated in changing strategies with patients:

> 'But I feel it just sort of comes around like, when you really reflect on your consultations and you go—ok well you know once you see 30 people you get an idea about what are some common things that come up with clients...and you sort of reflect on that and come up with some strategies that you know are going to help them.' (Dietitian 3)

One dietitian reflected on how she would react differently, if a similar situation happened in the future:

> 'So I guess that first consult, when I reflect back on it was really, you know, probably faced with somebody else in that situation I wouldn't have done anything, I would've said you know "this is what it is" maybe explained it—off to hospital you go.' (Dietitian 2)

Reflective practice as phronesis. The participants were able to reflect and respond within the consultation in response to cues, as well as reflect on previous circumstances involving patients. They used these reflective skills to help them respond appropriately, increase self-awareness, and improve future performance. In this way, phronesis, which is aligned with reflective practice, underpinned these actions. Phronesis is said to underscore reflection as a means to guide wise action, assist with navigating the various contexts of practice, and ultimately gain practical wisdom [29].

4. Discussion

The theoretical model of the philosophies of dietitians in private practice, integrates the experiences, practices, and perspectives of 11 dietitians working in private practices in Australia. It describes the key strategies and processes that dietitians use in the context of private practice and the therapeutic relationships which were found to be important mediators. It also highlights the underlying knowledge types that dietitians utilize when performing and learning these key strategies. Most studies exploring episteme, techne, and in particular, phronesis, as philosophies underpinning health care, concentrate on medicine and nursing [21,30,31,42,43]; they do not account for the context of private practice or the complexities faced by dietitians when helping patients choose and/or change lifelong eating habits.

The processes that the dietitians used in this study shared similarities with health care and counselling models that are a small part of dietetic student curricula [38,40]. This study supports the accepted notion that the counselling relationship is a fundamental aspect of a successful counselling relationship [41]. We extend and enhance this concept by exploring the processes specific to dietetics, as well as by identifying a philosophical/knowledge construct that may be useful in framing the explicated processes and strategies.

The key strategy, 'collaborative therapy', shares similarities with what is generally known as 'patient or client centered care' [14,44,45]. Nutrition and dietetics suffer from a lack of definition surrounding client-centered care, as it pertains to nutrition counselling [14,44]. The contextual and collaborative approach for applying interventions in this study was, at times, in conflict with applying a straight forward, evidence-based guideline. Despite a lack of time and skill being the most cited barriers to using EBP, the dietitians in this study described the client's contextual situation as the main driver, when deciding on intervention strategies ahead of EBP [15,46,47]. This disparity could be due to the longer consultation that private practice affords and the possibility of follow-up appointments affording a slower approach to education and therapy. Barriers cited when applying this contextual approach elsewhere, specifically professional norm and organizational culture, are not present in this study, which highlights the professional freedom that dietitians have in private practice, when delivering patient-centered care [44,48]. This contextual approach to intervention was strongly favored by clients of dietitians in a qualitative examination of client preferences [14]. This study confirms that dietitians in private practice are not only aware of the mitigating factors that affect the food choice and practices of their clients, but also strive to collaboratively develop interventions with these in mind. Hancock et al. (2012) found that most patients favored a non-prescriptive approach, although a small subset preferred a specific diet plan [14]. The dietitians in our study appeared aware of which approach their clients preferred and this is reflected in the strategies which they use in response to these perceived preferences.

Building a rapport was shown to be an important aspect of practice in our study. This finding is consistent with research that shows that building a rapport is important for establishing a counselling relationship [41,42]. The practice of building a rapport helps to build trust in clients, allowing for more positive outcomes and relationships [42]. Hancock et al. (2012) found that dietetic clients cited rapport building as being important in their dealings with dietitians [14]. Further to these findings, our study revealed that the context of private practice provided the motivation to establish a rapport with clients, and a rich learning environment in which to foster the skills to do so.

The practices of dietitians in this study support the findings by Cant and Aroni, who found that dietitians strive to show empathy in their consultations by listening, in order to understand the patient's situation [12]. This is further supported by Goodchild et al., who noted that empathic moments are common throughout dietetic consultations and that these moments are rarely missed by dietitians [49]. Patients reported a higher satisfaction in consultations where responses to emotional opportunities by dietitians were coded as more empathic [49]. Rogers (1940) contends that demonstrating empathy towards the client is an integral part of the counselling process [45]. The dietitians in this study also used their own experiences to relate to the patient empathically. It is suggested that using one's own experience to relate to the patient may optimize the empathic response and, in turn, improve the patient's satisfaction [14]. It is argued that empathy as a character trait is needed, to enable an understanding of the needs and wishes of patients [41]. To use empathy as a phronetic, the practitioner would need to seek to understand and desire ethical solutions that align with the patients' goals for the most beneficial outcome in that situation [41]. This requires the practitioner to be highly cognizant of the patients' version of what their own best health and wellbeing is. Further study on this concept within dietetics would be beneficial to ascertain levels of empathetic responses within consultations that take into account the patients' viewpoint of their own best health outcome.

Our study showed that nonverbal communication featured heavily in the way that dietitians responded to their patients. Further, the participants described using perception or intuition when dealing with their clients, and that perceptiveness was intrinsic to them. Nonverbal communication is largely involved with conveying feelings and attitudes, and is often beyond our conscious awareness [12]. Nonverbal communication may account for 65% of meaning in interpersonal communications [50]. The present study confirms the Cant and Aroni finding, that dietitians are aware of nonverbal communication and place an importance on this being nonthreatening [12]. Intuition and perception in dietitians has not been previously researched; however, research on nurses has recognized its presence in nursing practice. Intuition and perception in clinical practice is a form of understanding or knowing something about the situation or patient, without logical thought processes or being explicitly told by the patient [51,52]. Rew and Barrow, in the reviewing literature, found that intuition was vital for complex decision making [53]. A review by King and Appleton found evidence that nurses used intuition (i.e., gut feelings) to initiate action [54]. Rigid adherence to protocol tended to devalue intuition and perception in clinical reasoning [54]. Feasibly, due to having less procedural and departmental constraints, the dietitians in our study were able to recognize and verbalize that intuition and/or perception played an important role when interacting with their clients.

Dietitians in this study saw successful outcomes by providing long term support and accountability to their clients. Hancock et al. found that, in a community and hospital setting, patients reported that support felt limited, due to the length or frequency of the appointment, or the continuity of the dietitian [14]. In a private practice situation, this scenario is avoided and, as such, the dietitians in this study reported successful outcomes for patients that they had seen, or were seeing, long term, both in biomedical markers and habit changes. This indicates that private practice is well placed to provide successful outcomes to those clients who can access long term private practice dietetic support.

The sources of evidence that participants used in this study are in contrast to Thomas et al., who found that pediatric dietitians had access to Medline, Cochrane, and CINAHL, and that 39% used Medline as their main source of information [17]. Dietitians in this study report using online searches (google scholar), and online resources provided by DAA and DAA interest groups, as their main sources of information when sourcing evidence. This is most likely due to the lack of access that private practice dietitians have to other sources of literature that require payment. There are no studies documenting other types of information that are sourced, such as social media, and this study uncovers the phenomenon of dietitians in private practice being inundated by nutrition and food information.

The newer dietitians in this study reported that, upon entering the practice, their communication and counselling skills increased quickly with continuous consultation experience. This supports Cant et al., who found only a small variation in communication practices of recently qualified and more senior dietitians [12]. Situational or experiential learning is at the core of learning for professionals, and health professional training courses require a period of placement types within their profession before graduation [55,56]. This study supports the concept that skill acquisition for professionals is embedded in practice, and highlights the importance of ongoing exposure to clinical settings by professionals as a means to improve and maintain their skills.

As part of the accreditation process, new graduates must enter a mentoring partnership for one year [57]. Part of that process is reflective by design, as the mentoring partnership requires the graduate to explore his/her practice with the mentor [58]. There is little research on the mentoring partnerships in Australia; however, research has shown that the mentoring partnership can facilitate lifelong learning through supporting the habit of reflective practice [58]. Palermo et al. found that mentor attributes of facilitating trusting relationships and providing effective feedback, were important components of mentoring [59]. This study supports this finding, with dietitians in this study reporting positive relationships and experiences with their mentor, and this positive experience compelled some dietitians to seek ongoing mentoring after the mandatory period was over, throughout their career.

Reflective practice is an essential skill for being an APD and dietitians are expected to autonomously continue this practice throughout their career [6]. Reflective practice allows practitioners to learn from experience. Ajjawi et al. found that self-evaluation and reflection in allied health professionals were important for monitoring and correcting clinical reasoning and communication [60]. Proponents of including phronesis as a necessary element, along with episteme and techne, for a model of good practice, and the traits of an expert practitioner, contend that to be phronetic is to be reflective [18,21,29]. Schon and Benner posit that the ability to reflect in and on practice, and change actions within constant contextual shifts within practice, distinguishes an expert from a technically proficient practitioner [25,61]. Kinsella contends that merely reflecting on practice, such as journaling and blogging, is aligned towards techne, and that to aspire to expertise resultant change and critical judgments must be able to be processed and arrived at within the context of the moment [22]. It was evident in this study that dietitians use high level reflective practice both in and out of the consultation experience to improve their interpersonal skills, clinical judgement, and their business models. This study supports the implications that dietitians continue to reflect on practice throughout their career and use those skills to improve services to their clients. This indicates that private practitioners subscribe to the DAA's stipulations and agree with the value of reflective practice.

5. Episteme, Techne, and Phronesis

This model of private practice revealed that dietitians use intertwining and embedded forms of episteme, techne, and phronesis in their practice and throughout the consultation practice. It was clear in this study that the dietitians used episteme, techne, and phronesis when using key strategies and processes, and that these philosophies also underpinned how the participants improved and integrated these strategies into practice. The key strategies that the dietitians employed, although discussed separately, are used in a simultaneous manner in response to the environment. Similarly, it is not possible to separate episteme, techne, and phronesis as underpinning forms of knowledge skills in practice, although at times, one form of knowledge may be predominant over another, depending on the situation. In line with other studies, elements of practice that are not easily described or assessed were evident when dietitians adapted their approach to clients within consultations, in response to both extrinsic and intrinsic cues. This study supported the use of the concept of phronesis through the dietitian's practices of perception, empathy, and reflective practice.

Phronesis was useful in exploring the therapeutic relationship that is a complex interpersonal experience where dietitians use tacit, theoretical, and evidential knowledge, to appropriately respond to clients. In this space, dietitians simultaneously reflect, respond, and learn. These responses become intrinsically embedded over time. It is also clear that the therapeutic relationship was a crucial platform for using, learning, and integrating these strategies, and that the context of private practice is an important mediator of nurturing the therapeutic relationship. Episteme, techne, and phronesis as a framework for professional practice, provided a useful lens to view dietetic practice, particularly the contexts and elements of practice that are not easily described, but that are crucial to being an expert practitioner.

6. Strengths and Limitations of the Study

The study's findings reveal the key strategies and underpinning philosophies that dietitians use during private practice. To our knowledge, this is the first investigation of dietitians' philosophies in private practice and shows a unique perspective of private practice in Australia. A strength of this study is that it reveals the dynamics and intricacies within the consultation process, including facets within the therapeutic relationship and strategies used that are frequently invisible. An important strength of this study is that it provides in-depth knowledge of private practice issues and reveals how dietitians nurture and protect the therapeutic relationship. The therapeutic relationship was shown to be an important learning environment and mediator of successful outcomes for patients, as well as crucial for a successful private practice business. Notably, the context of private practice was revealed as a stimulus for developing key strategies to nurture the therapeutic relationship. Further study in these areas would greatly benefit the area of dietetic private practice in Australia. The aspects of practice that contributed to successful outcomes for patients, such as empathy, perception, and reflective practice, are scarce in nutrition and dietetic studies. This study contributed important information on key strategies that are understudied, and that are poorly understood in the context of dietetic private practice.

This study used a lens of episteme, techne, and phronesis, to understand the different types of knowledge that dietitians use when performing key strategies and processes. In addition to using evidence and techniques that meet competency standards, other aspects of practice, such as, perception, intuition, empathy, and reflection in and on practice were evident, and as such, phronesis is a useful lens with which to view these aspects. In this regard, phronesis could add valuable dimensions to dietetic practice when gauging the differences between competent and expert dietitians. The framework of episteme, techne, and phronesis as knowledge types, provided a useful lens to explain a patient-centered holistic practice style and to examine how these key strategies are learnt and integrated into practice. This grounded theory study produced a model of private practice that shows concepts and relationships that could be explored quantitatively.

These strengths are countered by the fact that the practice and nutrition strategies were only investigated from the dietitian's perspective. How patients experienced their care and approach was not a focus of this study, and there is a need for studies that consider the patients' perspective of their care. Another limitation is that, although terms such as 'client centred approach', 'mindfulness', and 'intuition' have been used by the dietitians in this study, no further enquiry was made as to how similar in meaning these were to each other, when used by another dietitian. Due to the interview question, this model depicts what usually happens, from the dietitians view of a 'case study'; that is, a long-term client. No data of how one-off 'Medicare' (public healthcare) patients were treated was included. Although the dietitians reported that these patients were treated similarly, the same outcomes were not seen with these short-term patients, due to the short length of care. The sample size ($n = 11$) was small; however, the sample represented a broad cross section of the profession and the concepts remained static across the sample, adding to the strength of the results. In this way, generality is plausible, but not possible with this sample size. Possibly due to the burden of the interview process on the participants, recruitment for this study was difficult, and the sample may be skewed towards dietitians who were interested in the subject matter and the trajectory of dietetics in Australia in general.

7. Conclusions

Dietetic private practice in Australia is a complex environment in which dietitians must employ high level professional, technical, and interpersonal skills. Private practice dietitians form collaborative relationships with their clients to nurture change over time and are able to provide continuity of care without departmental constraints. Thus, private practice is well placed to provide successful outcomes to those clients who can access long term private practice.

The context of private practice was revealed to be an important element of how and why dietitians develop and integrate knowledge over time. Further study aimed at uncovering more detailed information of how dietitians experience different aspects of private practice would be advantageous, to further develop our understanding of the challenges that dietitians face in private practice. The nuances that seem unique to private practice seem to facilitate a practitioner's ability to respond in a client-centered manner, over a short period of time. Dietitians used intertwined forms of episteme, techne, and phronesis, to collaboratively nurture change in clients.

Episteme, techne, and phronesis offer a broader model of practice that has considerable applicability for nutrition and dietetics. Framing practice research within these concepts could be useful for addressing the complex aspects that are specific to the nutrition and dietetic profession.

Acknowledgments: The author disclosed receipt of the following financial support for the research, authorship, and publication of this article: Honours Funding, University of the Sunshine Coast.

Author Contributions: Judith Maher conceived and designed the research; Claudia Harper performed the research; Claudia Harper and Judith Maher analyzed the data; Claudia Harper wrote the paper; Judith Maher edited the paper. This paper was undertaken as an Honours Project by Claudia Harper. Judith Maher acted as the supervisor. The Figure was produced by: Heather Ngata, QUT Art Student.

Conflicts of Interest: The authors declare no conflict of interest. The founding sponsors had no role in the design of the study; in the collection, analyses, or interpretation of data; in the writing of the manuscript, and in the decision to publish the results.

References

1. Sackett, D.L.; Rosenberg, W.M.C.; Muir Gray, J.A.; Haynes, R.B.; Richardson, W.S. Evidence based medicine: What it is and what it isn't. *BMJ* **1996**, *312*, 71–72. [CrossRef] [PubMed]
2. DAA. Available online: http://daa.asn.au/wp-content/uploads/2013/09/Dietitian-Scope-of-Practice-2015.pdf (accessed on 31 August 2014).
3. Hise, M.E.; Kattelmann, K.; Parkhurst, M. Evidence-Based Clinical Practice: Dispelling the Myths. *NCP* **2005**, *20*, 294–302. [CrossRef] [PubMed]
4. International Confederation of Dietetic Associations. ICDA Code of Ethics and Code of Good Practice. Available online: http://www.internationaldietetics.org/Downloads/ICDA-Code-of-Ethics-and-Code-of-Good-Practice.aspx (accessed on 28 August 2014).
5. Ball, L.; Larsson, R.; Gerathy, R.; Hood, P.; Lowe, C. Working profile of Australian private practice Accredited Practising Dietitians. *Nutr. Diet.* **2013**, *70*, 196–205. [CrossRef]
6. DAA. The National Competency Standards for Dietitians in Australia. Available online: http://daa.asn.au/wp-content/uploads/2015/12/NCS-Dietitians-Australia-1.0.pdf (accessed on 23 August 2014).
7. Freeland-Graves, J.H.; Nitzke, S. Position of the Academy of Nutrition and Dietetics: Total Diet Approach to Healthy Eating. *J. Acad. Nutr. Diet.* **2013**, *113*, 307–317. [CrossRef] [PubMed]
8. Grimmer, K.; Bialocerkowski, A.; Kumar, S.; Milanese, S. Implementing evidence in clinical practice: The 'therapies' dilemma. *Physiotherapy* **2004**, *90*, 189–194. [CrossRef]
9. Buchanan, D. Two Models for Defining the Relationship between Theory and Practice in Nutrition Education: Is the Scientific Method Meeting Our Needs? *J. Nutr. Educ. Behav.* **2004**, *36*, 146–154. [CrossRef]
10. Schubert, L.; Gallegos, D.; Foley, W.; Harrison, C. Re-imagining the 'social' in the nutrition sciences. *Public Health Nutr.* **2012**, *15*, 352–359. [CrossRef] [PubMed]
11. Swift, J.A.; Tischler, V. Qualitative research in nutrition and dietetics: Getting started. *J. Hum. Nutr. Diet.* **2010**, *23*, 559–566. [CrossRef] [PubMed]
12. Cant, R.; Aroni, R. Exploring dietitians' verbal and nonverbal communication skills for effective dietitian-patient communication. *J. Hum. Nutr. Diet.* **2008**, *21*, 502–511. [CrossRef] [PubMed]
13. Cant, R. Constructions of competence within dietetics: Trust, professionalism and communications with individual clients. *Nutr. Diet.* **2009**, *66*, 113–118. [CrossRef]
14. Hancock, R.E.E.; Bonner, G.; Hollingdale, R.; Madden, A.M. 'If you listen to me properly, I feel good': A qualitative examination of patient experiences of dietetic consultations. *J. Hum. Nutr. Diet.* **2012**, *25*, 275–284. [CrossRef] [PubMed]
15. Byham-Gray, L.D.; Gilbride, J.A.; Dixon, L.B.; Stage, F.K. Evidence-Based Practice: What Are Dietitians' Perceptions, Attitudes, and Knowledge? *J. Am. Diet. Assoc.* **2005**, *105*, 1574–1581. [CrossRef] [PubMed]
16. Taylor, M.A. Evidence-based practice: Are dietitians willing and able? *J. Hum. Nutr. Diet.* **1998**, *11*, 461–472. [CrossRef]
17. Thomas, D.E.; Kukuruzovic, R.; Martino, B.; Chauhan, S.S.; Elliott, E.J. Knowledge and use of evidence-based nutrition: A survey of paediatric dietitians. *J. Hum. Nutr. Diet.* **2003**, *16*, 315–322. [CrossRef] [PubMed]

18. Benner, P.; Hughes, R.; Sutphen, M. Clinical Reasoning, Decisionmaking and Action: Thinking Critically and Clinically. In *Patient Safety and Quality: An Evidence-Based Handbook for Nurses*; Hughes, R., Ed.; Agency for Healthcare Research and Quality: Rockville, MD, USA, 2008; Volume 1, pp. 1–109.
19. Beresford, M.J. Medical reductionism: Lessons from the great philosophers. *QJM Int. J. Med.* **2010**, *103*, 721–724. [CrossRef] [PubMed]
20. Braude, H.D. Conciliating cognition and consciousness: The perceptual foundations of clinical reasoning. *J. Eval. Clin. Pract.* **2012**, *18*, 945–950. [CrossRef] [PubMed]
21. Flaming, D. Using phronesis instead of 'research-based practice' as the guiding light for nursing practice. *Nurs. Philos.* **2001**, *2*, 251–258. [CrossRef]
22. Kinsella, E.A. Professional knowledge and the epistemology of reflective practice. *Nurs. Philos.* **2009**, *11*, 3–14. [CrossRef] [PubMed]
23. Miles, A. On a medicine of the whole person: Away from scientistic reductionism and towards the embrace of the complex in clinical practice. *J. Eval. Clin. Pract.* **2009**, *15*, 941–949. [CrossRef] [PubMed]
24. Thorgaard, K.; Jensen, U.J. Evidence and the end of medicine. *Med. Health Care Philos.* **2011**, *14*, 273–280. [CrossRef] [PubMed]
25. Benner, P. *From Novice to Expert: Excellence and Power in Clinical Nursing Practice*; Prentice Hall: Upper Saddle Rive, NJ, USA, 2001.
26. Aristotle. Metaphysics. In *The Complete Works of Aristotle*; Ross, W.D., Tr., Ed.; Princeton University Press: Princeton, NJ, USA, 1984; Volume 2.
27. Dreyfus, H.; Dreyfus, S. *Mind over Machine: The Power of Human Intuition and Expertise in the Era of the Computer*; Free Press: New York, NY, USA, 1986.
28. Dunne, J. Professional judgement and the predicaments of practice. *Eur. J. Mark.* **1999**, *33*, 707–720. [CrossRef]
29. Kinsella, E.A. Practitioner Reflection and Judgement as Phronesis: A Continuum of Reflection and Considerations for Phronetic Judgement. In *Phronesis as Professional Knowledge: Practical Wisdom in the Profession*; Kinsella, E.A., Pitman, A., Eds.; Sense Publishers: Rotterdam, The Netherlands, 2012.
30. James, I.; Andershed, B.; Gustavsson, B.; Ternestedt, B.-M. Knowledge Constructions in Nursing Practice: Understanding and Integrating Different Forms of Knowledge. *QHR* **2010**, *20*, 1500–1518. [CrossRef] [PubMed]
31. Nieminen, A.L.; Mannevaara, B.; Fagerstrom, L. Advanced practice nurses' scope of practice: A qualitative study of advanced clinical competencies. *Scand. J. Caring Sci.* **2011**, *25*, 661–670. [CrossRef] [PubMed]
32. Hirst, R.J. *Philosophy: An outline for the Intending Student*; Routledge & Kegan Paul Ltd.: London, UK, 1968.
33. Gadamer, H.G. Practical philosophy as a model of human sciences. *Res. Phenomol.* **1979**, *9*, 74–85. [CrossRef]
34. Gustavsson, B. What do we mean by lifelong learning and knowledge? *Int. J. Educ. Res.* **2002**, *21*, 13–23. [CrossRef]
35. Gustavsson, B. Revisiting the philosophical roots of practical knowledge. In *Developing Practice Knowledge for Health Professionals*; Higgs, J., Richardson, W.S., Abrandt Dahlgren, M., Eds.; Butterworth Heinemann: Edinburgh, UK, 2004; pp. 35–51.
36. Charmaz, K. *Constructing Grounded Theory: A Practical Guide Through Qualitative Analysis*; Sage Publications: London, UK, 2006.
37. Blumer, H. *Symbolic Interactionism*; Prentice-Hall: Englewood Cliffs, NJ, USA, 1969.
38. Bauer, K.; Sokolik, C. *Basic Nutrition Counselling Skill Development*; Wadsworth/Thomson Learning: Belmont CA, USA, 2002.
39. Aristotle. *The Ethics of Aristotle [Electronic Resource]: (the Nichomachean Ethics, Chase's Translation, Newly Revised)*; W. Scott: London, UK, 1890.
40. Gable, J. *Counselling Skills for Dietitians*; Blackwell Publishing: Oxford, UK, 2007.
41. Svenaeus, F. Hermeneutics of medicine in the wake of Gadamer: The issue of phronesis. *Theor. Med. Bioeth.* **2003**, *24*, 407–431. [CrossRef] [PubMed]
42. Daniel Davis, F. Phronesis, clinical reasoning, and Pellegrino's philosophy of medicine. *Theor. Med.* **1997**, *18*, 173–195. [CrossRef]
43. Tyreman, S. Promoting critical thinking in health care: Phronesis and criticality. *Med. Health Care Philos.* **2000**, *3*, 117–124. [CrossRef] [PubMed]
44. MacLellan, D.L.; Berenbaum, S. Dietitians' Opinions and Experiences of Client-Centred Nutrition Counselling. *Can. J. Diet. Pract. Res.* **2006**, *67*, 119–124. [CrossRef] [PubMed]

45. Rogers, C.R. The processes of therapy. *J. Consult. Psychol.* **1940**, *4*, 161–164. [CrossRef]
46. Metcalfe, C.; Lewin, R.; Wisher, S.; Perry, S.; Bannigan, K.; Moffett, J.K. Barriers to Implementing the Evidence Base in Four NHS Therapies: Dietitians, occupational therapists, physiotherapists, speech and language therapists. *Physiotherapy* **2001**, *87*, 433–441. [CrossRef]
47. Upton, D.; Upton, P. Knowledge and Use of Evidence-based Practice by Allied Health and Health Science Professionals in the United Kingdom. *J. Allied Health* **2006**, *35*, 127–133. [PubMed]
48. Deschênes, S.-M.; Gagnon, M.-P.; Légaré, F.; Lapointe, A.; Turcotte, S.; Desroches, S. Psychosocial Factors of Dietitians' Intentions to Adopt Shared Decision Making Behaviours: A Cross-Sectional Survey. *PLoS ONE* **2013**, *8*, e64523. [CrossRef] [PubMed]
49. Goodchild, C.E.; Skinner, T.E.; Parkin, T. The value of empathy in dietetic consultations. A pilot study to investigate its effect on satisfaction, autonomy and agreement. *J. Hum. Nutr. Diet.* **2005**, *18*, 181–185. [CrossRef] [PubMed]
50. Putnis, P.; Petelin, R. *Professional Communication: Principles and Applications*; Prentice Hall: Sydney, Australia, 1996.
51. Mitchell, G.J. Intuitive Knowing: Exposing a Myth in Theory Development. *Nurs. Sci. Q.* **1994**, *7*, 2–3. [CrossRef] [PubMed]
52. Young, C.E. Intuition and nursing process. *Holist. Nurs. Pract.* **1987**, *1*, 52–62. [CrossRef] [PubMed]
53. Rew, L.; Barrow, E.M. Intuition: A neglected hallmark of nursing knowledge. *Adv. Nurs. Sci.* **1987**, *10*, 49–62. [CrossRef]
54. King, L.; Appleton, J.V. Intuition: A critical review of the research and rhetoric. *JAN* **1997**, *26*, 194–202. [CrossRef]
55. Benner, P. Using the Dreyfus model of skill acquisition to describe and interpret skill acquisition and clinical judgment in nursing practice and education. *Bull. Sci. Technol. Soc.* **2004**, *24*, 188–199. [CrossRef]
56. O'Reilly, S.L.; Milner, J. Transitions in reflective practice: Exploring student development and preferred methods of engagement. *Nutr. Diet.* **2015**, *72*, 150–155. [CrossRef]
57. DAA. Guide to the APD Program, Continuing Professional Development and Mentoring. Available online: http://daa.asn.au/wp-content/uploads/2014/09/Guide-to-APD-September-2014.pdf (accessed on 16 July 2014).
58. Hawker, J.; McMillan, A.; Palermo, C. Enduring mentoring partnership: A reflective case study and recommendations for evaluating mentoring in dietetics. *Nutr. Diet.* **2013**, *70*, 339–344. [CrossRef]
59. Palermo, C.; Hughes, R.; McCall, L. An evaluation of a public health nutrition workforce development intervention for the nutrition and dietetic workforce. *J. Hum. Nutr. Diet.* **2010**, *23*, 244–253. [CrossRef] [PubMed]
60. Ajjawi, R.; Higgs, J. Learning to Reason: A Journey of Professional Socialisation. *Adv. Health Sci. Educ.* **2008**, *13*, 133–150. [CrossRef] [PubMed]
61. Schön, D.A. *The Reflective Practitioner: How Professionals Think in Action*; Basic Books: New York, NY, USA, 1983.

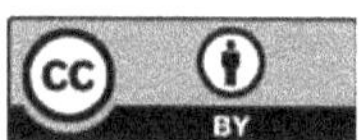

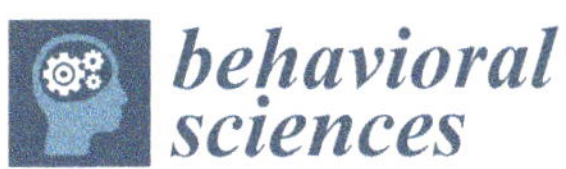

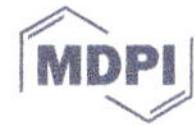

Article

Insights into the Experiences of Treatment for An Eating Disorder in Men: A Qualitative Study of Autobiographies

Priyanka Thapliyal [1,*], Deborah Mitchison [2] and Phillipa Hay [1]

1 Translational Health Research Institute, School of Medicine, Western Sydney University, Building 3.G.P9, Locked Bag 1797, Penrith NSW 2751, Australia; p.hay@ westernsydney.edu.au
2 Centre for Emotional Health, Department of Psychology, Macquarie University, Sydney 2109, Australia; deborah.mitchison@mq.edu.au
* Correspondence: p.thapliyal@westernsydney.edu.au; Tel.: +61-246-203-905

Academic Editors: Amanda Sainsbury and Felipe Q. da Luz
Received: 13 April 2017; Accepted: 8 June 2017; Published: 16 June 2017

Abstract: Eating disorders are increasingly recognized as a problem for men but help-seeking is low and little is known about their treatment experiences. This paper sought to determine the treatment experiences of men who have suffered from an eating disorder using autobiographical data. Inclusion criteria were autobiographies of men who had experienced an eating disorder and sought any form of treatment for this, written in the English language, published between 1995 and 2015, and available for purchase in 2016. The search resulted in six books that were thematically analyzed. Analysis of data resulted in two broad themes (1. Positive experiences; 2. Negative experiences) with sub-themes. With regards to the first theme, factors such as concern of staff members, therapist's expertise (in treating eating disorders in men), and a collaborative treatment approach were considered favorable for treatment. In contrast to the first theme, apathy of staff members, the authors' own negative preconceptions, treatment providers being perceived as prioritizing financial concerns, perceived as incompetent and judgmental behavior of therapist(s), and time limitations of sessions were considered unfavorable treatment experiences. In this study, the perceived success of treatment depended on therapist's features and the form of treatment provided. Further research examining these is indicated.

Keywords: eating disorder; men; treatment; experiences

---

1. Introduction

Eating disorders include anorexia nervosa (AN), bulimia nervosa (BN) and binge eating disorder (BED). AN is a condition in which an individual practices extreme food restriction to the point of self-starvation and excessive weight loss. By definition the person is underweight for their age and height. Two subtypes are defined: the restrictive/compulsive exercise and binge-eating/purging types [1]. BN is characterized as a condition in which an individual has episodes of overeating accompanied by a sense of loss of control (binge eating). These are followed by repeated compensatory behaviors that include self-induced vomiting, laxative misuse, excessive exercise, fasting, use of diuretics, and/or other medications to prevent weight gain [1]. BED is characterized as having recurrent and distressing binge eating episodes which may be characterized by eating more rapidly than normal, eating until uncomfortably full, eating large amounts even when not hungry, eating alone because of embarrassment and/or feeling disgusted or guilty after eating [1].

Despite the popular view of these as conditions suffered by women, eating disorders are not rare among men. Raevuori et al. [2] recently conducted a review of eating disorders in men. The paper emphasized the revised Diagnostic and Statistical Manual of Mental Disorders (DSM-5) published in 2013 as an important landmark in recognizing BED alongside AN and BN [1], a disorder almost as prevalent in adult men as in women. Further, the elimination of amenorrhea as a criterion improves conceptual inclusiveness of men with a diagnosis of AN. The overall prevalence of eating disorders in male and female Swedish twins born between 1935 and 1958 was 1.20% in women and 0.29% in men [3] and the lifetime prevalence in Finnish twin men born between 1975 and 1979 was 0.24% [4]. Carlat et al. [5] also conducted a review of prevalence literature and concluded that men account for 10–15% of all bulimic patients, and that 0.2% of all adolescent and young adult men meet strict criteria for BN. Similar prevalence figures have been reported for male patients with AN [6,7]. Hudson et al. [8] conducted a large population-based household survey in the US in 2001–2003 and estimated the lifetime prevalence of DSM-IV AN, BN, and BED as 0.3%, 0.5% and 2.0%, respectively, among men. A similar pattern to that seen in women, with BED prevalence higher than BN which in turn is higher in prevalence than AN, has been reported in men [9]. Despite this, men are excluded from the majority of epidemiological and other research studies, reinforcing the perception of eating disorders as a problem predominantly concerning women, and making it less likely for researchers to design future studies representative of men [10].

There may however be differences between men and women in regards to eating disorder epidemiology. For example, as reported by Mitchison et al. [11] the prevalence of extreme dietary restriction and purging behaviors are increasing at a faster rate in men (2008 vs. 1998 odds ratios = 4.9 and 6.2, respectively) compared to women (odds ratios = 1.7 and 0.9, respectively). While treatment approaches are based on interventions developed for women with eating disorders; there are no male-specific treatment guidelines [12]. Although treatment in predominantly "feminine" environments can be successful for men [13], issues of stigmatization and isolation have also been reported [14,15]. Men may have unique needs, including consideration of masculine identity, gender role conflict and emasculation [16,17]. Further, behavioral manifestations may differ (e.g., more emphasis on muscle-building and exercise in general).

Seeking help for an eating disorder is not common in general, however men with AN and BN have said that their willingness to seek professional help has been further thwarted by societal ideals that include notions of gender-specific illnesses [18]. A quantitative study by Ming et al. [19] evaluated service utilization in men with eating disorders in Singapore. The study reported that a significant proportion of men with an eating disorder had never been hospitalized (62.5%) or enrolled in specialized inpatient/outpatient treatment programs (68.1%). The low rate of treatment-uptake was associated with unwillingness among the men in this study to seek help.

In regard to men who do access treatment, a quantitative study [20] has reported on the experiences of 334 men in a residential center (23% binge/purge type, 24% BN, 23% EDNOS including n = 6 with BED). Overall treatment was reported to be effective. The authors surmised that the men's experiences of treatment did not appear to differ to that observed among women, but no specific similarities were reported. There were also distinctive aspects of the program perceived as particularly relevant to men. These included addressing excessive exercise, body image concerns with muscularity, sexual orientation, sexual identity, and spirituality. This study also emphasized the importance of "male only" group therapy to facilitate discussion of eating disorder symptoms that have been viewed as "female" problems.

In a recent systematic review [21] of qualitative studies exploring the treatment experiences of men with eating disorders, only four papers were eligible for review. Of the four included studies [22–25] only two had a primary focus on men's experiences of treatment [23,24]. Common themes that emerged across the studies were most often related to an understanding of the barriers to help-seeking with less about processes once treatment engagement had occurred. Key themes identified included: (1) delays in seeking treatment; (2) clinical features distinctive to men such as drive for muscularity; (3) feminine and other aspects of treatment services; and (4) a lack of consensus in views about the relevance of gender in treatment. Similarly, in some of the studies the participating men described feeling disappointed with the competency of the help they received and also expressed a wish for their maleness to be recognized when in the treatment setting [26,27].

Similar to studies of females [28,29], two studies [26,27] reported that some males perceived their treatment experience as being unsupportive, with professionals lacking time and experience. Men also reported feeling a loss of power and control when in treatment. The males in this review drew attention to a lack of care providers' appreciation of male issues. Male participants with AN or BN reported that female-oriented treatments for eating disorders were not entirely appropriate for them.

General stigmatization of eating disorders also affects men's treatment experiences. Robinson et al. [24] explored the experiences of men using eating disorder services and identified that the biggest challenge they had faced was admitting to themselves and others that they had an eating disorder and that it was a problem. This may be because of the stereotype that eating disorders only affects women. Similarly, a study by Griffiths et al. [30] supported this premise, as males with eating disorders reported that they were being more frequently stigmatized as "less of a man" than women experienced being stigmatized as "less of a woman".

2. Deficits in Previous Research

Whereas quantitative research aims to assess causal relationships between variables, qualitative research understands truth to be evolving, culturally constructed and derived from an interaction between experience and the human mind [31]. Qualitative methods are particularly suited to understanding a lived experience, as they target underlying processes and meaning that cannot be adequately conveyed in surveys or represented by numbers.

Qualitative literature pertaining to men's experiences of eating disorder treatment is scarce. Historically few men have been included as participants in such research designs. In a systematic review and meta-synthesis of qualitative studies [32] on patients' understanding of eating disorder treatment and recovery, the participants were almost exclusively women. Likewise, Bezance and Holliday [33] identified 11 qualitative studies of adolescents' experiences that included only one paper with a single male participant. In the eating disorder field men are either not being represented at all, or at best, studies have included only very small numbers [34–37]. Other limitations of previous qualitative studies include a narrow focus on a specific eating disorders or subset of eating disorders, such as AN [38] or AN and BN only [39]. This is problematic as we know that men are more likely to experience disorders such as BED, and are over-represented in the residual diagnostic category, Other/Unspecified Feeding or ED. To our knowledge there is no qualitative study to date that has focused primarily on treatment experiences of men with an eating disorder.

3. Aims

Eating disorders in men is an under-researched area, particularly with regards to the exploration of male experiences in treatment. The aim of this present study was to explore the experiences of men who ever had any form of treatment for an eating disorder. Given the relatively unexplored nature of this topic, a qualitative approach was deemed most suitable.

4. Methods

4.1. Study Sample: Men's Eating Disorder Autobiographies

The sample consisted of autobiographical accounts written by men who had experienced an eating disorder. Inclusion criteria were that the book should be an autobiography of a man, who had or has had a treatment experience with an eating disorder. Further, the books were to be written in the English language and published between the years 1995 and 2015.

4.2. Autobiographical Literature Search

Autobiography is referred to as a form of "personal document". At the core of personal document research is the life story—an account of one person's life in his or her own words. For example, oral interviews, testaments, literary biographies, and psychological case studies bring life stories into being that would not otherwise have happened in everyday life [40]. On the other hand, personal documents include "any first-person narrative that describes an individual's actions, experiences and beliefs" [41]. Autobiographies provide a complementary and rich source of qualitative data regarding authors' attitudes, beliefs and views of the world. It reflects the author's perspective, which is what most qualitative research is seeking, and it also provides a subjective account of the situation it records. In addition, autobiography as a source of unsolicited data in our view may reduce one element of investigator bias when compared to other commonly used forms of qualitative data, such as participant interviews, in which the investigator chooses the topic and questions to be posed. Aronson [42] analyzed around 270 book length stories, most written in the past 20 years, and concluded that more men than women write about their illness. He concluded that men write out of a desire to help other patients, and to come to terms with their own illnesses, and also for doctors to have a better understanding of their experiences. Thus men may primarily write to express repressed emotions and create awareness about male mental illness, and less often are driven to write their autobiography out of mercenary motivations.

The search for published autobiographies was conducted using Amazon.com and the keywords were ["biography" AND "man" AND "eating disorders"]. The search resulted in twelve books. Further scrutiny of the texts led to the exclusion of six books: one was written by a mother, two were concerned with recovering from obesity rather than an eating disorder, one was about the presentation of illness narratives, one did not mention treatment experience, and one was a collection of motivational stories on staying young. Additional searches of Booktopia and The Book Depository produced 4 and 31 books respectively, of which none were autobiographies of men with an eating disorder.

5. Procedure

The qualitative method employed was thematic analysis, according to the five phases in the Framework method outlined by Ritchie and Spencer [43] and Pope, Zeibland and Mays [44]. This comprised the following stages:

(1) *Familiarization* (reviewing a subsample of the raw data in detail). This involved the first (PT) and second (DM) authors reading the books two times completely to familiarize themselves with the content and to empathize with the authors.

(2) *Identifying a Thematic Framework*. This involved ascertaining all key issues and themes in the books by drawing both from the research aims and from the data itself. PT and DM undertook this separately and then discussed the themes identified until a consensus was reached on an overarching framework.

(3) *Indexing*. This phase was undertaken by PT and involved systematically applying the agreed upon thematic framework to the data by coding sections of text. Any newly emerging themes were identified and discussed at regular meetings with the other authors, and if agreed, added to the framework.

(4) *Charting*. This involved rearrangement of distilled summaries of the data according to the thematic framework. A thematic tree was formed to highlight the main themes that were identified by the first author (PT).

(5) *Mapping and Interpretation*. This involved finding associations between themes and mapping the range and nature of phenomena to find explanations for the findings. This was carried out by PT and DM with regular review by PH.

6. Results

6.1. Characteristics of Sample

The autobiographies of six men that suffered eating disorders formed the data sample. The age of authors ranged from 25 to 50 years. A brief description of each book follows and is also presented in Table 1.

(1) "Born Round" [45] presents a sufferer's account of binge eating and bulimia nervosa. In this book Frank Bruni describes his helplessness as a man with an eating disorder. Although he realized that he had a problem, it took him years to get help, due to self-stigma and shame. Frank eventually sought help from a therapist, the process of which he describes, and moves forward toward living a life free of binge eating.

(2) "Hiding Under the Table" [46] is authored by Dennis Henning who suffered from BED, BN and AN. This book is written from a recovered perspective and focuses on the barriers experienced in trying to access treatment. Dennis provides an account of his misery as a man who had eating disorder. He desperately tried seeking treatment but often found his gender denied him access. After recovering from his eating issues Dennis pursued his goal to create public awareness about eating disorders. He is also co-founder for the Lifestyle Institute for Eating Disorders.

(3) "Weightless" [47] is an autobiography written by Gary A. Grahl that presents a sufferer's perspective of BED. In this account Greg moves through the process of illness and recovery. Presently, he is involved in creating awareness through his blog JustStopEatingSoMuch.com, which focuses on weight loss and food addiction.

(4) Michael Krasnow authored the autobiography "My Life as a Male Anorexic" [48] from a suffering perspective. He suffered from severe AN and wrote with the intention to help other young people, as well as to assist health professionals to better understand and provide help to sufferers. His account is almost exclusively focused on his experiences in treatment. Michael died three days after writing the final epilogue of this book.

(5) "My Thinning Years" [49] was written by Jon Derek Croteau. In this book he presents an account of how his denial of his own homosexuality led to the development of AN, BN, and other obsessional behavior.

(6) Gary Grahl wrote "The Skinny Boy" [50] and now is a professional counselor in Wisconsin and also a resource person for ANAD (National Association of Anorexia Nervosa and Associated Disorders) in Illinois. The narrative of Skinny Boy is about a young man suffering from AN. In his book Gary described in detail the daily struggles of living with AN and experiences of treatment that he had in the inpatient psychiatric unit of a hospital.

Three of the autobiographies were about men with a history of AN, of which two (The Skinny Boy & My Life as a Male Anorexic) provided details of experiences within eating disorder specific inpatient treatment settings. The other autobiography (My Thinning Years) discussed experiences of outpatient Cognitive Behavioral Therapy. BED was reported in two of the books, where one author discussed outpatient therapy sessions (Weightless) and the other (The Good Eater) did not describe the type of treatment experienced, excepting that it included self-help strategies such as "changing mindset" and exercise. Only one (Hiding Under the Table) author identified himself as suffering from BN and he describes his experiences seeking and receiving treatment from an inpatient rehabilitation center for eating disorders. All of the autobiographies described eating problems that first emerged during childhood. Two of the six authors identified themselves as homosexual. All autobiographies included rich detail about the authors' experiences of suffering from an eating disorder, and all but one included details about the authors' journey to recovery from their eating disorders. Treatment experiences were described in detail in 4 books, where text about treatment appeared on at least 15% of pages. This included two books (The Skinny Boy and My Life as a Male Anorexic), which were almost entirely about the treatment experienced by the authors. The remaining two books focused more about the reasons and situations that led to the eating disorder and discussion of treatment appeared on around 5% of all pages.

The analysis of data resulted in two broad themes. (1) Negative experiences of treatment and (2) Positive experiences of treatment, under which emerged several sub-themes.

Table 1. A brief summary of each of the autobiographies analysed in the study.

Book	Author	Country (Year)	ED Diagnosis	Self-Perceived Status at Writing	Sexual Orientation	Occupation	Age of ED Onset; Duration
Born Round [45]	Frank Bruni	US (2010)	Binge Eating, Bulimia Nervosa	Recovered	Homosexual	Restaurant critic	5 years; 30 years
Hiding Under the Table [46]	Dennis Henning	US (2004)	Binge Eating, Bulimia Nervosa, Anorexia Nervosa	Recovered	Heterosexual	Salesperson	9 years; 30 years
Weightless [47]	Gregg McBride	US (2014)	Binge Eating Disorder	Recovered	Heterosexual	Writer & Producer †	8 years; 23 years
My Life as a Male Anorexic [48]	Michael Krasnow	US (1996)	Anorexia Nervosa	Not Recovered (Later deceased)	Heterosexual	Library staff	15 years; 13 years
My Thinning Years [49]	Jon Derek Croteau	US (2014)	Anorexia Nervosa, Bulimia Nervosa	Recovered	Homosexual	Consultant, Writer & Speaker †	14 years; 18 years
Skinny Boy [50]	Gary A Grahl	US (2007)	Anorexia Nervosa	Recovered	Heterosexual	Professional ED Counsellor †	15 years; 5 years

NB: ED = eating disorder. † Occupation following eating disorder recovery.

6.2. Negative Experiences of Treatment

The authors provided many reasons for a negative experience. These included the behavior of the treating staff, negative thoughts and preconceptions of the men themselves, the time constraint of treatment sessions and also a lack of expertise of the health professionals.

(1) Unhelpful Interactions with Health Professionals

Judgmental. Firstly, the perceptions of authors about health professionals being invasive emerged as an important issue, though it was not the case every time. The authors identified that it was quite challenging for them to visit a health professional due to what was perceived as a stigmatized and judgmental stance against the patient. For example, one author mentioned that whenever he visited the doctor he felt as if he was being judged, which heightened his self-consciousness about his weight.

> "I had finally gotten around to selecting and paying a visit to a doctor. I'd neglected it before because I always avoided doctors, whose poking and prodding and above all weighing of me amounted to a judgment I didn't want rendered. Doctors made you stand naked or half naked in front of them." [45] (p. 203)

In the quote above, the author refers to feeling "naked" in front of the doctor, which may be interpreted both literally as well as metaphorically as being exposed. The "prodding" and "poking" referred to also suggests that rather than feeling accepted and understood by the health professional during such exposure, the author felt threatened and critically examined. The attitude of a therapist as being judgmental about the men's past also emerged as a common issue. As described in the account below, the author felt that his own healthy intentions toward therapy and recovery were being thwarted by the judgmental nature of the therapist:

> "I entered an eating disorder clinic. The therapist told me I had to really work on things and share in groups and to take my medications. I felt nervous but open. I rebelled against some groups and a yoga class, so the doctor came to visit me one day. He was very judgmental about my past and what I had done to survive." [46] (p. 65)

Unfriendly Attitude of the Therapist. A few authors described an "unfriendly" attitude of therapists toward them, which was thought to sometimes emanate from an antipathy against males. This type of attitude in a clinical setting plays a particularly important role because the treatment provided, as well as the patient's response to treatment, are influenced by the preconceptions of the therapist, as well as those of the patient.

> "There are people and therapists who want to help others, but who cannot even help themselves. There was this therapist who had issues with men that are not resolved and she became a therapist to help women who suffered like her. It is sad because they still harbor anger toward men and while treating men they are not able to really separate their anger." [46] (p. 83)

Another example of unfriendly and stern behavior is exemplified in this quote by another author, below. This author felt that his attempts to build rapport with his therapist were unsuccessful, which negatively affected the therapeutic relationship.

> "I also didn't like that he never laughed at my jokes and that he always had a stoic expression on his face whenever I explained some of the circumstances of my upbringing. Where was this guy's compassion? Didn't he knows I was a victim and unable to help myself? That none of this was my fault?" [47] (p. 163)

(2) Thoughts and Behaviors Impeding Treatment

Apart from the attitude and behavior of health professionals, the mindset of the person in treatment is very crucial for a positive outcome. The analysis of data found that sometimes it was the preformed notions of patients that negatively affected treatment outcomes, such that they were slow to engage in therapy.

Low expectations of therapists. Authors sometimes described unhelpful negative beliefs about therapy and therapists that influenced their attempts to seek and engage in treatment. The following excerpt from an autobiography indicates the self-assertive thinking of an author along with denigration of the health professionals.

> "I went into rehab knowing—and I mean knowing—that I knew it all and that the professionals there did not know jack shit." [46] (p. 177)

Similarly, an unsparing disclosure by one of the authors demonstrated the extent of the negative perceptions of treatment providers that may occur. The author in the following excerpt claims that psychiatric help is of no use.

> "Psychiatrists and psychiatric hospitals are pointless, if not detrimental." [48] (p. 52)

Such beliefs are likely formed on the basis of prior experience, however clearly place individuals in a position "against" rather than "in alliance" with the treatment team even before treatment commences.

High expectations of therapists. In contrast to the low expectations of the competencies of health providers, sometimes it was the patients' overly high expectations of health professionals, and the health professionals' subsequent inability to fulfill such expectations, that led to negative treatment experiences. An author, who was severely ill with AN in particular used the term "miracle workers" for therapists/doctors and reported that while initially he thought highly of doctors, over time, as he did not recover, they were viewed less favorably.

> "To us doctors were miracle workers. We had the incorrect belief that when you go to a doctor with your problem, he can solve it with a snap of his fingers." [48] (p. 11)

This alternating idealizing and demeaning of health professionals may be symptomatic of an unhealthy attachment or interpersonal style, which serves to create strain and distance in the therapeutic relationship, and thus hinder recovery.

Self-sabotaging. The authors of the autobiographies wrote that they felt that they were being judged within treatment centers, and were not well understood by others, including staff and other patients. This often resulted in unhelpful or self-sabotaging behavior in an attempt to have their need for acceptance met. In one instance an author recalled how he intentionally lied to a therapist in order to gain acceptance from him:

> "Jeff asked me to tell the truth during our first meeting and I thought that even though I was in a rehab and they were there to help me, he would think that I was a freak, a loser, unworthy of love, a pathetic excuse for a human being. I thought I had to lie to him to be accepted, so I lied." [46] (p. 167)

(3) Therapist Limitations

In continuation to the first theme of author's perception about the treatment providers' behavior, their knowledge regarding eating disorders and their expertise in the field as perceived by the men in this study emerged as a significant issue. All the authors unanimously acknowledged the expertise of therapists as an important factor in determining their treatment outcomes.

Lack of expertise in treating eating disorders. Perceived incompetency of therapists emerged as an important and critical issue in the study. After a person becomes sure that he is suffering from a health problem, the primary concern becomes the need for it to be resolved. In the case of an eating disorder this is not always simple, as exemplified in the following quote in which an author reported the inadequacy and unavailability of accurate treatment in men:

> "Some places tell me that they have a program for men, but the truth is they have no idea how to work with men, nor do they understand the differences between men and women who had eating disorders." [46] (p. 80)

The same author further added that the claims made by treatment centers that they were capable of treating eating disorders in men were false and there is a notable scarcity of centers that know how to treat a man with eating disorder.

> "Until this stay I had seen eight different professionals who tried to help me and at the same time only two knew how to work with someone who suffered from an eating disorder." [46] (p. 67)

Contradictory to his expectations that treatment providers would understand eating disorder issues, one author reported feeling misunderstood by the staff. Perceptions that eating disorders occur in women only may explain such disregard of the male author's symptoms.

> "The doctor and nurses made me feel as if I was crazy. None of them asked why I'd dropped so much weight." [49] (p. 172)

The experience of rehabilitation for men varied. One of the authors described his rehabilitation stay as a "real eye-opener" because of the conduct displayed by the staff members.

> "The one thing that was really an eye opener was to me in my last stay in rehab is that the people treating me were no healthier than I was." [46] (p. 67)

Ignorance of eating disorders in men. Furthermore, another author declared the therapist as ignorant and unaware of the occurrence of eating disorders in men. Interestingly, this author, who was severely underweight at the time, discussed how even though he was displaying excessive distress about fatness, the health professionals did not assess him for an eating disorder. To this author, such an experience spoke to the dismissal of the fact that eating disorders exist in men:

> "I was freaking out about how much fat was in the intravenous fluids they were giving me, but ironically, it never occurred to anyone to ask whether I had any kind of eating issues. It probably never occurred to them that a male could be anorexic. Even though I told the doctor I was running twelve miles or more a day on a bowl of cereal or a bagel and a handful of fat burners, he never asked about an eating disorder." [49] (p. 172)

Money-mindedness. Half of the men mentioned the money-mindedness of therapists. They quoted many instances where they felt their individual needs were neglected because the therapist prioritized monetary gains. This finding was similar, irrespective of the place of treatment (e.g., residential care, inpatient setting, or counseling session). The following excerpt clearly stated the frustration and misery of an author in this regard:

> "He was getting paid around sixty dollars per hour and we were staring at each other. That's all. No talking. I frequently told my parents that I wanted to stop seeing Dr P. He did not help and was a complete waste of time. I could be wrong but I believe he was more interested in money than anything else (either that or he was totally incompetent)." [48] (p. 24)

Ineffective Communication. Staff members have a critical role in the treatment setting of a clinic or hospital. According to the majority of authors the staff members were expected to be more authoritative, as opposed to authoritarian, in order to bring a subtle and long-lasting change in their behavior. For example in the following quote the author wished to have a tangible plan for recovery.

> "I needed something more concrete, something that was going to hold me accountable and responsible for my behaviors and actions." [46] (p. 170)

(4) Feeling Ostracized as a Man

By staff members. The role of staff members in the treatment setting was duly acknowledged. Being a man with an eating disorder is itself very challenging. A few men in treatment reported feeling unwanted in the treatment setting by the staff members due to their male gender.

> "Some of the staff had a problem with a male in the group and they did not have a problem letting me know." [46] (p. 67)

By other patients. Some men in treatment described feeling misunderstood and targeted by the prejudiced behavior of female patients towards men. For example, one author stated that women in the group could not accommodate his presence and wanted him to leave because they had some personal issues with men in their lives:

> "The meetings I first went to were all women and young girls - maybe a man once in a while. In these meetings, I was looked at as an outsider. In one OA (Overeaters Anonymous) meeting, a woman went as far as to ask me to leave because they had issues with men in their lives and a man in group was hard for them to deal with." [46] (p. 170)

(5) Treatment Side Effects

Two out of six authors wrote that antidepressants and electroconvulsive therapy were deleterious to their health. In particular, authors discussed unwanted side effects and/or ineffectiveness of medication:

> "Dr C prescribed antidepressant medication. Some were stopped because of side effects, such as drowsiness, light-headedness, fidgetiness (the most bothersome - like the jitters), and uncontrollable shaking. Others were stopped because they had no effect one way or the other." [48] (p. 11)

> "Prozac hadn't given me the speedy buzz it gave some people. It had given me the opposite: a gauzy lethargy." [45] (p. 200)

One author who described his treatment with electroconvulsive therapy, reported concern regarding memory loss that occurred following therapy:

> "One of the possible side effects of ECT is memory loss and this was the most prevalent result of my treatment." [48] (p. 11)

6.3. Positive Experiences of Treatment

The autobiographies focused very seldom on positive, as opposed to negative, treatment experiences. However in contrast to negative experiences, which were at times a result of the author's own thoughts and behaviors, it is interesting to note that the factors that were considered as positive in treatment were usually external, such as the behavior of staff members in hospital, therapists, or other patients in the treatment center.

(1) Therapist

Non-judgmental empathic behavior. Three of the six authors described non-judgmental behavior of therapists as an important positive experience in treatment. For example, one of the men felt encouraged to continue his therapy sessions because of the uncritical attitude of the therapist. In fact, he admitted that he actually liked being in her company.

> "She was the first therapist who took the time to help me and not judge me. I liked seeing her and listening to her." [46] (p. 92)

When the authors of the autobiographies perceived that the health professional was being empathic, this was important to them in regarding the treatment as positive. This is opposed to the negative treatment experience themes discussed above where the therapist was perceived as being judgmental or unfriendly. Thus, an understanding nature, non-judgmental behavior, and a caring and gentle attitude were therapist qualities that were discussed by authors as contributing to the success of their treatment. The following quote reflects on how a therapist who had a gentle nature was appreciated.

> "He had a careful, gentle way of helping me, as if he were carefully removing a bandage that had covered a massive wound for years. He didn't tear it off; he pulled back the adhesive slowly but steadily." [49] (pp. 228–229)

Expertise. The therapist had a very important role in defining the treatment outcome. Trust in the treatment aligned with the perceived expertise of the health professional, as exemplified in the following quote:

> "Once I started to work with the idea that the therapists knew more than I did at the same time, and I began to trust their input in my life, I began to trust myself and how I really felt." [46] (p. 86)

Interestingly, this theme appears to be in contrast to the negative treatment experience theme where authors described how their preconceptions of the treatment providers' incompetence at times sabotaged their ability to engage in therapy. Other authors acknowledged the expertise of therapists in helping them to address their symptoms.

> "I learned from Jeff R. and Jeff S. how to look at situations and handle them from a positive and realistic point of view, rather than turning to food, sex or the other dysfunctional behaviors I turned to as treatment for my emotional pain." [46] (p. 167)

Effective communication style. The adage that "one rule applies to all" defies for eating disordered patients, as is evident from the varied views presented by the authors regarding the style of communication they preferred from their treatment providers. Whereas some authors described a desire for a "tough" approach from their therapist, others clearly desired a more gentle approach. This demonstrates the need for therapists to assess the communication and relationship needs of their clients in informing their own interaction style.

Under the "non-judgmental" theme above, an example is provided of an author who appreciated a gentle and slow approach from his therapist: "*carefully removing a bandage*". On the other hand, for several of the authors, an authoritative nature of the doctor was considered as a welcoming effort to men in treatment. Perhaps this approach instilled confidence in the men, or gave them the permission to relinquish control over their eating to an authoritative figure. The metaphor of the bandage is used again here.

> "I have to admit that it was some of the best (and toughest) therapy I'd ever received. I'm not knocking whatever kind of therapy may work for someone else. But for me, this quick, tough love, rip-off-the-bandage-fast approach was really powerful." [47] (p. 168)

> "Dr X was making a major difference in my life. After he had earned my trust, he challenged me and never let me off easy. I liked that he pushed me." [49] (p. 263)

(2) Effect of Others in Hospital

Staff members. The role of staff members as being friendly and considerate had an important influence in forming the treatment experience as positive. One of the men in this study stated that being able to accept help from staff proved beneficial to him.

> "I have learned to let people into my life and trust them to help me, rather than to try to do everything alone and fail." [46] (p. 188)

Other patients. In addition to this, the supportive nature of group members emerged as a positive aspect of treatment.

> "We listen. We share pain and heartache. We ask questions. We empathize without feeling sorry for each other. We find the support to heal and gather strength to go on." [50] (p. 95)

(3) Treatment forms

There was lack of consensus in men with regards to the most effective form of treatment provided for an eating disorder.

Group therapy vs. individual therapy. In a hospital, the usual form of treatment includes medicine, counseling sessions, group therapy and behavioral therapy. In most of the instances being a part of group therapy was considered as an effective measure by the authors while in treatment. This could be attributed to the fact that talking about their eating disorder openly in group with other members with similar issues provided a sense of normalization and empathy. The following extract clearly outlines the perceived benefits of group therapy:

> "Sitting there in groups and slowly discussing my issues with a mind open for feedback made it easier to confront my fears, shame, guilt, anger, low, low, low self-esteem, self-hatred, and lack of self-respect. I no longer believed I had to hide and numb my pain." [46] (p. 175)

In contrast to this, other authors reported that they felt more supported in individual therapy. For example, in the following excerpt the author clearly stated that he felt safe and secure in therapy sessions where he does not have to acknowledge the presence of others as in group therapy:

> "I preferred the quiet safety and the anonymity of the one-on-one therapy." [49] (p. 213)

This clearly indicates that understanding the individual needs of men is central to tailoring an effective treatment regime.

Cognitive Behavioral Therapy. The effectiveness of treatment provided was frequently the primary concern of these men when discussing treatment experiences. In the majority of cases, cognitive behavioral therapy was followed and this approach was perceived as helpful.

> "After months of gaining my trust and respect through listening to my story, and understanding my past to help me move forward, she introduced me to cognitive behavioral therapy. This approach and other tools she gave me were meant to help me notice the behaviors I was engaging in and stop them." [49] (p. 214)

(4) Hospital Environment

The general atmosphere of the hospital environment was also mentioned as important. Although at times isolating, as reflected by one of the men, this characteristic of hospitalization was appreciated. This may in part be due to a desire to maintain control of the eating disorder, which may be threatened by the interference of others, as expressed here:

> "This hospital thing will fit my lifestyle quite nicely since I've recently become allergic to people. Social interaction makes me break out in a terrible rash called guilt; I simply can't seem to please enough people, no matter how hard I try." [50] (p. 9)

Maintaining a restrictive-type eating disorder requires significant self-control and determination, which is taxing for an individual. Quite a few men mentioned that being hospitalized provided temporary relief from this self-imposed control, which could be relinquished to staff.

"My feelings about the hospital were similar to those I had when I was taken out of the school. Deep down I think that I wanted to be hospitalized. It was a relief. Again it was a control issue." [48] (p. 14)

7. Discussion

The present study examined the treatment experiences of men who had or have had an eating disorder and engaged in any form of treatment. The analysis found that the factors that most commonly contributed to a negative experience were judgmental behavior of professionals and their perceived lack of expertise. The findings regarding the judgmental behavior of health professionals are commensurate with those reported in previous studies by women [28,29]. Additional themes also emerged however, such as the ulterior motives of therapists, like money-mindedness. Though financial cost of treatment had been discussed earlier [51–54], the putative "mercenary" attitudes of therapists has not been cited previously. Unexpectedly, a few of the men reported an antipathy of female practitioners towards them in treatment. This biased treatment was made sense of by the authors who assumed that some female practitioners had unresolved conflicts with men in their own lives and projected these towards the males they encountered in their treatment centers. All the negative experiences encountered by males thwarted their further engagement in therapy, as has been reported by women in other studies [55]. In contrast, an empathizing nature, non-judgmental behavior, good understanding and expertise with eating disorders in men, and a trustworthy relationship with the health professional formulated a positive experience of treatment. This finding is in consensus with studies in women [28].

Interestingly, the study found that sometimes men's own thoughts and behaviors impacted on treatment experiences. For example, having very high expectations of the therapist as a "miracle worker" led to disappointment when treatment was not progressing. Also, one author reported intentionally misleading therapists at times, to the detriment of their own outcomes. This self-sabotaging behavior may have occurred due to a fear of criticism, or a fear of losing the perceived positive aspects of an eating disorder, indicative of a lack of readiness to change [55]. Also, it was interesting that sometimes different approaches were preferred, for example some preferred a female therapist while others had no issues with the gender of the therapist. This highlights the importance of individualized or person-centered care [24] and increased availability of male providers.

In treatment, the role of group members and staff was recognized as important by the men in the present study and consistent with men reporting feelings of isolation in prior studies [14]. The study identified that men in the present study felt misunderstood and unwanted by staff members [26,27]. Some authors endorsed the desire for healthcare staff to be authoritative (expressing confidence in their expertise) but to also provide an equal distribution of power and to be empathic and friendly. Feminization of the disorder in society by referring it as women's disease or a "gay problem" [18] and also the stigma attached to men with eating disorders discouraged the male authors in this study to seek help [24,30]. Also, the sexuality of the authors was not a major theme as only 2 of 6 was identified as homosexual.

The study supports the limited literature that treatment approaches should consider men also and not only women [12]. However, it should be acknowledged that there are efforts being made to improve the situation and to provide educational material (e.g., videos) to clinicians. Examples include ways to ask questions to men about their eating patterns and exercise as described by Hildebrandt and Craigen [56].

In this study, there was a gender disparity in the number of treatment centers available to the men and there appeared to be a deficit in male-only treatment facilities. The men in treatment had varied opinions about the form of therapy. However, the majority of them promoted group therapy because of the supportive environment experienced within the group, as stated by Weltzin et al., [20]. In contrast to group therapy, there were few that reported positive experiences within individual therapy. Regarding the environment of the hospital, there was no consensus, as some pointed to the "stillness" of hospital as scary, whereas others preferred the isolation of the unit as a way to escape societal pressures. For these latter authors, the ability to relinquish control to hospital staff members in regards to diet and exercise schedules was experienced as a temporary relief from the pressures of the eating disorder.

8. Strengths and Limitations

Strengths of the study include autobiographical accounts of the men with eating disorders about their treatment experiences and broad inclusion criteria of all forms of eating disorders. Further strengths include that a systematic search was employed to identify autobiographies; two investigators read the autobiographies and coded themes, increasing the validity of the emergent themes; and the coding of themes by the authors continued until saturation was achieved. However, this study also has some limitations including: the very small sample size that consisted of a highly specific group of men who (1) decided to write an autobiography about their experiences and (2) found a publisher for it; selection of autobiographies to one language (English); and defined dates (years 1995–2015). It is possible that relevant autobiographies in other languages and/or from different (non-Western) cultures, or other time periods were missed. In addition the study did not include men younger than 18 years of age, so it was not possible to discuss how this age group reflect on their treatment experiences. On the other hand, all authors included in this study wrote about their childhood and adolescent experiences of eating disorder symptoms. In addition, while two authors who identified as homosexual were included in this study, it is possible that the treatment experiences of men with varied sexual identities differ and it would be relevant to include more men with homosexual or transgender identities in future studies. Autobiographies are also limited in that there are unknown motivations for writing (including income from royalties) although research [42] suggests several altruistic motivations for men who write about an eating disorder such as AN. Thus, it would be also important to follow this research with larger samples and with face-to-face interviews that would support the validity of these preliminary findings. Finally, while all authors wrote about treatment experience in the US, people's experiences may differ in other countries where health care services are government-funded, and where doctors are salaried (e.g., there may be less perceived "money mindedness" of the doctors).

9. Conclusions

This is the first study that used autobiographical accounts of men with eating disorders to understand their treatment experiences. The study identified that the behaviors and attitudes of both treatment providers and male patients may influence the outcome of treatment defining it as a positive or negative experience. Furthermore, the study provides a platform for designing further research and consideration of treatment strategies with a primary focus on attending to patients' perspectives. In particular, the findings highlight the importance of specialized expertise and a non-judgmental understanding in healthcare providers caring for men with eating disorders. Pre-treatment strategies aimed at educating patients as to expectations of treatment, and practitioner training interventions may be helpful to address barriers to positive treatment experiences.

Acknowledgments: Financial support was provided to PT from a Western Sydney University doctoral scholarship.

Author Contributions: P.H. designed the study. Data collection, analysis and interpretation was done by P.T. and D.M. P.T. drafted the article that is critically revised by D.M. and P.H. All the authors (P.T., D.M. and P.H.) gave their approval to publish this article.

Conflicts of Interest: The authors declare no conflict of interest.

References

1. American Psychiatric Association. *Diagnostic and Statistical Manual of Mental Disorders (DSM-5®)*; American Psychiatric Pub: Arlington, VA, USA, 2013.
2. Raevuori, A.; Keski-Rahkonen, A.; Hoek, H.W. A review of eating disorders in males. *Curr. Opin. Psychiatry* **2014**, *27*, 426–430. [CrossRef] [PubMed]

3. Bulik, C.M.; Sullivan, P.F.; Tozzi, F.; Furberg, H.; Lichtenstein, P.; Pedersen, N.L. Prevalence, heritability, and prospective risk factors for anorexia nervosa. *Arch. Gen. Psychiatry* **2006**, *63*, 305–312. [CrossRef] [PubMed]
4. Keski-Rahkonen, A.; Hoek, H.W.; Susser, E.S.; Linna, M.S.; Sihvola, E.; Raevuori, A.; Bulik, C.M.; Kaprio, J.; Rissanen, A. Epidemiology and course of anorexia nervosa in the community. *Am. J. Psychiatry* **2007**, *164*, 1259–1265. [CrossRef] [PubMed]
5. Carlat, D.J.; Camargo, C.A., Jr.; Herzog, D.B. Eating disorders in males: A report on 135 patients. *Am. J. Psychiatry* **1997**, *154*, 1127. [PubMed]
6. Hall, A.; Delahunt, J.W.; Ellis, P.M. Anorexia nervosa in the male: Clinical features and follow-up of nine patients. *J. Psychiatr. Res.* **1985**, *19*, 315–321. [CrossRef]
7. Crisp, A.H.; Burns, T.; Bhat, A.V. Primary anorexia nervosa in the male and female: A comparison of clinical features and prognosis. *Psychol. Psychother. Theory Res. Pract.* **1986**, *59*, 123–132. [CrossRef]
8. Hudson, J.I.; Hiripi, E.; Pope, H.G.; Kessler, R.C. The prevalence and correlates of eating disorders in the National Comorbidity Survey Replication. *Biol. Psychiatry* **2007**, *61*, 348–358. [CrossRef] [PubMed]
9. Taylor, J.Y.; Caldwell, C.H.; Baser, R.E.; Faison, N.; Jackson, J.S. Prevalence of eating disorders among Blacks in the National Survey of American Life. *Int. J. Eat. Disord.* **2007**, *40*, S10–S14. [CrossRef] [PubMed]
10. Striegel, R.H.; Bedrosian, R.; Wang, C.; Schwartz, S. Why men should be included in research on binge eating: results from a comparison of psychosocial impairment in men and women. *Int. J. Eat. Disord.* **2012**, *45*, 233–240. [CrossRef] [PubMed]
11. Mitchison, D.; Hay, P.; Slewa-Younan, S.; Mond, J. The changing demographic profile of eating disorder behaviors in the community. *BMC Public Health* **2014**, *14*, 943. [CrossRef] [PubMed]
12. National Collaborating Centre for Mental Health. *Eating Disorders: Core Interventions in the Treatment and Management of Anorexia Nervosa, Bulimia Nervosa and Related Eating Disorders*; British Psychological Society: Leicester, UK, 2004.
13. Woodside, D.B.; Kaplan, A.S. Day hospital treatment in males with eating disorders—Response and comparison to females. *J. Psychosom. Res.* **1994**, *38*, 471–475. [CrossRef]
14. Andersen, A.E.; Holman, J.E. Males with eating disorders: Challenges for treatment and research. *Psychopharmacol. Bull.* **1997**, *33*, 391. [CrossRef] [PubMed]
15. Weltzin, T.E.; Weisensel, N.; Franczyk, D.; Burnett, K.; Klitz, C.; Bean, P. Eating disorders in men: Update. *J. Men's Health Gend.* **2005**, *2*, 186–193. [CrossRef]
16. Fernández-Aranda, F.; Krug, I.; Jiménez-Murcia, S.; Granero, R.; Núñez, A.; Penelo, E.; Solano, R.; Treasure, J. Male eating disorders and therapy: A controlled pilot study with one year follow-up. *J. Behav. Ther. Exp. Psychiatry* **2009**, *40*, 479–486. [CrossRef] [PubMed]
17. Greenberg, S.T.; Schoen, E.G. Males and eating disorders: Gender-based therapy for eating disorder recovery. *Prof. Psychol. Res. Pract.* **2008**, *39*, 464. [CrossRef]
18. Olivardia, R.; Pope, H.G., Jr.; Borowiecki, J.J., III; Cohane, G.H. Biceps and Body Image: The Relationship Between Muscularity and Self-Esteem, Depression, and Eating Disorder Symptoms. *Psychol. Men Masc.* **2004**, *5*, 112. [CrossRef]
19. Ming, T.S.; Lin Miao Shan, P.; Kuek Shu Cen, A.; Lian, L.E.; Boon Swee Kim, E. Men do get it: Eating disorders in males from an asian perspective. *ASEAN J. Psychiatry* **2014**, *15*, 72–82.
20. Weltzin, T.E.; Cornella-Carlson, T.; Fitzpatrick, M.E.; Kennington, B.; Bean, P.; Jefferies, C. Treatment issues and outcomes for males with eating disorders. *Eat. Disord.* **2012**, *20*, 444–459. [CrossRef] [PubMed]
21. Thapliyal, P.; Hay, P.J. Treatment experiences of males with an eating disorder: A systematic review of qualitative studies. *Transl. Dev. Psychiatry* **2014**, *2*. [CrossRef]
22. De Beer, Z.; Wren, B. Eating Disorders in Males. In *Eating and its Disorders*; Fox, J.R.E., Goss, K.P., Eds.; John Wiley & Sons, Ltd.: Chichester, UK, 2012.
23. Dearden, A.; Mulgrew, K.E. Service provision for Men with eating issues in Australia: An analysis of Organisations', Practitioners', and Men's experiences. *Aust. Soc. Work* **2013**, *66*, 590–606. [CrossRef]
24. Robinson, K.J.; Mountford, V.A.; Sperlinger, D.J. Being men with eating disorders: Perspectives of male eating disorder service-users. *J. Health Psychol.* **2013**, *18*, 176–186. [CrossRef] [PubMed]
25. Drummond, M.J. Men, body image, and eating disorders. *Int. J. Men's Health.* **2002**, *1*, 89. [CrossRef]
26. Drummond, M. Life as a male 'anorexic'. *Aust. J. Prim. Health* **1999**, *5*, 80–89. [CrossRef]
27. Copperman, J. *Eating Disorders in the United Kingdom: Review of the Provision of Health Care Services for Men with Eating Disorders*; Eating Disorders Association Norwich: Norwich, UK, 2000.

28. Evans, E.J.; Hay, P.J.; Mond, J.; Paxton, S.J.; Quirk, F.; Rodgers, B.; Jhajj, A.K.; Sawoniewska, M.A. Barriers to help-seeking in young women with eating disorders: A qualitative exploration in a longitudinal community survey. *Eat. Disord.* **2011**, *19*, 270–285. [CrossRef] [PubMed]
29. Rich, E. Anorexic dis (connection): Managing anorexia as an illness and an identity. *Sociol. Health Illn.* **2006**, *28*, 284–305. [CrossRef] [PubMed]
30. Griffiths, S.; Mond, J.M.; Murray, S.B.; Touyz, S. The prevalence and adverse associations of stigmatization in people with eating disorders. *Int. J. Eat. Disord.* **2015**, *48*, 767–774. [CrossRef] [PubMed]
31. Marchel, C.; Owens, S. Qualitative research in psychology: Could William James get a job? *Hist. Psychol.* **2007**, *10*, 301. [CrossRef] [PubMed]
32. Espindola, C.R.; Blay, S.L. Anorexia nervosa's meaning to patients: A qualitative synthesis. *Psychopathology* **2009**, *42*, 69–80. [CrossRef] [PubMed]
33. Bezance, J.; Holliday, J. Adolescents with anorexia nervosa have their say: A review of qualitative studies on treatment and recovery from anorexia nervosa. *Eur. Eat. Disord. Rev.* **2013**, *21*, 352–360. [CrossRef] [PubMed]
34. Lamb, J.; Bower, P.; Rogers, A.; Dowrick, C.; Gask, L. Access to mental health in primary care: A qualitative meta-synthesis of evidence from the experience of people from 'hard to reach' groups. *Health* **2012**, *16*, 76–104. [CrossRef] [PubMed]
35. Tierney, S. The individual within a condition: A qualitative study of young people's reflections on being treated for anorexia nervosa. *J. Am. Psychiatr. Nurses Assoc.* **2008**, *13*, 368–375. [CrossRef] [PubMed]
36. Nakamura, H. Overcoming bulimia nervosa: A qualitative study of recovery in Japan. *Proceedings* **2012**, *17*, 101–109.
37. Reid, M.; Burr, J.; Williams, S.; Hammersley, R. Eating disorders patients' views on their disorders and on an outpatient service: A qualitative study. *J. Health Psychol.* **2008**, *13*, 956–960. [CrossRef] [PubMed]
38. Hay, P.J.; Cho, K. A qualitative exploration of influences on the process of recovery from personal written accounts of people with anorexia nervosa. *Women Health* **2013**, *53*, 730–740. [CrossRef] [PubMed]
39. Malson, H.; Finn, D.; Treasure, J.; Clarke, S.; Anderson, G. Constructing 'The Eating Disordered Patient' 1: A discourse analysis of accounts of treatment experiences. *J. Community Appl. Soc. Psychol.* **2004**, *14*, 473–489. [CrossRef]
40. Plummer, K. *Documents of Life 2: An Invitation to A Critical Humanism*; Sage: Newcastle upon Tyne, UK, 2001; Volume 2.
41. Bogdan, R.C.; Biklen, S.K. *Qualitative Research for Education*; Allyn and Bacon: Boston, MA, USA, 1992.
42. Aronson, J.K. Autopathography: The patient's tale. *Br. Med. J.* **2000**, *321*, 1599. [CrossRef]
43. Ritchie, J.; Spencer, L.; Bryman, A.; Burgess, R. *Analysing Qualitative Data*; Routledge: London, UK, 1994.
44. Pope, C.; Ziebland, S.; Mays, N. Analysing qualitative data. *Br. Med. J.* **2000**, *320*, 114. [CrossRef]
45. Bruni, F. *Born Round: The Story of Family Food and a Ferocious Appetite*; Penguin Book: New York, NY, USA, 2009.
46. Henning, D.; Woods, P. *Hiding Under the Table*; Americana Publishing Inc.: Albuquerque, NM, USA, 2004.
47. McBride, G. *Weightless: My Life as a Fat Man and How I Escaped*; Central Recovery Press: Las Vegas, NV, USA, 2014.
48. Krasnow, M. *My Life as a Male Anorexic*; Harrington Park Press: New York, NY, USA, 1996.
49. Croteau, J.D. *My Thinning Years: Starving the Gay Within*; Hazelden Publishing: Center City, MN, USA, 2014.
50. Grahl, G.A. *The Skinny Boy: A Young Man's Battle and Triumph over Anorexia*; American Legacy Media: Clearfield, UT, USA, 2007.
51. Becker, A.E.; Franko, D.L.; Nussbaum, K.; Herzog, D.B. Secondary prevention for eating disorders: The impact of education, screening, and referral in a college-based screening program. *Int. J. Eat. Disord.* **2004**, *36*, 157–162. [CrossRef] [PubMed]
52. Hepworth, N.; Paxton, S.J. Pathways to help-seeking in bulimia nervosa and binge eating problems: A concept mapping approach. *Int. J. Eat. Disord.* **2007**, *40*, 493–504. [CrossRef] [PubMed]
53. Escobar-Koch, T.; Banker, J.D.; Crow, S.; Cullis, J.; Ringwood, S.; Smith, G.; van Furth, E.; Westin, K.; Schmidt, U. Service users' views of eating disorder services: An international comparison. *Int. J. Eat. Disord.* **2010**, *43*, 549–559. [CrossRef] [PubMed]
54. National Eating Disorder Association, 2015. Available online: http://www.nationaleatingdisorders.org/ (accessed on 13 September 2016).

55. Leavey, G.; Vallianatou, C.; Johnson-Sabine, E.; Rae, S.; Gunputh, V. Psychosocial barriers to engagement with an eating disorder service: A qualitative analysis of failure to attend. *Eat. Disord.* **2011**, *19*, 425–440. [CrossRef] [PubMed]
56. Hildebrandt, T.; Craigen, K. Eating-Related Pathology in Men and Boys. In *Handbook of Assessment and Treatment of Eating Disorders*; Walsh, B.T., Attia, E., Glasofer, D.R., Sysko, R., Eds.; American Psychiatric Publishing, Inc.: Arlington, VA, USA, 2015; Chapter 6, pp. 105–118.

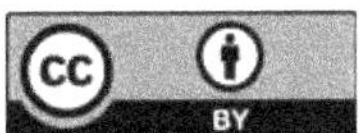

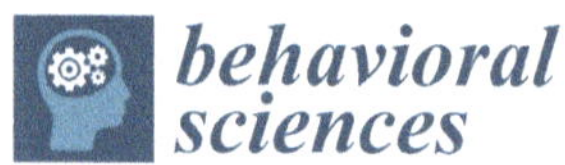

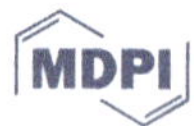

Article

Cognitive Remediation Therapy for Adolescents with Anorexia Nervosa—Treatment Satisfaction and the Perception of Change

Camilla Lindvall Dahlgren * and Kristin Stedal

Regional Department for Eating Disorders, Division of Mental Health and Addiction, Oslo University Hospital, Ullevål HF, Postboks 4950 Nydalen, 0424 Oslo, Norway; post.psykiskhelse@oslo-universitetssykehus.no

* Correspondence: camilla.lindvall@dahlgren.no; Tel.: +47-4729-1950

Academic Editors: Amanda Sainsbury and Felipe Luz

Received: 20 March 2017; Accepted: 10 April 2017; Published: 18 April 2017

Abstract: Cognitive remediation therapy (CRT) has recently been developed for children and adolescents with anorexia nervosa (AN). It focuses on decreasing rigid cognitions and behaviors, as well as increasing central coherence. Overall, CRT has been proven feasible for young individuals with AN, but little is known regarding the specifics of its feasibility, and the perception of change associated with the intervention. Consequently, the aim of the current study was to explore service users' perspective on CRT with a specific focus on treatment delivery, treatment content, and perceived change. Twenty adolescents (age 13–18) with AN participated in a 10-session course of CRT. A 20-item treatment evaluation questionnaire was administered at the end of treatment, focusing on four aspects of the intervention: (1) general attitudes towards treatment, (2) treatment specifics, (3) the perception of change and (4) the patient-therapist relation. The main findings suggest high levels of treatment satisfaction, but somewhat limited perceptions of change. The current study is one of the most detailed accounts of adolescents' perspective on CRT published on eating disorders, and highlights several important aspects of the treatment viewed through the eye of the receiver.

Keywords: anorexia nervosa; cognitive remediation therapy; eating disorders; treatment satisfaction; neuropsychology; rigidity; cognitive flexibility; central coherence

---

1. Introduction

Anorexia nervosa (AN) is an eating disorder (ED) characterized by a persistent restriction of energy intake which leads to significant low body weight, an intense fear of gaining weight or becoming fat, a distorted experience of one's own body and an amplified sense of the body's influence on self-worth [1]. Individuals with AN often display rigid behaviors and cognitions characterized by preoccupation with details [2]. Such behaviors and cognitions are predominantly linked to core ED symptoms such as food restriction and preoccupancy with weight and shape, but are also commonly seen in the individual's approach to exercise routines, work or school, or in relation to family and friends [3]. Inflexibility and preoccupation with details are often explained in terms of neuropsychological dysfunction. Studies in adults with AN have yielded consistent evidence of suboptimal executive functioning, especially in cognitive flexibility [4,5], and in information processing which is often characterized by weak central coherence [6]. Cognitive function in children and adolescents with AN has received less attention, and the extant literature report mixed findings with a number of studies failing to find evidence of poor neuropsychological functioning, whereas others have replicated results similar to those reported in adults [7].

Following the introduction of cognitive remediation therapy (CRT) for EDs in 2005 [8], a number of case and feasibility studies have supported its utility in adults with AN [9], and four randomized controlled trials (RCTs) [10–13] have sought to investigate the effect of the intervention. For individuals with AN, CRT aims to decrease rigidity and increase the balance between local and global information processing [14–16]. It is hypothesized that by alleviating some of these cognitive difficulties, ambivalence towards engaging in other psychological interventions might decrease, rendering the individual more open to the prospect of change [8]. In 2010, the original, adult CRT manual [17] was adapted for children and adolescents [18], and although a number of studies have established its feasibility for this younger group [14,19–22], there are no published RCT. There is also a paucity in studies evaluating the treatment from the receiver's perspective. This is in contrast with the increased focus on assessment of client satisfaction in ED health services [23,24]. Additionally, it is well known that that treatment dissatisfaction may lead to treatment delay, failure to engage and, ultimately, to treatment withdrawal [25,26]. The aim of this study is to present post-intervention feedback from a feasibility study of CRT for adolescents with AN, and to examine the results through the aspects of treatment satisfaction and perception of change.

2. Materials and Methods

2.1. Participants

A total of 20 inpatients (N = 10) and outpatients (N = 10) aged 13–18 (mean = 15.9, SD = 1.6) were recruited from Oslo University Hospital HF, Ullevål, and took part in a CRT feasibility trial [14]. All participants were female and in treatment for AN at the time of inclusion. Based on self-reports of binge eating and compensatory behaviors, 18 participants were classified as having a restricting subtype of AN (AN-R). The two remaining participants fitted the description for a binge-purge subtype (AN-BP). Intelligence was assessed using the Wechsler Adult Intelligence Scale—Third Edition (WAIS-III) [27], the Wechsler Abbreviated Scale of Intelligence (WASI) [28] or the Wechsler Intelligence Scale for Children-Third Edition (WISC-III) [29]. All participants scored within the normal range. There were no significant differences between in- and out-patients in any of the baseline assessment variables. Descriptive data at baseline is presented in Table 1.

Table 1. Descriptive data for the sample (N = 20) at baseline.

	N	Mean (SD)	Range
Age (years)	20	15.9 (1.6)	13.1–18.7
BMI Percentile	20	10.2 (17.2)	0.0–28.0
Duration of illness [1]	19	2.7 (2.1)	1–7
Global EDE-Q [2]	20	3.4 (1.4)	0.6–5.4
BDI	20	32.2 (15.1)	7–58
STAI	20	58.6 (9.7)	43–78

Note. SD = Standard Deviation; BMI = Body Mass Index; [1] = Years, self-reported; [2] = Eating Disorder Examination Questionnaire Global Score [30]; BDI = Beck Depression Inventory [31]; STAI = State Trait Anxiety Inventory [32].

2.2. Procedure

Participants were assessed using an extensive neuropsychological and psychiatric test battery both before and after receiving CRT. The neuropsychological assessment battery included tests focusing primarily on set-shifting and central coherence, whereas the psychiatric assessment included self-reported measures of depression, anxiety and ED psychopathology. A more detailed account of the assessment procedure and content have been presented elsewhere [3,14,33]. After the initial assessment, participants received, on average, 10 once- or twice-weekly individually delivered sessions, and were then re-tested using the same measures as before the treatment started. In addition, participants were asked to fill out a treatment evaluation questionnaire, allowing for exploration of treatment acceptability and the perception of change after treatment. The study was conducted at the Regional Department for Eating Disorders at Oslo University Hospital, Ullevål, HF. All necessary ethical procedures were followed; the data protection service approved the project, and the Regional Committees for Medical and Health Research Ethics granted us ethical approval. Informed consent was sought from all participants as well as from their parents when below the age of 16.

2.3. The Intervention—Cognitive Remediation Therapy

All CRT sessions were delivered face-to-face, and followed the structure and content outlined in a CRT manual specifically developed for children and adolescents with AN [34]. In accordance with previous CRT studies [14,35], no efforts were made to explore themes normally addressed in ED treatment such as food, weight or shape. One to two tasks were administered each session followed by discussion. The selection of tasks was based on the therapist's clinical judgment, and chosen to address particular cognitive styles or difficulties specific to each individual. To help participants to engage in the meta-cognitive process, all tasks were accompanied or followed by questions encouraging the patients to reflect on their thinking processes. As an important part of CRT is to explore how experiences acquired in therapy can be transferred to real-life settings, homework tasks were introduced around session three or four. The aim of these tasks was for participants to use the knowledge acquired during CRT sessions, and to experiment with this knowledge outside the therapy context (e.g., in social settings, at school, or at work). Examples of these homework tasks can be found in the CRT Resource Pack [34,36].

2.4. Assessment—The CRT Treatment Evaluation Questionnaire

A treatment evaluation questionnaire was developed to investigate various aspects of treatment satisfaction and the participants' perspective of change (see Table 2). The questionnaire combines CRT-specific items generated by clinicians and researchers at the unit where CRT was delivered, and items derived from treatment satisfaction questionnaires published by Kunnskapssenteret (the Knowledge Center for Health Services) [37] and RIKSÄT (a Swedish national register for ED treatment) [38]. The 20-item questionnaire was divided into four sections each exploring different aspects of treatment: (1) general attitudes towards CRT (items 1–5), (2) treatment-specific items (items 7–10), (3) the perception of change (items 6, 11–16c), and (4) the relationship to the CRT therapist (items 17–20). Aspects 1, 2 and 4 were labelled *treatment satisfaction* and aspect 3 was labelled *perceived change*. All but one item (item 13) were closed questions, and with one exception (item 9), response options were rated on a 5-point Likert scale. Response options differed depending on the wording of each item, i.e. where the response options to the question *"How do you feel about the number of sessions"* (item 8) were "Way too few", "A little few", "Just enough", "A little too many" or "Way too many", the corresponding response options to the question "How did you experience the collaboration between you and your CRT therapist?" were "Very poor", Quite poor", "Both", "Quite good" or "Very good".

Table 2. The CRT Treatment Evaluation Questionnaire.

Item No.	Question
1.	Overall, how satisfied or dissatisfied are you with the course of CRT you have received? [1]
2.	Before you initiated CRT, you were informed about the treatment. Was this information useful? [1]
3.	How did your CRT experiences match the expectations you had prior to treatment initiation? [1]
4.	To what extent did you feel that the CRT sessions were useful to you? [1]
5.	Did you experience CRT as being relevant to your situation? [1]
6.	Did you acquire any skills during CRT that might be useful in your everyday life? [3]
7.	How do you feel about the length of the sessions? [2]
8.	How do you feel about the number of sessions? [2]
9.	How did you experience the division between practical exercises and discussion during the session (you can check as many boxes as you like)? [2]

Table 2. *Cont.*

Item No.	Question
10.	What is your opinion on the tasks used during the sessions? [2]
11.	How has the way you reflect on your own thinking changed during the course of CRT? [3]
12.	To what extent do you experience distress in relation to your eating disorder now, compared to before you started the CRT treatment program? [3]
13.	Are there other areas in your life which have become more or less difficult now, compared to before you started the CRT program? a) Example no. 1, b) Example no. 2
14.	What is your relationship to your family like now compared to before you started the CRT program? [3]
15.	How are things working out in your everyday life now, compared to before you entered the CRT treatment program? a) School/work? b) Leisure time/friends? [3]
16.	Do you think the CRT sessions have had an impact on your ability to change with regards to: a) Your eating disorder? b) School/work? c) Leisure time/friends? [3]
17.	How did you experience the collaboration between you and your CRT therapist? [4]
18.	Did you feel that you were treated with respect during the course of CRT? [4]
19.	Did the CRT therapist listen to you? [4]
20.	Did your therapist explain the tasks in a way that was easy to understand? [4]

Note: [1] = Items assessing general aspects of treatment; [2] = Items assessing treatment-specific aspects; [3] = Items assessing the perception of change; [4] = items assessing the participants' view of the CRT therapist. Items 1–5, 7–10 and 17–20 represent items specific *to treatment satisfaction*. Items 6, 11–15, and 16a,b represent items specific to *perceived change*. CRT = cognitive remediation therapy.

2.5. Analyses

Results are presented using bar graphs (see Appendix A), with the response option being presented on the x axis, and number of responses on the y axis. As response options differed depending on the wording of each item, it was not possible to create bar graphs reporting collated results. Items were therefore divided into the following four categories: (1) General attitudes towards treatment (items 1–5), (2) Treatment-specific items (items 7–10), (3) The perception of change (items 6 and 11–16c) and (4) The relationship to the CRT therapist (items 17–20) and presented as individual item graphs. Item 13a-b was excluded due to the low response rate ($N^{13a} = 5$, $N^{13b} = 9$), and large variations in examples of areas that had become more or less difficult after the course of CRT.

3. Results

A detailed overview of the results from the CRT treatment evaluation questionnaire is presented in Appendix A. There were no voluntary drop-outs, and 19 out of 20 participants completed the entire course of treatment. Eighteen out of the 20 participants completed the treatment evaluation questionnaire post-CRT.

3.1. Treatment Satisfaction

In terms of the general assessment, 16 participants (89%) were either "very satisfied" or "satisfied" with the course of CRT they had received. Seventeen participants (94%) reported that the course of treatment had matched their expectations, and the same number of participants also reported having acquired skills that could be useful in their everyday life (with answers ranging from "very few" to "many"). All participants (N = 18) reported that the CRT sessions had been useful. As for treatment-specific items, 100% of the participants (N = 18) were either "very satisfied" or "extremely satisfied" with the tasks used during the sessions. Thirteen participants (72%) felt that the session length and the division between practical exercises and discussion were "just right". Ten participants (56%) reported the total number of sessions to be "a little few", whereas seven participants (39%) reported that the number of sessions were "just enough". Overall, participants responded highly affirmative with regards to the therapist-specific items (items 17–20). For example, 15 (83%) participants reported that the collaboration between the patient and therapist was "very good", and an equal number felt they had been treated with respect during the intervention and that the therapist had listened to them. Seventy-eight percent of the participants (N = 14) reported that the therapist had explained the tasks in a way that was easy to understand (item 20).

3.2. The Perception of Change

The perception of change was evaluated in relation to ED-specific items, but also in terms of other aspects of life, such as school or work, leisure time, friends and family. Eleven out of 18 participants (61%) reported that they were either slightly, or much more aware of their thinking style post CRT. Fifty-nine percent of the participants (N = 10) reported that ED-related distress was "more or less the same as before" CRT, and seven participants (41%) chose the same response when probed to appraise their relationship to their family post-CRT. Eight participants (47%) reported a "slightly better" relationship to their family after the intervention. As for items related to everyday functioning (item 15a-b), the majority of participants (61%, N = 11) reported that school/work was "more or less the same as before" CRT. Corresponding numbers for leisure time/friends was N = 8 (44%). Whereas 10 participants (56%) reported that the CRT sessions had had "a little" (N = 7), "quite a lot" (N = 2) or "a lot" (N = 1) of impact on their ability to change with regards to the ED, 44% of the patients (N = 8) reported that CRT had had either "very little" (N = 5) or "none not at all" (N = 3) impact on ED-related change. Results were almost identical with regards to perceived change in relation to school and/or work. The intervention appeared to have had limited impact on the participants' perceived change with regards to leisure and/or social activities with six participants (40%) choosing the response option "very little", five participants (33%) "little", three participants (20%) quite a lot and one patient (7%) "a lot".

4. Discussion

The aim of the current study was to investigate post-intervention feedback from a feasibility study on CRT for adolescents, and to delineate the individuals' perspective in terms of general and specific attitudes towards treatment, and the relationship to the CRT therapist. Perceived change post-CRT was also investigated using ED-specific and non-ED-specific items. Overall, results indicate high levels of treatment satisfaction, both in terms of general attitudes towards treatment, treatment specifics (e.g., treatment length, content, tasks, etc.), and the relationship to the therapist, but somewhat limited perceptions of change.

4.1. Treatment Satisfaction

Tasks used in CRT are based on their potential playful capacity, and it is hypothesized that their simple, non-threatening nature help engage patients in treatment, and encourage curiosity rather than resistance [14,39,40]. This was supported in the current study where the majority of patients reported being either slightly or very satisfied with the tasks used to identify and challenge cognitive styles. Our results regarding task specifics are also in line with those recently published by Giombini et al. [20] supporting the use of board games and puzzles presented in the CRT Resource Pack [36]. Ten sessions is the length of treatment most commonly provided in both adult, child and adolescent CRT delivery. However, the results presented here call into question whether ten sessions are enough. More than half of the patients in our study reported that the number of sessions was "a little few", and similar to the study by van Noort et al. [22], some of the patients actually requested additional sessions, an underreported phenomenon in patients with AN. In contrast to patient feedback in Wood et al.'s study from 2011 [40] where sessions exceeding 30 minutes were felt as being too long, the majority of patients in the current study reported the session length to be "just right", and a few patients actually thought the sessions were a little short. In addition, the majority of patients in the current study communicated that they were satisfied with the treatment that they had received, and on an overall level, patients reported that the CRT sessions were both useful and relevant to their situation. Thus, in stark contrast to other treatment studies in EDs where adolescents with AN often report negative recollections of their treatment [41], CRT appears to provide a positive framework for this particular patient group.

High levels of dropout is a recurrent issue in treatment of AN, suggesting that a number of patients are either unwilling or unable to engage in treatment. Dropout rates for adolescents with AN who are hospitalized are reported as high as 24% [42], and even though dropout rates are less frequent in adolescents than in adults, a 95% completion rate, as reported in the current study, is unusual—and highly promising—for this group of patients. As treatment compliance has been shown to be a facilitator for recovery and a predictor of a successful outcome [43], it is paramount that we identify therapies that increase compliance and therapy adherence.

CRT for adolescents has been administered in a variety of modes including individual delivery [19,22,35], family-CRT [44], CRT delivered in collaboration with carers [45] and in groups [39,40]. In the current study, CRT was provided individually with one therapist delivering all treatment. One major advantage of individually delivered CRT is the possibility to tailor the treatment to each specific patient. In our case, CRT sessions were dedicated exclusively to the specific needs and circumstances of each individual, and it is not unlikely that such exclusivity could have had a positive effect in strengthening the therapist–patient bond. A good therapeutic alliance is known to predict treatment adherence and better outcomes in patients with EDs [46], especially young patients [47], and previous research in eating disorders suggests that treatment satisfaction is closely related to the way in which care is delivered [48]. In the current study, the vast majority of patients chose the most favorable response outcome ("very good") when asked about the collaboration between the patient and the therapist, and the remaining therapist-specific items were answered equally, positively affirmative. Favourable outcomes, such as these, might reflect a number of aspects specific to CRT. Firstly, it is likely that the very nature of the intervention plays an important role in this type of feedback. In contrast to traditional ED treatment, CRT does not focus on core ED psychopathology such as weight, shape or eating. The lack of focus on ED symptomatology, which is often emotionally charged, might have rendered patients curious, rather than reluctant, and motivated rather than discouraged to engage and remain in treatment.

4.2. Perception of Change

In line with a recently published study by Giombini et al. [20], individuals in the current study experienced limited transferability of skills from the therapy context to their everyday lives. In Giombini et al.'s study [20], patients were asked to provide feedback on the CRT sessions as a way of evaluating the program. Although CRT was positively received by the majority of patients, a group of patients reported difficulties in understanding how CRT might be helpful in their everyday life, and what impact it would have on their recovery. In an adult CRT study by Easter and Tchanturia [49], similar findings are reported. This study used therapists' feedback letter to investigate the implementation of CRT in the patients' day-to-day life. Comparable to the current study, these patients also found it challenging when attempting to relate skills acquired in CRT to their everyday lives. A similar methodological approach, with comparable findings, was presented in a recently published study by Giombini et al. [50]. In their qualitative appraisal of young peoples' experience of individual CRT, only 13% (N = 9) of the patients were able to describe how they could use knowledge acquired during CRT sessions in their daily life. In the current study, more than half of the patients reported that they had acquired either quite a few or many skills during CRT sessions that could be useful in their everyday life. However, when probed more specifically on whether CRT had impacted the ability to change—either with regards to the eating disorder or their everyday life—the majority of patients reported "Not at all", "Very little" or "Little". These results call into question the direct transferability of in-session learning, suggesting that more work needs to be done in order to help patients to channel new insights and behaviors from the inside to the outside of the therapy room.

To the authors' knowledge, this is one of two [51] existing studies to explicitly investigate how individuals perceive everyday life and ED-related changes post CRT. Despite the majority of participants reporting being slightly more, or more, aware of how they reflect on their own thinking after CRT, our results indicate that they find the impact of CRT on the ability to change to be fairly limited. It could be argued that this is due to difficulties in evaluating one's own change. In a previous study investigating self-reported executive functioning before and after CRT, Dahlgren and colleagues [3] showed that parents reported a greater extent of change in their child's everyday behaviors, in comparison to the patients' own reports. This could be due to biased post-intervention ratings based on anticipation or wishful thinking, or it could be because adolescents have difficulties in evaluating their own behavior and potential changes in behavior and attitudes. Another explanation is that changes in cognitions and behaviors require far more than ten CRT sessions to appear, or in our case, perceived by patients themselves.

5. Strengths and Limitations

Altogether, the participants in the current study appeared to find CRT useful and relevant, and the vast majority of patients reported being very satisfied with the relationship to the CRT therapist. However, since it is well documented that a good alliance between the patient and the therapist is central to engaging patients and motivating them to stay in treatment [46,47], it is possible that the role of the therapist played an important part in treatment adherence. For example, it is difficult to differentiate "treatment satisfaction" from "therapist satisfaction". It is unknown whether the results would have changed if more than one therapist had delivered the CRT, and that such changes had been independent of the treatment per se. Further, we cannot exclude a therapist-specific contribution to the observed low dropout rate. Thus, it remains to be investigated if the results from the current study can be reproduced in other contexts with a number of therapists delivering the intervention remains. The study is also limited in terms of its sample size and the age range. It is likely that the perspective of change more easily can be reflected on and self-assessed by an individual at age 18 compared to someone at age 13. Further, as response options differed between items, it was not possible to report summary scores or merged data from the four different sections of the questionnaire. In-depth interviews could have served as an important adjunct to our questionnaire, allowing for qualitative analyses of the service user's perspective.

Finally, the study is limited by not providing anonymous feedback forms. This is a limitation not just for the current study, but for all studies that have so far been published on patients' perception of CRT. Patients' reports are likely to be biased as all patients knew that the therapist would read their feedback forms. In addition, as AN patients often have a tendency of seeking social approval [52,53], this is especially important to take into consideration when evaluating patient feedback.

6. Conclusions

The current study provides one of the most detailed accounts of the patient's perspective on CRT published for adolescent patients with AN. The findings highlight several important intervention aspects viewed through the eye of the receiver. On an overall level, patients reported CRT sessions as being both useful and relevant to their situation, and the majority of patients communicated that they were satisfied with the treatment they had received. On the other hand, and in line with a number of previous studies, the findings also indicate that patients perceived limited impact of CRT in terms of changes in their everyday-life functioning and their eating disorder. Such results warrant further investigation and a critical evaluation of treatment content, as well as of outcome measures used. Future studies might want to place an emphasis on crystalizing the primary purpose of CRT for adolescents with AN, and choose outcome measures appropriate to assess expected outcomes. If, as pointed out by Dahlgren and Rø [9], the main aim of CRT is to prepare the patients for subsequent treatment, future CRT studies should place further emphasis on motivational aspects of treatment and its likelihood of preventing drop-out, rather than focusing on the direct effect of CRT on measurable cognitive or behavioral changes.

Acknowledgments: This work was funded, in its entirety, by the Regional Department for Eating Disorders (RASP), Oslo University Hospital HF, Ullevål. Costs associated with open access publishing were also funded by RASP.

Author Contributions: Dahlgren, C.L. conceived and designed the experiments; Dahlgren, C.L. performed the experiments; Dahlgren, C.L. and Stedal, K. analyzed the data; Oslo University Hospital contributed materials/analysis tools; Dahlgren, C.L. and Stedal, K. wrote the paper.

Conflicts of Interest: The authors declare no conflict of interest.

Appendix A

Item-Specific Results from the Treatment Evaluation Questionnaire (N = 18). *Note.* Response options are presented on the x axis, and number of responses are presented on the y axis. Items with an asterisk (*) indicate fewer than N = 18 responses.

Appendix A.1 General Attitudes towards Treatment (Item 1–5)

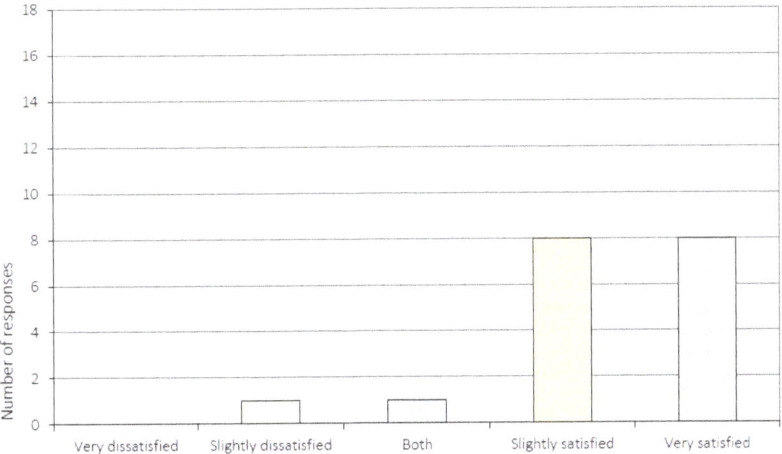

Figure A1. Overall, how satisfied or dissatisfied are you with the course of CRT that you have received?

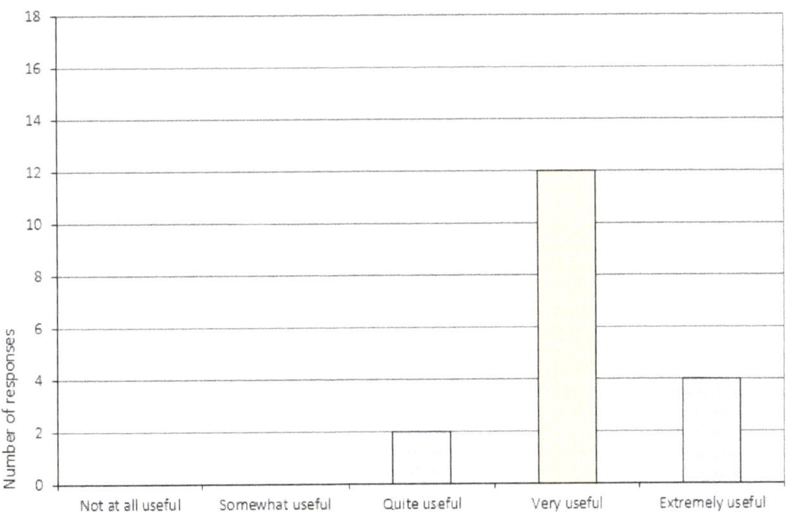

Figure A2. Before initiating CRT you were informed about the treatment. Was this information useful?

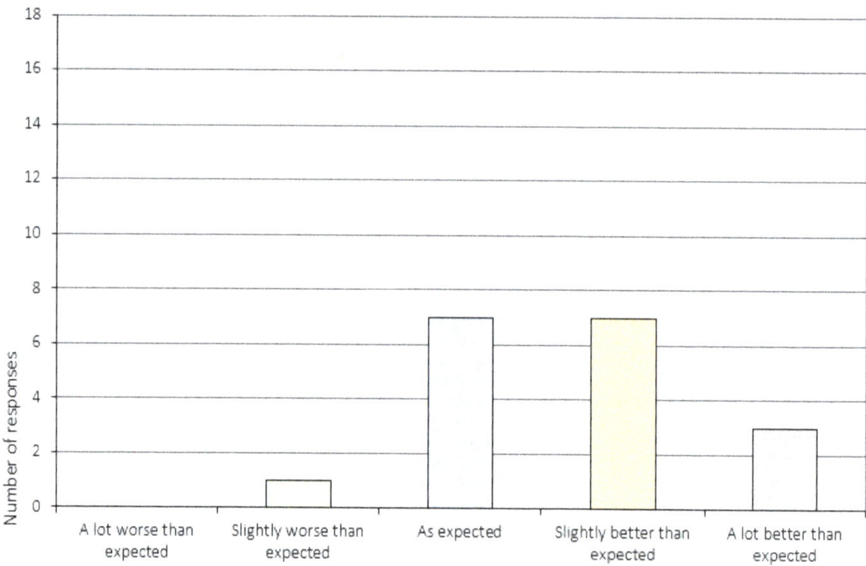

Figure A3. How did your CRT experience match the expectancies you had prior to treatment initiation?

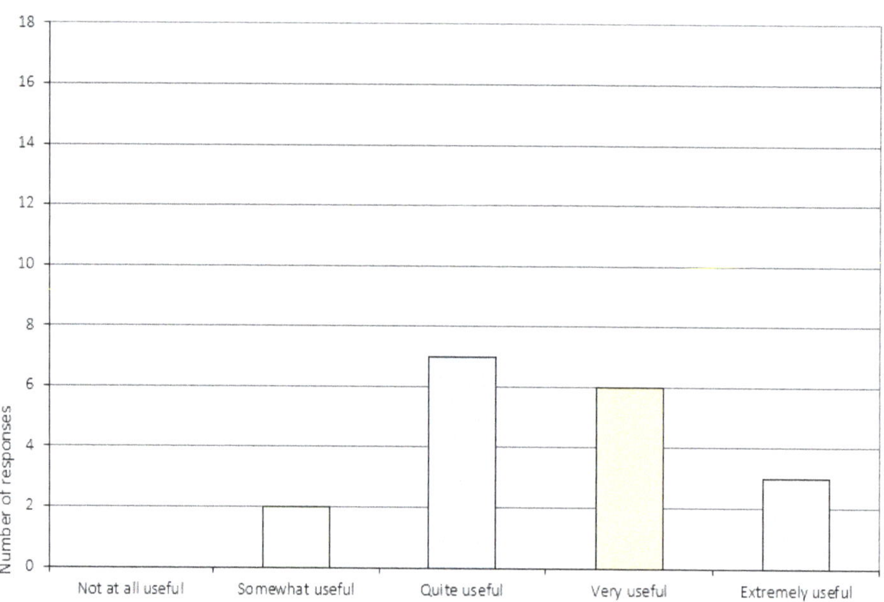

Figure A4. To what extent did you feel that the CRT sessions were useful to you?

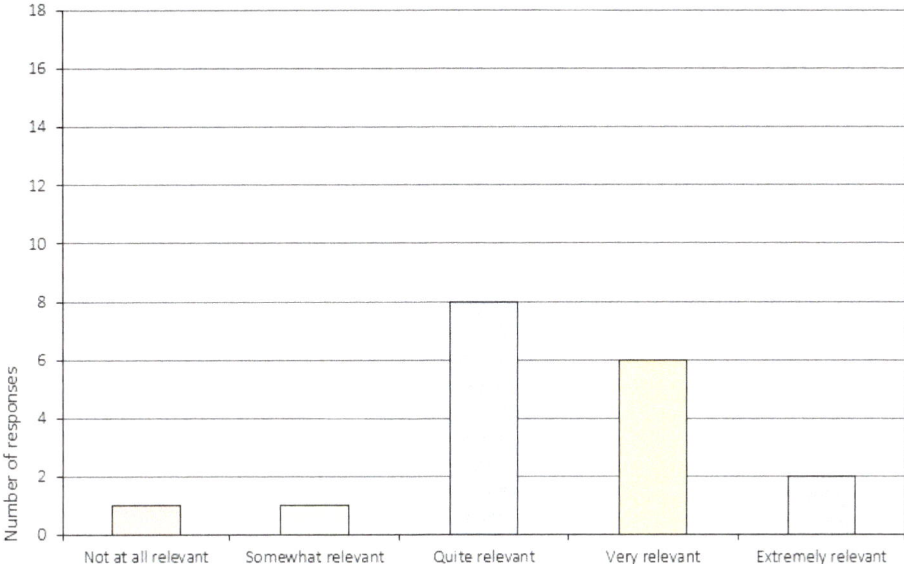

Figure A5. Did you experience CRT as being relevant to your situation?

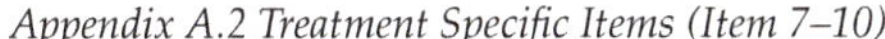

Appendix A.2 Treatment Specific Items (Item 7–10)

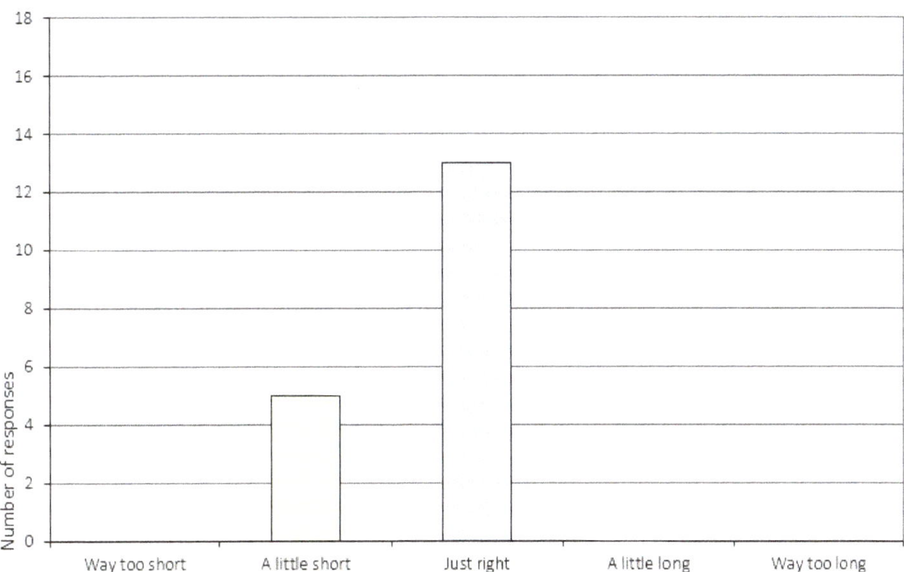

Figure A7. How did you feel about the the length of the sessions?

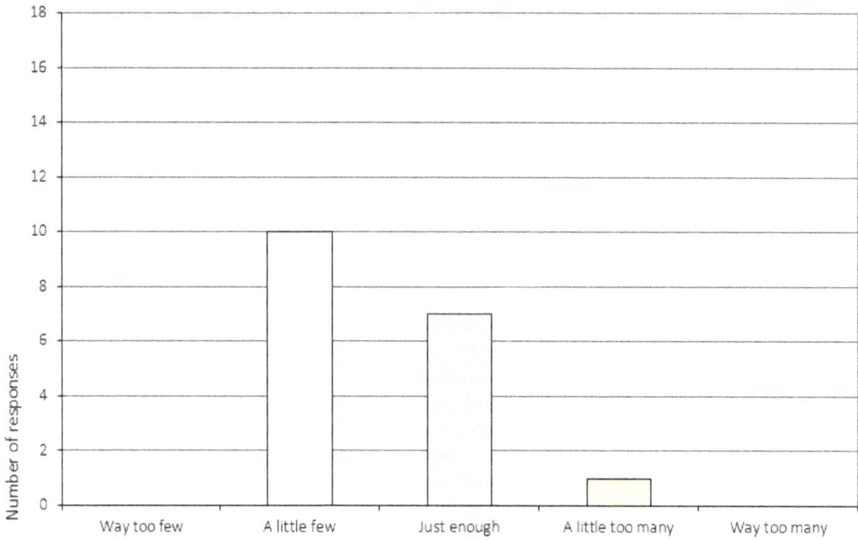

Figure A8. How did you feel about the number of session?

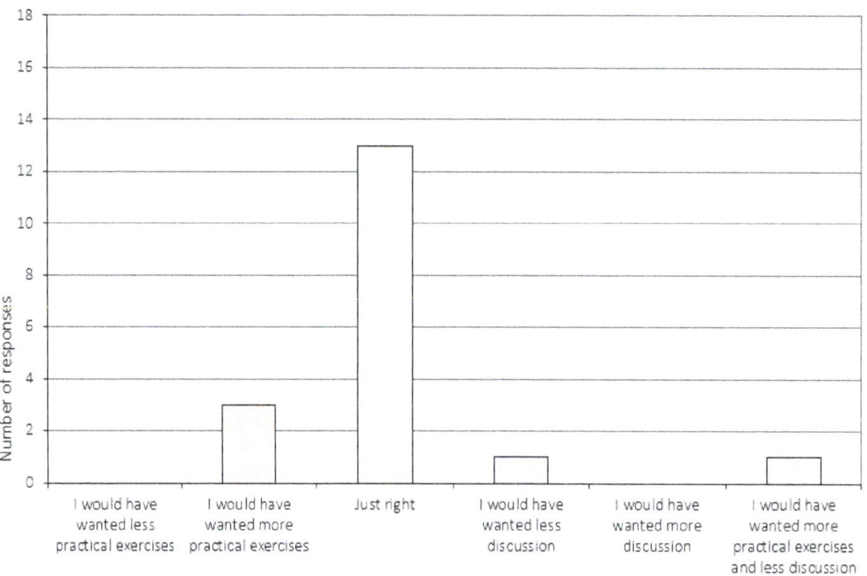

Figure A9. How did you experience the division between practical exercises and discussion during the sessions?

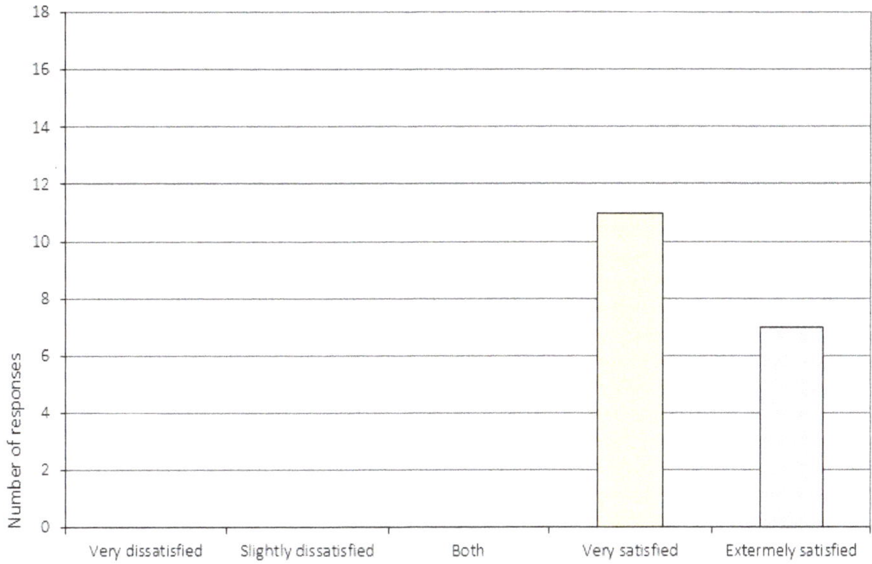

Figure A10. All in all, how satisfied or dissatisfied are you with the course of CRT that you have received?

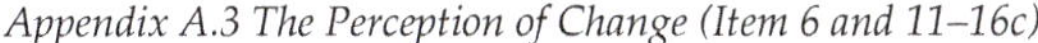

Appendix A.3 The Perception of Change (Item 6 and 11–16c)

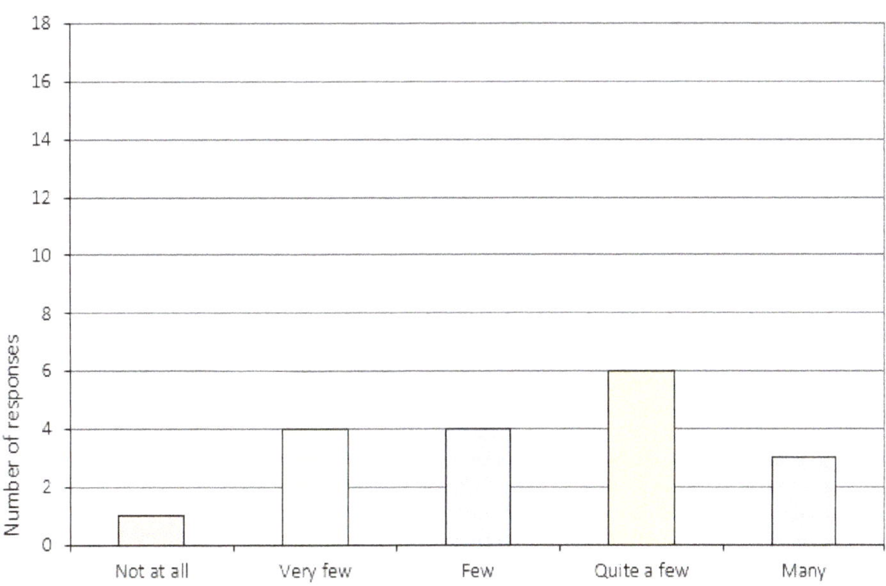

Figure A6. Did you acquire any skills during the CRT sessions that might be useful in your everyday life?

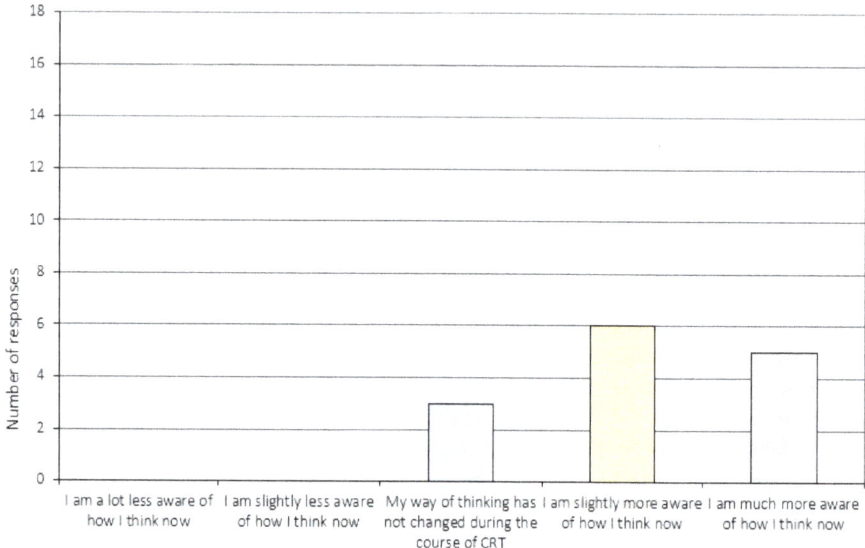

Figure A11. How has the way you reflect on your own thinking changed during the course of CRT? (*N = 14).

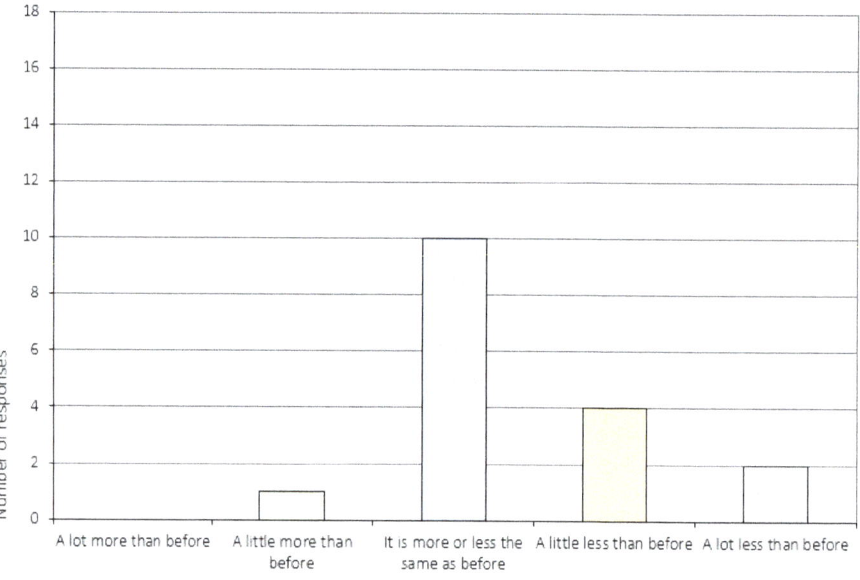

Figure A12. To what extent do you experience distress in relation to your eating disorder now, compared to before you started the CRT treatment program? (*N = 17).

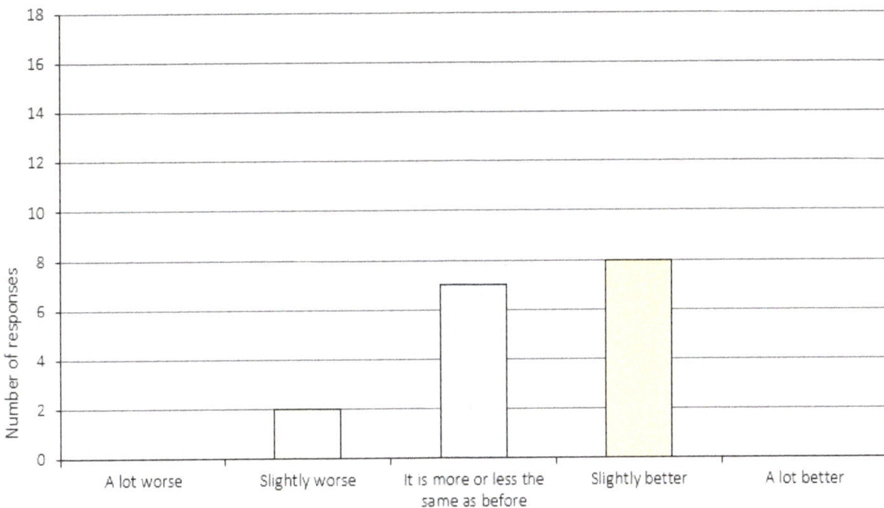

Figure A14. How is your relationship to your family now, compared to before you started the CRT treatment program? (*N = 17).

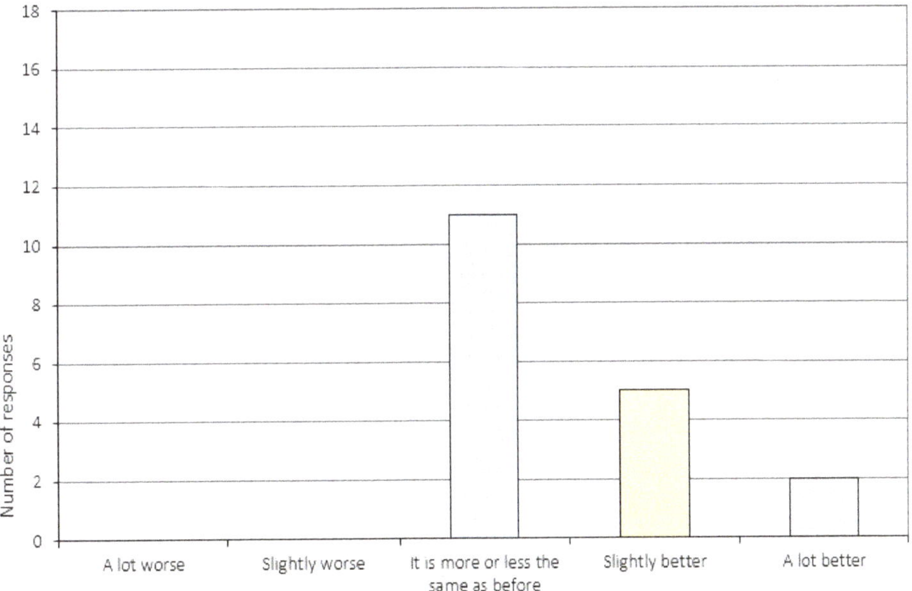

Figure A15a. How are things working out in your daily life now, compared to before you started the CRT treatment program? (**a**) School/Work.

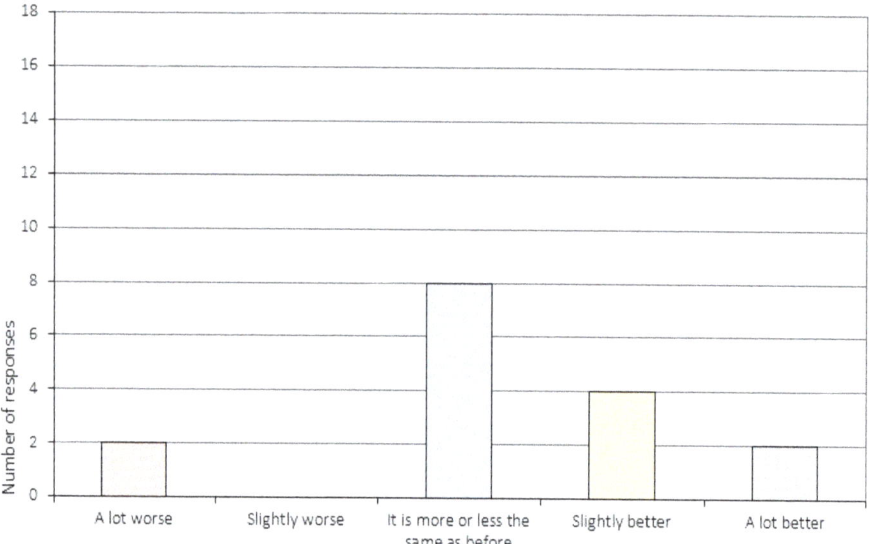

Figure A15b. How are things working out in your daily life now, compared to before you started the CRT treatment program? (b)Leisure time/friends (*N = 16).

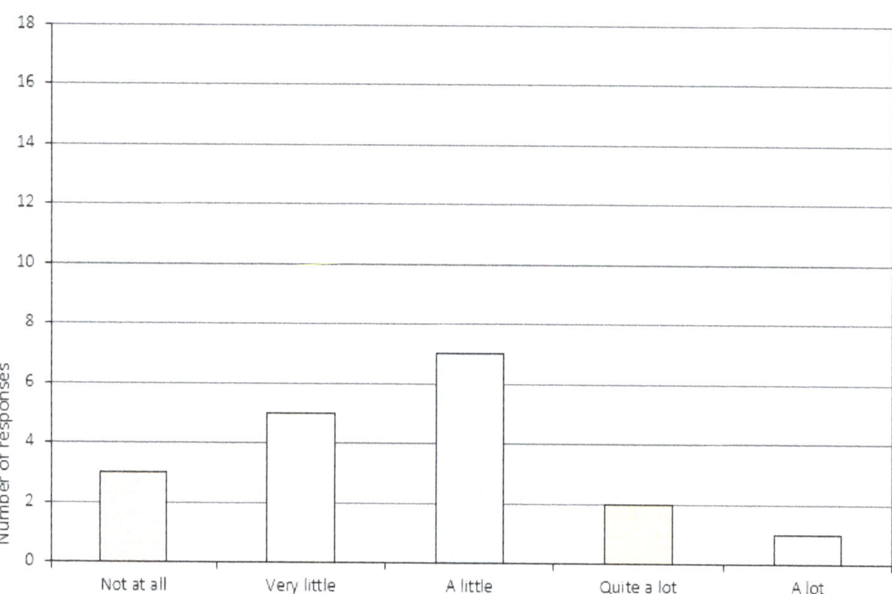

Figure A16a. Do you think the CRT sessions have had an impact on your ability to change with regards to your eating disorder?

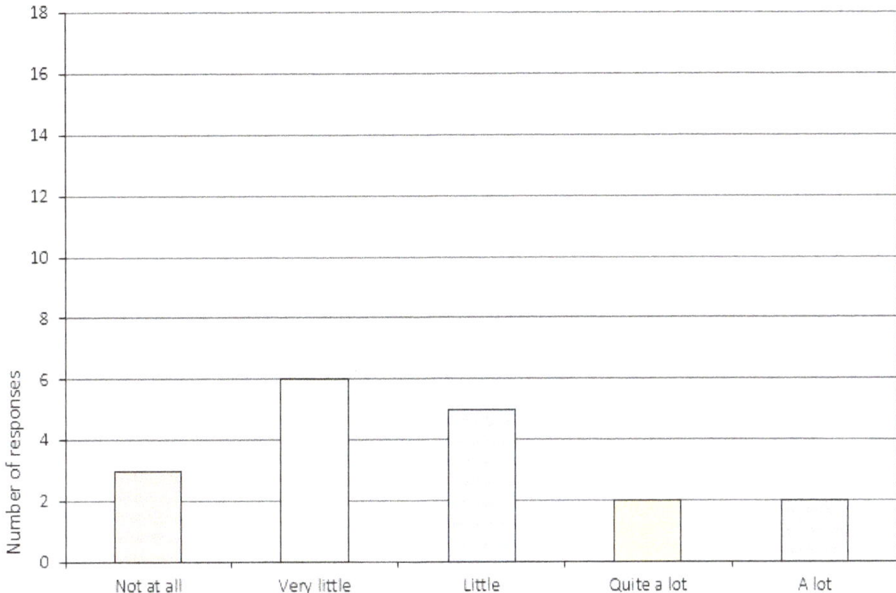

Figure A16b. Do you think the CRT sessions have had an impact on your ability to change with regards to school/work?

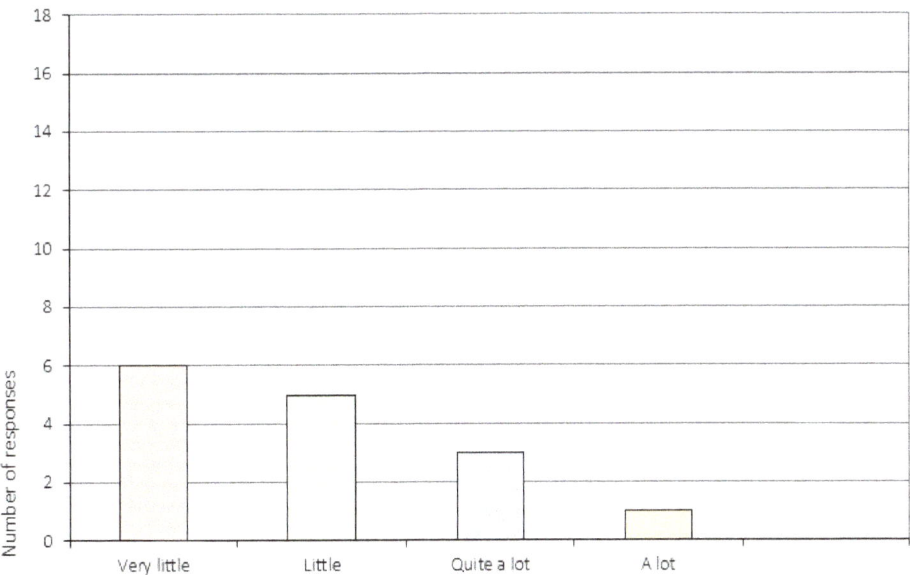

Figure A16c. Do you think the CRT sessions have had an impact on your ability to change with regards to leisure time/friends? (*N = 15).

Appendix A.4 The Relationship to the CRT Therapist (Item 17–20)

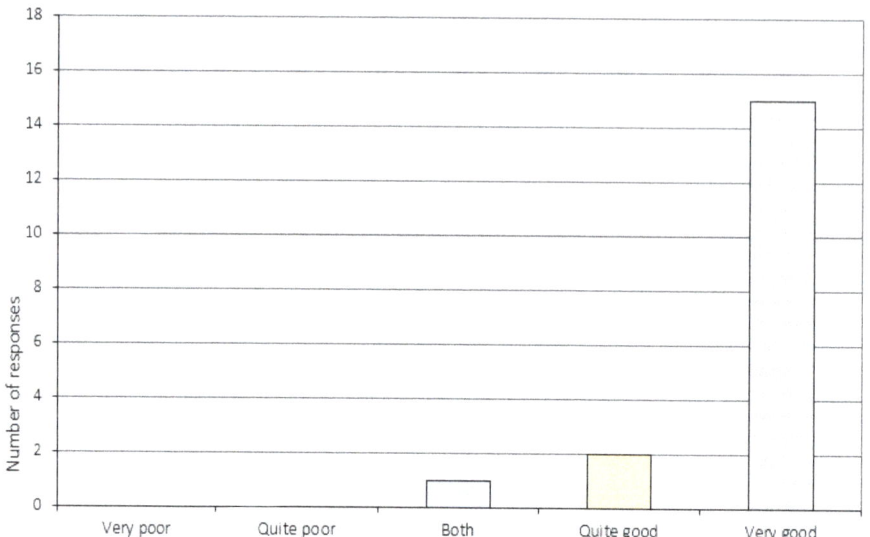

Figure A17. How did you experience the collaboration between you and your CRT therapist?

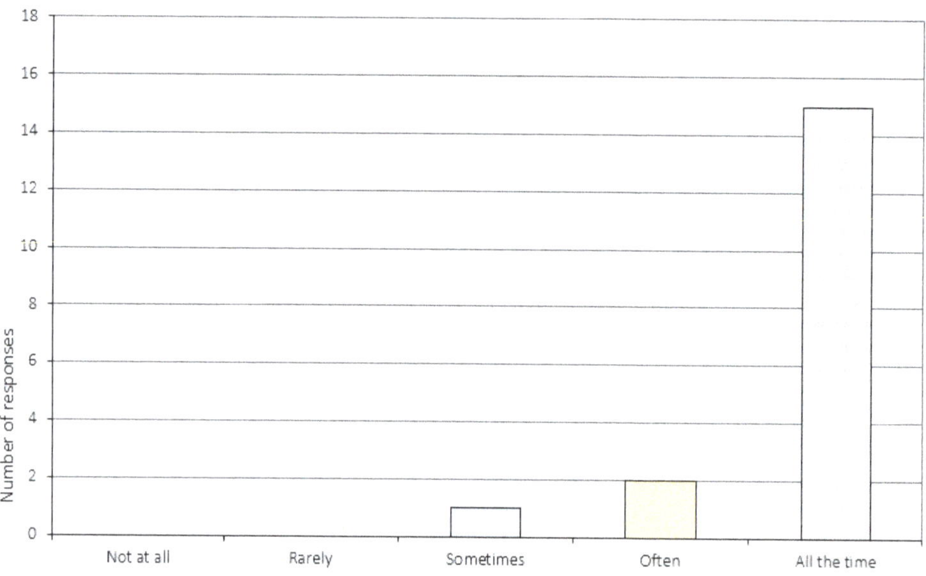

Figure A18. Were you treated with respect during the course of CRT?

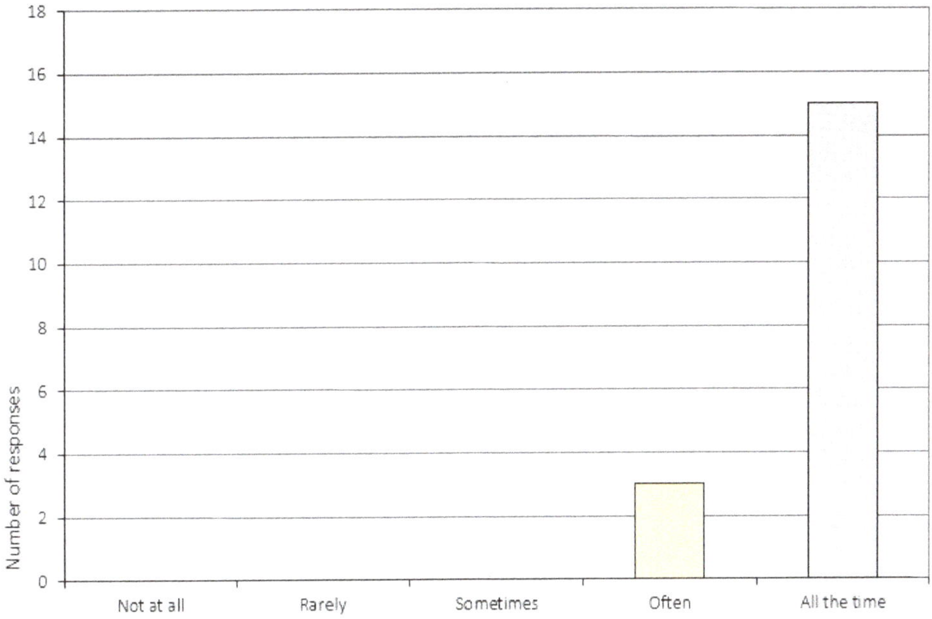

Figure A19. Did the CRT therapist listen to you?

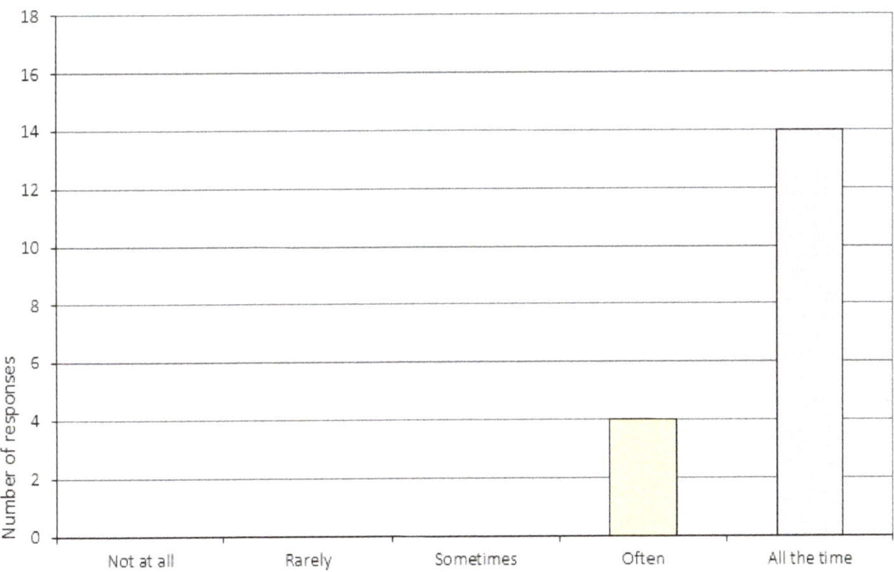

Figure A20. Did your therapist explain the tasks in a way that was easy to understand?

References

1. American Psychological Association. *Diagnostic and Statistical Manual of Mental Disorders*, 5th ed.; American Psychiatric Association: Washington, DC, USA, 2013.

2. Stedal, K.; Frampton, I.; Landrø, N.I.; Lask, B. An Examination of the Ravello Profile—A Neuropsychological Test Battery for Anorexia Nervosa. *Eur. Eat. Disord. Rev.* **2012**, *20*, 175–181.
3. Dahlgren, C.L.; Lask, B.; Landrø, N.I.; Rø, Ø. Patient and Parental Self-reports of Executive Functioning in a Sample of Young Female Adolescents with Anorexia Nervosa Before and After Cognitive Remediation Therapy. *Eur. Eat. Disord. Rev.* **2014**, *22*, 45–52. [CrossRef] [PubMed]
4. Perpina, C.; Segura, M.; Sanchez-Reales, S. Cognitive flexibility and decision-making in eating disorders and obesity. *Eat Weight Disord.* **2016**. [CrossRef]
5. Aloi, M.; Rania, M.; Caroleo, M.; Bruni, A.; Cauteruccio, M.A.; De Fazio, P.; Segura-Garcia, C. Decision making, central coherence and set-shifting: a comparison between Binge Eating Disorder, Anorexia Nervosa and Healthy Controls. *BMC Psychiatr.* **2015**, *15*, 6. [CrossRef]
6. Lang, K.; Lopez, C.; Stahl, D.; Tchanturia, K.; Treasure, J. Central Coherence in Eating Disorders: A Synthesis of Studies Using the Rey Osterrieth Complex Figure Test. *PLoS ONE* **2016**, *11*, e0165467. [CrossRef] [PubMed]
7. Lang, K.; Tchanturia, K. A systematic review of central coherence in children and adolescents with anorexia nervosa. *J. Child. Adolesc. Behav.* **2014**, *2*, 140. [CrossRef]
8. Davies, H.; Tchanturia, K. Cognitive Remediation Therapy as an Intervention for Acute Anorexia Nervosa: A Case Report. *Eur. Eat. Disord. Rev.* **2005**, *13*, 311–316. [CrossRef]
9. Dahlgren, C.; Rø, Ø. A systematic review of cognitive remediation therapy for anorexia nervosa-development, current state and implications for future research and clinical practice. *J. Eat. Disord.* **2014**, *2*, 26.
10. Brockmeyer, T.; Ingenerf, K.; Walther, S.; Wild, B.; Hartmann, M.; Herzog, W.; Bents, H.; Friederich, H.C. Training cognitive flexibility in patients with anorexia nervosa: A pilot randomized controlled trial of cognitive remediation therapy. *Int. J. Eat. Disord.* **2013**, *47*, 24–31. [CrossRef] [PubMed]
11. Lock, J.; Agras, W.S.; Fitzpatrick, K.K.; Bryson, S.W.; Jo, B.; Tchanturia, K. Is outpatient cognitive remediation therapy feasible to use in randomized clinical trials for anorexia nervosa? *Int. J. Eat. Disord.* **2013**, *46*, 567–575. [CrossRef] [PubMed]
12. Brockmeyer, T.; Ingenerf, K.; Walther, S.; Wild, B.; Hartmann, M.; Herzog, W.; Bents, H.; Friederich, H.C. Training cognitive flexibility in patients with anorexia nervosa: A pilot randomized controlled trial of cognitive remediation therapy. *Int. J. Eat. Disord.* **2014**, *47*, 24–31. [CrossRef] [PubMed]
13. Dingemans, A.E.; Danner, U.N.; Donker, J.M.; aardoom, J.J.; van Meer, F.; Tobias, K.; van Elburg, A.A.; van Furth, E.F. The effectiveness of cognitive remediation therapy in patients with a severe or enduring eating disorder: A randomized controlled trial. *Psychother. Psychosom.* **2014**, *83*, 29–36. [CrossRef] [PubMed]
14. Dahlgren, C.L.; Lask, B.; Landrø, N.I.; Rø, Ø. Developing and evaluating cognitive remediation therapy (CRT) for adolescents with anorexia nervosa: a feasibility study. *Clin. Child. Psychol. Psychiatry* **2014**, *19*, 476–487. [CrossRef] [PubMed]
15. Tchanturia, K.; Lounes, N.; Holttum, S. Cognitive remediation in anorexia nervosa and related conditions: A systematic review. *Eur. Eat. Disord. Rev.* **2014**, *22*, 454–462. [CrossRef] [PubMed]
16. van Noort, B.M.; Kraus, M.K.A.; Pfeiffer, E.; Lehmkuhl, U.; Kappel, V. Neuropsychological and Behavioural Short-Term Effects of Cognitive Remediation Therapy in Adolescent Anorexia Nervosa: A Pilot Study. *Eur. Eat. Disord. Rev.* **2016**, *24*, 69–74. [CrossRef] [PubMed]
17. Tchanturia, K.; Davies, H.; Reeder, C.; Wykes, T. Cognitive Remediation Therapy for Anorexia Nervosa. 2010. Available online: www.katetchanturia.com (accessed on 2 March 2017).
18. Owen, I.; Lindvall, C.L.; Lask, B. Cognitive Remediation Therapy. In *Eating Disorders in Childhood and Adolescence*; Lask, B., Bryant-Waugh, R., Eds.; Routledge: New York, NY, USA, 2013; pp. 301–318.
19. Giombini, L.; Moynihan, J.; Turco, M.; Nesbitt, S. Evaluation of individual cognitive remediation therapy (CRT) for the treatment of young people with anorexia nervosa. *Eat. Weight. Disord.* **2016**. [CrossRef] [PubMed]
20. Giombini, L.; Turton, R.; Turco, M.; Nesbitt, S.; Lask, B. The use of cognitive remediation therapy on a child adolescent eating disorder unit: Patients and therapist perspectives. *Clin. Child. Psychol. Psychiatry* **2017**, *22*, 288–300. [CrossRef] [PubMed]
21. van Noort, B.M.; Pfeiffer, E.; Ehrlich, S.; Lehmkuhl, U.; Kappel, V. Cognitive performance in children with acute early-onset anorexia nervosa. *Eur. Child. Adolesc. Psychiatry.* **2016**, *25*, 1233–1244. [CrossRef] [PubMed]
22. van Noort, B.M.; Pfeiffer, E.; Lehmkuhl, U.; Kappel, V. Cognitive Remediation Therapy for Children with Anorexia Nervosa. *Z. Kinder. Jugendpsychiatr. Psychother.* **2015**, *43*, 351–355. [CrossRef] [PubMed]

23. Doran, D.; Smith, P. Measuring service quality provision within an eating disorders context. *Int. J. Health. Care Qual. Assur. Inc. Leadersh. Health Serv.* **2004**, *17*, 377–388. [CrossRef] [PubMed]
24. Newton, T. Consumer involvement in the appraisal of treatment for people with eating disorders: A neglected area of research? *Eur. Eat. Disord. Rev.* **2001**, *9*, 301–308. [CrossRef]
25. Bell, L. What can we learn from consumer studies and qualitative research in the treatment of eating disorders? *Eat. Weight Disord.* **2003**, *8*, 181–187. [CrossRef] [PubMed]
26. de la Rie, S.; Noordenbos, G.; Donker, M.; van Furth, E. Evaluating the treatment of eating disorders from the patient's perspective. *Int. J. Eat. Disord.* **2006**, *39*, 667–676. [CrossRef] [PubMed]
27. Wechsler, D. *Wechsler Adult Intelligence Scale-Third Edition (WAIS-III)*; Harcourt Assessment: London, UK, 1997.
28. Wechsler, D. *Wechsler Abbreviated Scale of Intelligence (WASI)*; NCS Pearson Inc.: San Antonio, TX, USA, 1999.
29. Wechsler, D. *Wechsler Intelligence Scale for Children-Third Edition (WISC-III)*; The Psychological Corporation Europe: London, UK, 1992.
30. Fairburn, C.G.; Beglin, S.J. Assessment of Eating Disorders, Interview or Self-Report Questionnaire. *Int. J. Eat. Disord.* **1994**, *16*, 363–370. [PubMed]
31. Beck, A.T.; Steer, R.A.; Brown, G.K. *Manual for the Beck Depression Inventory-II*; Psychological Corporation: San Antonio, TX, USA, 1996.
32. Spielberger, C.D.; Goursuch, R.; Lushene, R. *Manual for the State Trait Anxiety Inventory*; Consulting Psychologists Press: Mountain View, CA, USA, 1983.
33. Dahlgren, C.L. *Cognitive Remediation Therapy for Young Female Adolescents with Anorexia Nervosa—Assessing the Feasibility of a Novel Eating Disorder Intervention*; Oslo University Hospital: Oslo, Norway, 2014.
34. Lindvall, C.; Owen, I.; Lask, B. *The CRT Resource Pack for Children and Adolescents with Anorexia Nervosa*; Oslo University Hospital: Ullevål HF, Oslo, Norway, 2010; Available online: http://www.researchgate.com (accessed on 1 April 2016).
35. Dahlgren, C.L.; Lask, B.; Landrø, N.I.; Rø, Ø. Neuropsychological functioning in adolescents with anorexia nervosa before and after cognitive remediation therapy: A feasibility trial. *Int. J. Eat. Disord* **2013**, *46*, 576–581.
36. Dahlgren, C.L.; van Noort, B.M.; Lask, B. *The Cognitive Remediation Therapy (CRT) Resource Pack for Children and Adolescents with Feeding and Eating Disorders*, 2nd ed.; Oslo University Hospital: Oslo, Norway, 2015; Available online: http://www.rasp.no/ (accessed on 1 January 2017).
37. Holmboe, O.; Groven, G.; Olsen, R.V. *Brukererfaringer med poliklinikker for voksne i det psykiske helsevernet 2007*; PasOpp-rapport nr 6-2008 fra Kunnskapssenteret; Norwegian Knowledge Centre for the Health Services: Olso, Norway, 2008.
38. Lago, C.; Norring, C.; Engström, I. Enkät om behandlingstillfredsställelse: RIKSÄT: Nationellt Kvalitetsregister för Ätstörningsbehandling. Available online: http://kcp.se/kvalitetsregister/riksat/arbetsmaterial-dokument/ (accessed on 15 January 2010).
39. Pretorius, N.; Dimmer, M.; Power, E.; Eisler, I.; Simic, M.; Tcanturia, K. Evaluation of a cognitive remediation therapy group for adolescents with anorexia nervosa: Pilot study. *Eur. Eat. Disord. Rev.* **2012**, *20*, 321–325. [CrossRef] [PubMed]
40. Wood, L.; Al-Khairulla, H.; Lask, B. Group cognitive remediation therapy for adolescents with anorexia nervosa. *Clin. Child Psychol. Psychiatry* **2011**, *16*, 225–231. [CrossRef] [PubMed]
41. Halvorsen, I.; Heyerdahl, S. Treatment perception in adolescent onset anorexia nervosa: Retrospective views of patients and parents. *Int. J. Eat. Disord.* **2007**, *40*, 629–639. [CrossRef] [PubMed]
42. Roux, H.; Ali, A.; Lambert, S.; Radon, L.; Huas, C.; Curt, F.; Berthoz, S.; Godart, N. Predictive factors of dropout from inpatient treatment for anorexia nervosa. *BMC Psychiatr.* **2016**, *16*, 339. [CrossRef] [PubMed]
43. Towell, D.B.; Woodford, S.; Reid, S.; Rooney, B.; Towell, A. Compliance and outcome in treatment-resistant anorexia and bulimia: A retrospective study. *Br. J. Clin. Psychol.* **2001**, *40*, 189–195. [CrossRef] [PubMed]
44. Lask, B.; Roberts, A. Family cognitive remediation therapy for anorexia nervosa. *Clin. Child Psychol. Psychiatr.* **2015**, *20*, 207–217. [CrossRef] [PubMed]
45. Lang, K.; Treasure, J.; Tchanturia, K. Acceptability and feasibility of self-help Cognitive Remediation Therapy for anorexia nervosa delivered in collaboration with carers: A qualitative preliminary evaluation study. *Psychiatry Res.* **2015**, *225*, 387–394. [CrossRef] [PubMed]

46. Graves, T.A.; Tabri, N.; Thompson-Brenner, H.; Franko, D.L.; Eddy, K.T.; Bourion-Bedes, S.; Brown, A.; Constantino, M.J.; Fluckiger, C.; Forsberg, S.; et al. A meta-analysis of the relation between therapeutic alliance and treatment outcome in eating disorders. *Int. J. Eat. Disord.* **2017**, *50*, 323–340. [CrossRef] [PubMed]
47. Zaitsoff, S.; Pullmer, R.; Cyr, M.; Aime, H. The role of the therapeutic alliance in eating disorder treatment outcomes: A systematic review. *Eat. Disord.* **2015**, *23*, 99–114. [CrossRef] [PubMed]
48. Gulliksen, K.S.; Espeset, E.M.; Nordbø, R.H.; Skårderud, F.; Geller, J.; Holte, A. Preferred therapist characteristics in treatment of anorexia nervosa: The patient's perspective. *Int. J. Eat. Disord.* **2012**, *45*, 932–941. [CrossRef] [PubMed]
49. Easter, A.; Tchanturia, K. Therapists' experiences of cognitive remediation therapy for anorexia nervosa: Implications for working with adolescents. *Clin. Child Psychol. Psychiatr.* **2011**, *16*, 233–246. [CrossRef] [PubMed]
50. Giombini, L.; Nesbitt, S.; Waples, L.; Finazzi, E.; Easter, A.; Tchanturia, K. Young people's experience of individual cognitive remediation therapy (CRT) in an inpatient eating disorder service: A qualitative study. *Eat. Weight Disord.* **2017**. [CrossRef]
51. Whitney, J.; Easter, A.; Tchanturia, K. Service users' feedback on cognitive training in the treatment of anorexia nervosa: A qualitative study. *Int. J. Eat. Disord.* **2008**, *41*, 542–550. [CrossRef] [PubMed]
52. Strober, M. Personality and symptomatological features in young, nonchronic anorexia nervosa patients. *J. Psychosom. Res.* **1980**, *24*, 353–359. [CrossRef]
53. Amianto, F.; Abbate-Daga, G.; Morando, S.; Sobrero, C.; Fassino, S. Personality development characteristics of women with anorexia nervosa, their healthy siblings and healthy controls: What prevents and what relates to psychopathology? *Psychiatr. Res.* **2011**, *187*, 401–408. [CrossRef] [PubMed]

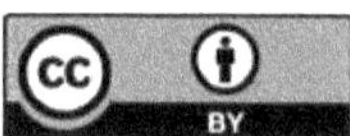

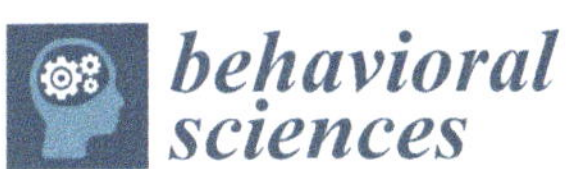
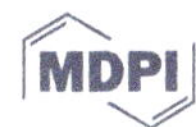

Article

Efficacy of Web-Based Weight Loss Maintenance Programs: A Randomized Controlled Trial Comparing Standard Features Versus the Addition of Enhanced Personalized Feedback over 12 Months

Clare E. Collins [1,2,*], Philip J. Morgan [2,3], Melinda J. Hutchesson [1,2], Christopher Oldmeadow [4,5], Daniel Barker [4,5] and Robin Callister [2,6]

1 Nutrition and Dietetics, School of Health Sciences, Faculty of Health and Medicine, The University of Newcastle, Callaghan, NSW 2308, Australia; Melinda.Hutchesson@newcastle.edu.au
2 Priority Research Centre in Physical Activity and Nutrition, The University of Newcastle, Callaghan, NSW 2308, Australia; Philip.Morgan@newcastle.edu.au (P.J.M.); Robin.Callister@newcastle.edu.au (R.C.)
3 School of Education, Faculty of Education and Arts, The University of Newcastle, Callaghan, NSW 2308, Australia
4 Clinical Research Design, IT and Statistical Support Unit, Hunter Medical Research Institute, Level 3 Pod, HMRI building Lot 1, Kookaburra Circuit, New Lambton Heights, NSW 2305, Australia; Christopher.Oldmeadow@hmri.org.au (C.O.); Daniel.Barker@newcastle.edu.au (D.B.)
5 School of Medicine and Public Health, Faculty of Health and Medicine, The University of Newcastle, Callaghan, NSW 2308, Australia
6 School of Biomedical Sciences and Pharmacy, Faculty of Health and Medicine, The University of Newcastle, Callaghan, NSW 2308, Australia
* Correspondence: Clare.Collins@newcastle.edu.au; Tel.: +61-2-4921-5646

Received: 31 July 2017; Accepted: 2 November 2017; Published: 8 November 2017

Abstract: Few randomized controlled trials (RCT) have evaluated the efficacy of web-based programs targeting maintenance of lost weight. The aims of this study were to evaluate two versions of a commercially available web-based weight loss maintenance (WLM) program and examine whether the provision of enhanced feedback was associated with better WLM. The study was an assessor-blinded RCT of change in body mass index (BMI) over 12 months WLM. Participants were 227 adults (44% male, 42.3 ± 10.1 years, BMI 30.4 ± 4.1 kg/m^2) randomized to either a basic (Basic WLM) or enhanced program with additional support (Enhanced WLM). Analysis was intention-to-treat with imputation using last observation carried forward. There was no significant weight rebound from the start of weight loss maintenance to 12 months for either group (mean: basic 1.3%, enhanced 1.5%) and limited change in secondary outcomes for either program. There were no significant between-group differences in the primary outcome of change in BMI (basic −0.5 (1.9) kg/m^2, enhanced −0.5 (1.6) kg/m^2, $p = 0.93$). In conclusion, a web-based WLM program was effective in preventing weight regain over one year following weight loss. However, the addition of personalized e-feedback provided limited additional benefits compared to a standard program. Given the potential reach of web-based approaches, further research examining which web-based program components optimize weight outcomes long-term is required.

Keywords: intervention; weight loss; web-based; randomized controlled trial; calorie restriction; eHealth

---

1. Introduction

Obesity rates are continuing to rise globally [1] in contrast to the limited access to treatment programs. While web-based approaches to treatment could potentially have broad reach, especially as households gain access to broadband internet, their evaluation in the context of longer-term follow-up has been limited.

Studies have shown that passive follow-up with no active intervention after weight loss is associated with weight gain [2], with 50–80% of participants gradually regaining weight lost following treatment, with most regain occurring in the first year [3–6]. A systematic review of weight loss maintenance (WLM) trials found that active WLM interventions facilitated a 1.56 kg (95% CI −2.27 to −0.86 kg) lower weight regain compared with passive follow-up after 12 months. Most WLM studies have required attendance at group sessions and have been hampered by methodological issues, such as mainly recruiting females or mid-aged adults and including only those with a good response to an initial weight loss phase, while excluding those with low adherence. [7]. Few studies have evaluated the use of eHealth technologies (e.g., websites, smartphone applications, text messages) to deliver WLM interventions. Furthermore, most research in this area has looked at short-term interventions (<6 months) without longer-term follow-up [8,9]. The small number of longer-term studies have reported a gradual regain of weight lost following treatment, with regain occurring after the first six months [10,11]. A recent randomized controlled trial examined the effectiveness of a 12-week short message service (SMS) based WLM program following an initial 12-week commercial weight loss program. At three and nine months follow-up, there was no significant difference in weight maintenance between the usual care control group who received a brief telephone call providing lifestyle information and a mailed leaflet with advice on weight loss maintenance and the intervention group who received a weekly SMS to remind them to self-weigh in addition to the call [12].

A systematic review published in 2017, evaluated the efficacy of web-based interventions on weight loss or WLM in adults with overweight or obesity and found web-based interventions were more effective than minimal treatments but less effective than face-to-face interventions [13]. Furthermore, a recent systematic review concluded that there was insufficient evidence to recommend the use of eHealth interventions for WLM [14]. There were however promising results from the eHealth weight loss trials with the addition of newer technologies including text messages, self-monitoring devices, and mobile applications, with meta-analysis demonstrating significantly greater weight loss (1.46 kg [0.80, 2.13], $p < 0.001$) in interventions with enhanced behavioral features (e.g., individualized counselling, feedback on dietary intake or weight change) or technologies (e.g., addition of text messaging) than standard eHealth interventions.

There is some evidence to suggest that these 'enhanced' interventions positively impact participant engagement, retention, and behavior change. We have previously published results of an online commercially available weight loss maintenance (WLM) program which demonstrated limited between-group differences for the basic and enhanced versions of the program after six months [15].

While the enhanced version resulted in greater retention (81.0% vs. 68.5%) and usage of the web-program, it did not result in a difference in weight loss [15].

A study using a 12-month intervention program (6-month weight loss plus a 6-month WLM) compared a self-directed web-based commercial program to a therapist-led behavioral web-based program and found greater weight loss in the behavioral web-based program than the therapist-led program at 12 months [16]. We have previously reported that adults randomized to this therapist-led web-based weight loss program initially lost more weight compared to wait list controls [17], and that there was no difference in weight loss between basic or enhanced versions of the weight loss program after either 12 weeks [17] or after 24 weeks [15] of participation.

To date, no WLM trials have specifically evaluated the inclusion of enhanced behavioral features in an eHealth WLM program, including those outlined in Table S1, such as automatically-generated personalized reports; personalized feedback on diet, physical activity, and weight loss, as well as reminders to use the online diary, visit the website, and weigh-in.

Therefore, the aim of the current study was to evaluate the impact of two versions of a WLM program on BMI in adults with overweight or obesity who had previously completed a weight loss program. The secondary aim was to compare differences in waist circumference and clinical measures including cholesterol, triglycerides, glucose and insulin between a standard version of a web-based WLM program (basic) and an enhanced version that provided additional personalized e-support.

2. Materials and Methods

2.1. Participants

Adults (BMI 25–40 kg/m^2), aged 18–60 years were initially recruited into a weight loss trial in 2009 from the Hunter community in NSW, Australia [18]. Written informed consent was obtained from all participants for the weight loss maintenance trial. The study was approved by the University of Newcastle Human Ethics Research Committee (H-2009-0245) on 10 September 2009. The trial was registered with the Australian New Zealand Clinical Trials Registry, anzctr.org.au ACTRN12610000197033.

2.2. Study Design

Participants who completed an initial 24-week web-based weight loss intervention (The Biggest Loser Club, SP Health Co Pty Ltd., North Sydney, Australia) were randomly assigned into one of two weight loss maintenance groups for 12 months using a stratified randomized block design. Participants were allocated to either a basic weight loss maintenance program (Basic WLM) or an enhanced version of the weight loss maintenance program (Enhanced WLM) (see Figure 1). Both participants and the outcome assessors were blinded to group allocation. Detailed methods of the RCT have been published elsewhere [18]. The WLM programs were developed to follow on directly after completion of 24 weeks of a web-based weight loss program [15]. Program features and differences between groups are summarized in Table S1 and also described in detail elsewhere [18]. The Basic WLM group received free access to the weight loss program, but the weekly meal plans were based on an energy intake target equivalent to weight maintenance. The Enhanced WLM group received access to these same meal plans and dietary information, but they also received personalized system-generated feedback on their progress. The feedback on progress was provided using system-generated personalized reports that were populated with the data entered into the platform by the participant. Feedback included progress in relation to weight maintenance goals; usage of the online diet and physical activity diary (which was recommended but not mandated); usage patterns for website features; and level of success with weight loss. Those allocated to the enhanced group also received an escalating scale of email reminders followed by SMS text message reminders (if no response) to use the diary, visit the website, to 'weigh-in' by recording their weekly weight in the online program, and a relapse phone call if their recorded weight rebounded by $\geq$3% to remind them to return to weight loss mode (Table S1).

2.3. Measures

Participants were assessed at baseline and 12 months [18] by blinded research assistants. Height, weight, waist circumference, and blood pressure were measured using standardized procedures [18] and BMI calculated. Following an overnight fast, blood samples were collected and analyzed for total cholesterol, low density lipoprotein (LDL), high density lipoprotein (HDL) cholesterol, triglycerides, glucose, and insulin by a single National Association of Testing Authorities accredited pathology service using standard automated techniques.

2.4. Data Analysis

Baseline variables were compared between treatment groups using analysis of variance (ANOVA) for continuous variables and chi-square tests for categorical variables. Analysis of covariance (ANCOVA) was used to test for group differences in outcomes at 12 months after adjusting for the baseline values of the outcome and sex. Analyses were performed in Stata v11 or SAS v9.2 (StataCorp, College Station, TX, USA). Intention-to-treat (ITT) analyses included all participants randomized at the weight loss management phase baseline, with missing follow-up data imputed using the last observation carried forward (LOCF).

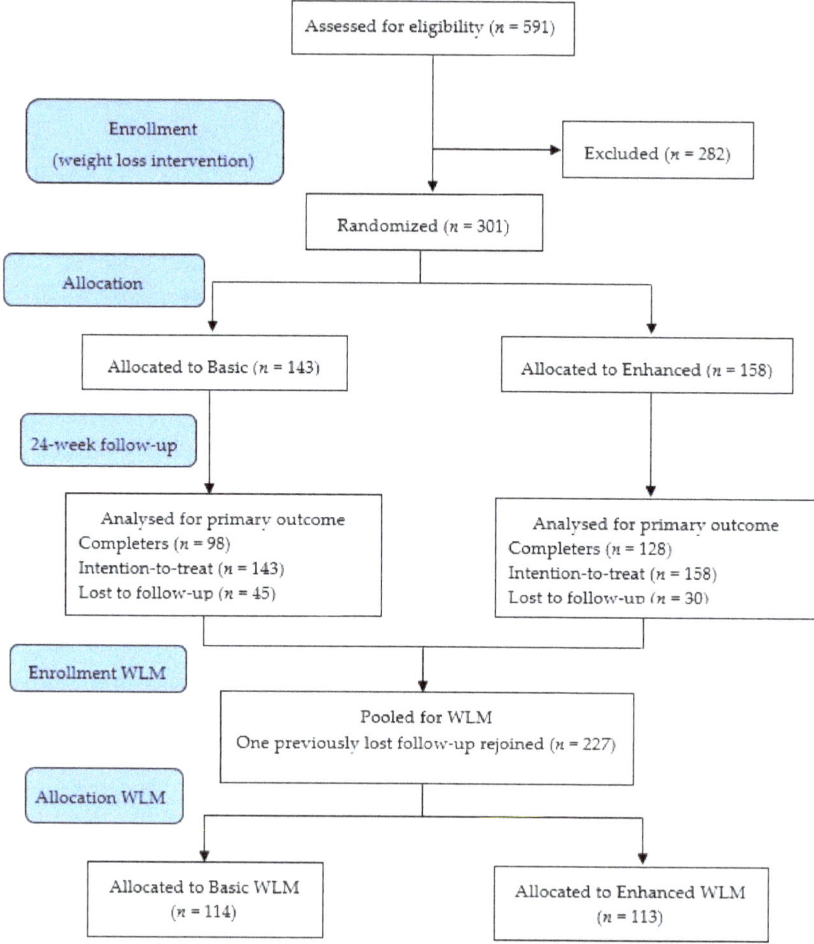

Figure 1. Participant flow from baseline of initial 24-week web-based weight loss intervention to group allocation in the WLM program. Further detail regarding participant flow has been published [15].

3. Results

At entry into WLM 227 participants were randomized to Basic WLM (n = 114) or Enhanced WLM (n = 113) program versions, with demographic data summarized in Table 1. Mean age was 43.3 (±9.7) years, with a mean BMI of 30.6 (±4.1) kg/m^2, 42% were male and 95% were Australian-born (Table 1). There was no significant between-group difference in attrition after 12 months, basic 18.4% and enhanced 23.9%, p = 0.31.

Both the Basic and Enhanced WLM groups successfully achieved WLM after 12 months with no significant rebound in weight. There were no significant between-group differences ($p > 0.05$) for the primary outcome of BMI with mean weight change (12 months—baseline) similar between the basic (−0.5 (1.9) kg/m^2) and enhanced groups (−0.5 (1.6) kg/m^2), $p > 0.05$ (Table 2). Table 2 shows that there were no significant differences in secondary outcomes between groups up to 12 months ($p > 0.05$).

Table 1. Demographic and other baseline characteristics of those randomized to 12 months of either a basic or enhanced features weight loss maintenance (WLM) web-based program.

Characteristic	Subgroup or Mean (SD)	Treatment Group			*p*-Value
		Basic WLM (n = 114)	Enhanced WLM (n = 113)	All (n = 227)	
Sex	Men	48 (42%)	52 (46%)	100 (44%)	0.55
Country of birth	Australia	108 (95%)	100 (88%)	208 (92%)	0.23
Highest level of education	School	37 (32%)	28 (25%)	65 (29%)	0.49
	Trade/Diploma	41 (36%)	40 (35%)	81 (35%)	
	University Degree	24 (21%)	28 (25%)	52 (23%)	
	Higher University Degree	12 (11%)	17 (15%)	29 (13%)	
Weekly household income (AUS$)	<$700	12 (11%)	7 (6.4%)	19 (8.8%)	0.60
	$700 to <$1000	6 (5.7%)	5 (4.5%)	11 (5.1%)	
	$1000 to <$1400	13 (12%)	11 (10%)	24 (11%)	
	$1500 or more	71 (67%)	84 (76%)	155 (72%)	
Age (years)	mean (SD)	43.3 (9.7)	41.3 (10.3)	42.3 (10.1)	0.14
Height (m)	mean (SD)	1.70 (0.09)	1.72 (0.09)	1.71 (0.09)	0.17
Weight (kg)	mean (SD)	88.5 (14.5)	89.3 (15.6)	88.9 (15.1)	0.70
Body mass index (kg/m^2)	mean (SD)	30.6 (4.1)	30.1 (4.1)	30.4 (4.1)	0.45
Waist circumference at umbilicus (cm)	mean (SD)	100.6 (11.1)	98.5 (11.7)	99.6 (11.4)	0.18
Waist circumference at narrowest point (cm)	mean (SD)	93.2 (11.5)	92.2 (11.9)	92.7 (11.7)	0.52
Waist to height ratio at umbilicus	mean (SD)	0.59 (0.07)	0.57 (0.07)	0.58 (0.07)	0.04
Waist to height ratio at narrowest point	mean (SD)	0.55 (0.07)	0.54 (0.06)	0.54 (0.06)	0.15
Weight loss at baseline entry to study (24 weeks)	mean (SD)	−4.38 (5.30)	−4.47 (6.37)	−4.42 (5.84)	0.91
Systolic blood pressure (mmHg)	mean (SD)	117.5 (13)	117.7 (12)	117.6 (12.5)	0.92
Diastolic blood pressure (mmHg)	mean (SD)	77.6 (10.6)	77.2 (9.2)	77.4 (9)	0.76
Resting heart rate (bpm)	mean (SD)	64.6 (9.5)	64.7 (10.2)	64.6 (9.8)	0.94
Total serum cholesterol (mmol/L)	mean (SD)	5.2 (1.1)	4.8(1.0)	5.0 (1.1)	0.03
LDL cholesterol (mmol/L)	mean (SD)	3.1 (1.0)	2.9 (0.8)	3.0 (0.9)	0.08
HDL cholesterol (mmol/L)	mean (SD)	1.3 (0.3)	1.3 (0.3)	1.3 (0.3)	0.41
Triglycerides (mmol/L)	mean (SD)	1.5 (1.0)	1.3 (0.7)	1.4 (0.9)	0.16
Glucose (mmol/L)	mean (SD)	4.6 (0.6)	4.5 (0.7)	4.6 (0.7)	0.08
Insulin (mIU/L)	mean (SD)	6.6 (5.5)	6.9 (6.2)	6.7 (5.9)	0.73

Table 2. Mean (SD) change in a anthropometric and clinical variables from WLM baseline to 12-month follow-up within each treatment group and least square mean (LSM) difference (95% CI) in change between treatments groups (Completed the six month Baseline, ITT/LOCF approach).

Characteristic	Treatment Group Mean Change (SD)		Absolute Difference between Groups LSM (95% CI)	p Values for Group Effect
	Basic	Enhanced	Enhanced vs. Basic	Difference at Specified Time
Weight (kg)	1.3 (5.1)	1.5 (4.4)	0.15 (−1.09, 1.39)	0.81
Systolic blood pressure (mmHg)	1.1 (12.1)	1.1 (10.2)	0.24 (−2.59, 3.08)	0.87
Diastolic blood pressure (mmHg)	−1.5 (8.1)	−0.1 (6.5)	1.15 (−0.76, 3.06)	0.24
Body mass index (kg/m^2)	0.5 (1.9)	0.5 (1.6)	0.02 (−0.46, 0.50)	0.93
Pulse rate (bpm)	−0.3 (6.7)	0.5 (5.8)	0.74 (−0.88, 2.35)	0.37
Waist circumference at umbilicus (cm)	3.8 (5.4)	3.3 (4.9)	0.76 (−0.63, 2.16)	0.28
Waist circumference at narrowest point (cm)	2.6 (4.6)	2.6 (4.6)	0.11 (−1.12, 1.35)	0.86
Waist to height ratio at umbilicus	0.0 (0.0)	0.0 (0.0)	0.01 (−0.00, 0.01)	0.21
Waist to height ratio at narrowest point	0.0 (0.0)	0.0 (0.0)	0.00 (−0.01, 0.01)	0.80
Total serum cholesterol (mmol/L)	0.1 (0.8)	0.2 (0.7)	0.07 (−0.12, 0.26)	0.50
LDL cholesterol (mmol/L)	0.0 (0.6)	0.1 (0.5)	0.01 (−0.15, 0.16)	0.94
HDL cholesterol (mmol/L)	0.0 (0.2)	0.0 (0.2)	0.00 (−0.06, 0.06)	0.88
Triglycerides (mmol/L)	0.0 (0.5)	0.2 (0.5)	0.13 (−0.02, 0.27)	0.10
Glucose (mmol/L)	0.1 (0.5)	0.2 (0.5)	0.08 (−0.05, 0.22)	0.20
Insulin (mIU/L)	1.6 (4.2)	0.89 (6.5)	0.61 (−0.719, 2.01)	0.39

4. Discussion

Whilst participants in both intervention arms of the current trial successfully maintained weight over one year of participating in a web-based program design to support maintenance of lost weight, those with access to the additional features designed to provide support and personalized feedback on diet, physical activity, and weight loss did not achieve better outcomes compared to those receiving access to the online program with minimal support. Both groups regained approximately one-and-a-half kilograms over the 12-month maintenance period, which was not significantly different between groups. This is comparable to results of the active intervention arms from a recent systematic review of all WLM intervention modes that included both food intake and physical activity advice, including group programs, face-to-face, and internet interventions [7]. The review included almost 3000 participants across 25 comparisons and found that the active intervention arms were associated with less weight regain of approximately 1.56 kg, up to 12 months [7]. This suggests that both active intervention arms in the current study were successful in achieving WLM. In our study, it appears that doing 'anything' was enough to support WLM, compared to the no-intervention arms in the systematic review, which also found no evidence that specific modes of intervention delivery were more effective than others. This suggests that having access to the level support provided in both the basic and enhanced versions of the current web-based WLM intervention, following a weight loss intervention did facilitate maintenance of lost weight. Given that it is well established that weight regain is common following initial weight loss [19], the results of the current study are important.

Our systematic review evaluating effectiveness of 56 interventions that included a specific dietary component within the WLM intervention found that 14 achieved significant between-group differences at follow-up [2]. Furthermore, our recent systematic review and meta-analysis which evaluated the effectiveness of 84 e-Health interventions, found that e-Health weight loss interventions that include extra support strategies including counselling, personalized feedback, motivational interviewing and/or personal contact, appear to achieve significantly greater weight loss compared with standard eHealth interventions [13]. However, five studies which focused specifically on WLM interventions found no significant difference in weight change between eHealth WLM programs vs. control [14]. The authors concluded that there is currently insufficient evidence to recommended eHealth interventions for WLM and that further high-quality research is required to determine their effectiveness [14]. Although the included studies were heterogeneous the typical intervention characteristics were WLM interventions that lasted 39 weeks on average, had approximately 180 participants and attrition of 26% compared to the current WLM study which lasted 52 weeks had 227 participants and an attrition rate of 21%.

The current study is important because individual studies to date suggest that face-to-face contact involving either weekly or monthly individual or group counseling sessions are more likely to achieve WLM than internet support in studies lasting 18 to 30 months. Recent systematic reviews on WLM interventions [7,14] suggest that there is a need for extended support for weight management following participation in weight loss programs internationally, as in-person attendance is not likely to be viable long-term. Hence, prolonged WLM support using eHealth technologies need to be evaluated for both feasibility, engagement, and cost-effectiveness in the long-term.

Limitations include the lack of a wait list control group, which is similar to the majority of WLM maintenance studies to date [2]. Although the small sample size and attrition likely reduced the power to detect significant differences between groups for the secondary outcomes, it is similar to other WLM trials lasting 12 or more months which had an average drop-out of 20% [7]. Furthermore. results from the current study need to be interpreted with caution given the meta-analysis within the systematic review [14] indicates that there is no significant difference between the support methods during WLM. This is also supported by our review of web-based interventions which also reported no difference between these two methods of delivery [20]. Strengths include the RCT design, use of blinded assessors, and the comparison of two versions of the WLM program for 12 months, following an initial period of weight loss. Future studies should consider evaluating cost-effectiveness and efficacy in specific population groups for whom access services may be a challenge, based on a range of issues related to time, cost, convenience, rurality, health conditions, or other socio-economic factors.

In conclusion, a commercial web-based weight loss maintenance program, with a specific intervention component targeting maintenance of lost weight can be effective at preventing weight re-gain up to one year following 24 weeks of weight loss. While the addition of enhanced features that provide additional feedback and social support did not provide additional benefits during maintenance, health professionals should advise clients that a specific WLM strategy does facilitate WLM up to one year following weight loss. Further research addressing level of feedback and support required to optimize weight status long-term in an online environment is required.

Supplementary Materials: The following are available online at www.mdpi.com/2076-328X/7/4/76/s1, Table S1: Description of the basic and enhanced commercial web-based weight loss maintenance programs.

Acknowledgments: This trial was funded by an Australian Research Council Linkage Project grant (2009–2012) (LP0990414, G0189752), with SP Health as the Industry Partner Organization (G0189753). Clare E. Collins is supported by an NHMRC Senior Research Fellowship and a University of Newcastle, Faculty of Health and Medicine Senior Brawn Fellowship. Melinda J. Hutchesson is a University of Newcastle, Faculty of Health and Medicine Gladys M Brawn Career Development Fellow. We would like to thank the study subjects for participating in the trial and the research assistants for helping with data collection and D. Coyle for assistance with formatting the manuscript.

Author Contributions: Clare E. Collins, Philip J. Morgan., and Robin Callister were responsible for the design of study. Christopher Oldmeadow and Daniel Barker conducted the statistical analysis. Clare E. Collins drafted the paper, Melinda J. Hutchesson was responsible for data collection and management and critically reviewing the manuscript and providing feedback on intellectual content. All authors were responsible for revising the manuscript and have approved the final version.

Conflicts of Interest: The authors declare no conflict of interest. The funding sponsors had no role in the design of the study; in the collection, analyses, or interpretation of data; in the writing of the manuscript, or in the decision to publish the results.

References

1. NCD Risk Factor Collaboration. Worldwide trends in body-mass index, underweight, overweight, and obesity from 1975 to 2016: A pooled analysis of 2416 population-based measurement studies in 128·9 million children, adolescents, and adults. *Lancet* **2017**. [CrossRef]
2. Collins, C.E.; Neve, M.J.; Williams, R.; Young, M.; Morgan, P.J.; Fletcher, K.R.C. Effectiveness of interventions with a dietary component on weight loss maintenance: A systematic review. *JBI Database Syst. Rev. Implement. Rep.* **2013**, *11*, 317–414. [CrossRef]
3. Bond, D.S.; Phelan, S.; Leahey, T.M.; Hill, J.O.; Wing, R.R. Weight-loss maintenance in successful weight losers: Surgical vs non-surgical methods. *Int. J. Obes.* **2009**, *33*, 173–180. [CrossRef] [PubMed]
4. Burke, L.E.; Steenkiste, A.; Music, E.; Styn, M.A. A descriptive study of past experiences with weight-loss treatment. *J. Am. Diet. Assoc.* **2008**, *108*, 640–647. [CrossRef] [PubMed]
5. Douketis, J.D.; Macie, C.; Thabane, L.; Williamson, D.F. Systematic review of long-term weight loss studies in obese adults: Clinical significance and applicability to clinical practice. *Int. J. Obes.* **2005**, *29*, 1153–1167. [CrossRef] [PubMed]
6. Wadden, T.A.; Crerand, C.E.; Brock, J. Behavioral treatment of obesity. *Psychiatr. Clin. N. Am.* **2005**, *28*, 151–170. [CrossRef] [PubMed]
7. Dombrowski, S.; Knittle, K.; Avenell, A.; Araujo-Soares, V.; Sniehotta, F. Long term maintenance of weight loss with non-surgical interventions in obese adults: Systematic review and meta-analyses of randomised controlled trials. *BMJ* **2014**, *348*. [CrossRef] [PubMed]
8. Painter, S.L.; Ahmed, R.; Hill, J.O.; Kushner, R.F.; Lindquist, R.; Brunning, S.A.M. What matters in weight loss? An in-depth analysis of self-monitoring. *J. Med. Internet Res.* **2017**, *19*, e160. [CrossRef] [PubMed]
9. Balk-Møller, N.C.; Poulsen, S.K.; Larsen, T.M. Effect of a nine-month web- and app-based workplace intervention to promote healthy lifestyle and weight loss for employees in the social welfare and health care sector: A randomized controlled trial. *J. Med. Internet Res.* **2017**, *19*, e108. [CrossRef] [PubMed]

10. Watson, S.; Woodside, J.V.; Ware, L.J.; Hunter, S.J.; McGrath, A.; Cardwell, C.R.; Appleton, K.M.; Young, I.S.; Mckinlev, M.C. Effect of a web-based behavior change program on weight loss and cardiovascular risk factors in overweight and obese adults at high risk of developing cardiovascular disease: Randomized controlled trial. *J. Med. Internet Res.* **2015**, *17*, e177. [CrossRef] [PubMed]
11. Hageman, P.A.; Pullen, C.H.; Hertzog, M.; Pozehl, B.; Eisenhauer, C.; Boeckner, L.S. Web-based interventions alone or supplemented with peer-led support or professional email counseling for weight loss and weight maintenance in women from rural communities: Results of a clinical trial. *J. Obes.* **2017**, *2017*. [CrossRef] [PubMed]
12. Sidhu, M.S.; Daley, A.; Jolly, K. Evaluation of a text supported weight maintenance programme 'lighten up plus' following a weight reduction programme: Randomised controlled trial. *Int. J. Behav. Nutr. Phys. Act.* **2016**, *13*. [CrossRef] [PubMed]
13. Sorgente, A.; Pietrabissa, G.; Manzoni, G.M.; Re, F.; Simpson, S.; Perona, S.; Rossi, A.; Cattivelli, R.; Innamorati, M.; Jackson, J.B.; et al. Web-based interventions for weight loss or weight loss maintenance in overweight and obese people: A systematic review of systematic reviews. *J. Med. Internet Res.* **2017**, *19*, e229. [CrossRef] [PubMed]
14. Hutchesson, M.J.; Rollo, M.; Krukowski, R.; Ells, L.; Harvey, J.; Morgan, P.J.; Callister, R.; Plotnikoff, R.; Collins, C.E. Ehealth interventions for the prevention and treatment of overweight and obesity in adults: A systematic review with meta-analysis. *Obes. Rev.* **2015**, *16*, 376–392. [CrossRef] [PubMed]
15. Collins, C.E.; Morgan, P.J.; Neve, M.J.; Callister, R. Efficacy of standard versus enhanced features in a web-based commercial weight-loss program for obese adults, part 2: Randomized controlled trial. *J. Med. Internet Res.* **2013**, *15*, e140. [CrossRef] [PubMed]
16. Gold, B.; Burke, S.; Pintauro, S.; Buzzell, P.; Harvey-Berino, J. Weight loss on the web: A pilot study comparing a structured behavioral intervention to a commercial program. *Obesity* **2007**, *15*, 155–164. [CrossRef] [PubMed]
17. Collins, C.E.; Morgan, P.J.; Jones, P.; Fletcher, K.; Martin, J.; Aguiar, E.J.; Lucas, A.; Neve, M.J.; Callister, R. A 12-week commercial web-based weight-loss program for overweight and obese adults: Randomized controlled trial comparing basic versus enhanced features. *J. Med. Internet Res.* **2012**, *14*, e57. [CrossRef] [PubMed]
18. Collins, C.E.; Morgan, P.J.; Jones, P.; Fletcher, K.; Martin, J.; Aguiar, E.J.; Lucas, A.; Neve, M.; McElduff, P.; Callister, R. Evaluation of a commercial web-based weight loss and weight loss maintenance program in overweight and obese adults: A randomised controlled trial. *BMC Public Health* **2010**, *10*, 669. [CrossRef] [PubMed]
19. Bamia, C.; Orfanos, P.; Ferrari, P.; Overvad, K.; Hundborg, H.H.; Tjønneland, A.; Olsen, A.; Kesse, E.; Boutron-Ruault, M.; Clavel-Chapelon, F.; et al. Dietary patterns among older europeans: The epic-elderly study. *Br. J. Nutr.* **2005**, *94*, 100–113. [CrossRef] [PubMed]
20. Neve, M.; Morgan, P.J.; Jones, P.R.; Collins, C.E. Effectiveness of web-based interventions in achieving weight loss and weight loss maintenance in overweight and obese adults: A systematic review with meta-analysis. *Obes. Rev.* **2010**, *11*, 306–321. [CrossRef] [PubMed]

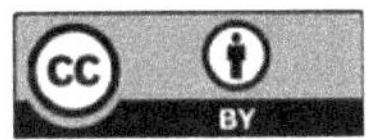

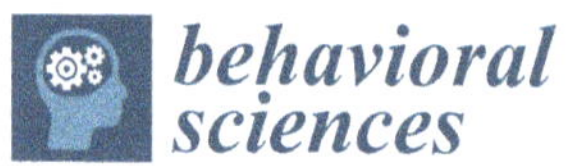

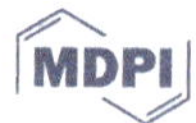

Article

The Role of Regular Eating and Self-Monitoring in the Treatment of Bulimia Nervosa: A Pilot Study of an Online Guided Self-Help CBT Program

Sarah Barakat [1,*], Sarah Maguire [2], Lois Surgenor [3], Brooke Donnelly [4], Blagica Miceska [2], Kirsty Fromholtz [2], Janice Russell [5], Phillipa Hay [6] and Stephen Touyz [1]

1 School of Psychology, University of Sydney, Sydney, NSW 2006, Australia; stephen.touyz@sydney.edu.au
2 Centre for Eating and Dieting Disorders, Boden Institute, University of Sydney, Sydney, NSW 2006, Australia; servicedevelopmentofficer@gmail.com (S.M.); bm405@uowmail.edu.au (B.M.); kfromholtz@gmail.com (K.F.)
3 Department of Psychological Medicine, University of Otago at Christchurch, Christchurch 8140, New Zealand; lois.surgenor@otago.ac.nz
4 Sydney Local Health District, Sydney, NSW 2006, Australia; brooke.donnelly@sswahs.nsw.gov.au
5 School of Medicine, University of Sydney, Sydney, NSW 2006, Australia; janice.russell@sydney.edu.au
6 Translational Health Research Institute, School of Medicine, Western Sydney University, Sydney, NSW 2751, Australia; p.hay@westernsydney.edu.au
* Correspondence: sbar1821@uni.sydney.edu.au; Tel.: +61-422-047-689

Received: 28 April 2017; Accepted: 21 June 2017; Published: 26 June 2017

Abstract: *Background*: Despite cognitive behavioural therapy (CBT) being regarded as the first-line treatment option for bulimia nervosa (BN), barriers such as its time-consuming and expensive nature limit patient access. In order to broaden treatment availability and affordability, the efficacy and convenience of CBT could be improved through the use of online treatments and selective emphasis on its most 'potent' components of which behavioural techniques form the focus. *Method:* Twenty-six individuals with BN were enrolled in an online CBT-based self-help programme and 17 completed four weeks of regular eating and food-monitoring using the online Food Diary tool. Participants were contacted for a weekly check-in phone call and had their bulimic symptom severity assessed at five time points (baseline and weeks 1–4). *Results*: There was a significant decrease in the frequency of self-reported objective binge episodes, associated loss of control and objective binge days reported between pre- and post-treatment measures. Significant improvements were also observed in most subscales of the Eating Disorder Examination-Questionnaire. *Conclusion*: This study provides encouraging preliminary evidence of the potential of behavioural techniques of online CBT in the treatment of BN. Online therapy with this focus is potentially a viable and practical form of treatment delivery in this illness group. These preliminary findings support the need for larger studies using control groups.

Keywords: bulimia nervosa; online treatment; self-monitoring; regular eating; cognitive behavioural therapy; objective binge episodes; purging

---

1. Introduction

Therapist-led cognitive behavioural therapy (CBT) currently forms the most empirically validated treatment for bulimia nervosa (BN), and accordingly is widely recommended as the first line treatment for adults with BN [1,2]. However, the empirical support which this "gold-standard" treatment enjoys is challenged by the statistic that on average only 23.2% of eating disorder (ED) sufferers actually access treatment [3], with this figure substantially lower in some urban and rural regions with no specialist ED services [4]. Importantly, the quality of CBT delivered in the community is inconsistent. Tobin, Banker, Weisberg and Bowers [5] report that only 6% of clinicians adhere to an evidence-based manualised version of CBT for eating disorders (EDs), concluding that therapist 'drift' from CBT is the norm rather than the exception [6]. Moreover, CBT for BN is a specialist treatment, which for a routine delivery costs US$6000.00 per individual case [7], with the Australian healthcare system rebating less than half of the CBT sessions for a routine case treated by a psychologist [4].

Modification of CBT-BN structure and delivery is vital to ensure treatment is accessible [8]. Broadening the format of CBT delivery beyond the current therapist-led structure to an online, self-help program will offset the shortage of ED specialist clinicians. Additionally, overcoming the lengthy nature of CBT-BN can be achieved through investigation of the most powerful therapeutic components of CBT-BN, of which behavioural techniques are a promising candidate [9].

1.1. Treatment Delivery Formats to Increase Access

In order to address barriers to accessing treatment, a number of alternative treatment formats have evolved. These are briefly reviewed.

1.1.1. Guided Self-Help

Various forms of guided self-help for BN have been available for several decades now, allowing a body of research to have evolved assessing its effectiveness. People who receive professional therapeutic support throughout their self-help treatment program display superior treatment outcomes to those independently engaging in self-help, producing equivalent outcomes to therapist led CBT for one-third of BN patients [10]. Accordingly, the addition of monthly thirty-minute guidance sessions for patients' observing Fairburn's *Overcoming Binge Eating* self-help manual [11] raised symptomatic improvement from 25% for those receiving no guidance, to 36% for telephone guidance and 50% for face-to-face guidance [12]. Supervision requirements for self-help treatment options are one-fifth of that required for a complete CBT course [13], advocating for a "stepped-care" approach which allows for the appropriate allocation of therapeutic skills according to one's clinical severity [14,15].

1.1.2. Online Self-Help

The successful application of CBT's primary principles into recent technological advancements has been demonstrated across a range of formats including online programs [16–21], email correspondence [22,23], text messaging [24] and CD-ROM programs [25]. Pretorius et al. [19] recently evaluated a web-based CBT intervention consisting of eight 30–40 min interactive online sessions for a sample of 101 patients diagnosed with BN or eating disorder not otherwise specified (EDNOS) with bulimic features. In addition to weekly email support, completion of the eTherapy program resulted in a significant improvement in the frequency of objective binge episodes (OBEs), purge episodes and global Eating Disorder Examination (EDE) [26] maintained at the six-month follow up. Additional support for eTherapy has been provided by a study of 75 BN or EDNOS patients of whom 25.8% displayed abstinence from bulimic behaviours following engagement in an eight-session online CBT-based program [21]. These findings are comparable to the 20% and 30% post-treatment abstinence from bulimic behaviours observed following the use of manual-based CBT self-help books and face-to-face CBT treatment, respectively [10,14].

Self-monitoring via a technological device upholds numerous benefits to traditional pen and paper methods, including in-built reminders to prompt higher completion, more ecologically valid data, real-time monitoring and personalised, immediate feedback on one's entries [27,28]. The recent popularity of a smartphone application for ED self-monitoring, known as 'Recovery Record', has seen 108,000 downloads across a two-year period, of which the majority of users logged their daily meals on the application for a thirty-day period [28]. However, Walsh and colleagues [27] found that while people with EDs viewed the idea of online monitoring favourably, they did not experience any benefit in practising the technique themselves.

1.2. Behavioural Components of CBT

Despite the extensive number of clinical trials assessing CBT as an entire treatment package, little empirical evidence exists on the effectiveness of CBT's individual therapeutic techniques [29]. Component analyses of CBT treatment for depression and anxiety demonstrate that therapy consisting purely of behavioural techniques produces equivalent outcomes to therapy involving both behavioural and cognitive techniques [30]. Moreover, in a comparative treatment trial for BN, CBT produced a greater shift in patients' distorted attitudes regarding shape, weight and extreme dieting as compared to a simplified behavioural version of CBT, yet was equivalent in all other treatment outcomes [31]. Key behavioural components of CBT for BN are briefly reviewed below.

1.2.1. Self-Monitoring

Self-monitoring is one of the first behavioural tasks introduced in CBT whereby patients record a target behaviour and any associated antecedents as they occur within their natural context [32]. Self-monitoring allows the clinician and patient to jointly evaluate problematic behavioural patterns, work to reduce them and can spark reactive effects due to the inherently reinforcing or punishing nature of self-records [32].

In CBT-BN, daily self-monitoring is introduced in the first session and requires patients to record their food and drink intake, including binge or compensatory behaviours, time, meal type and associated feelings at each meal [33]. A number of experts credit self-monitoring as the most powerful therapeutic intervention in the treatment of BN [9,34]. In support of this, investigations of the temporal effectiveness of CBT reveal the largest reduction in key bulimic behaviours occurs within the first four to six weeks of treatment, while self-monitoring and regular eating are being introduced, and is the best predictor of short and long term treatment outcomes for BN patients [35–39].

Latner and Wilson [9] conducted one of the very few studies examining the effect of self-monitoring in BN treatment. Following six to seven days of food-monitoring, 30 individuals diagnosed with either BN or binge eating disorder (BED) reported a significant decrease in OBEs. It has also been found that in addition to a reduction in OBEs, self-monitoring produces a simultaneous increase in subjective binge episodes (SBEs). Such a response was termed 'binge drift', with Hildebrandt and Latner [34] claiming that although food monitoring allows for greater awareness of one's eating behaviours, it may not target the destructive thoughts and negative affect, characteristic of the loss of control (LOC) experienced during binges. Other studies have examined the efficacy of self-monitoring alone in small or non-clinical samples, also suggesting its effectiveness [40,41].

1.2.2. Regular Eating: The Three-Hour Rule

Paired with food monitoring is another behavioural activity known as the three-hour rule whereby patients are instructed to consume three planned meals and two or three planned snacks daily to ensure food deprivation does not exceed three to four hours [42,43]. Regular eating interrupts the heavy dietary restriction practiced by individuals with BN, reducing vulnerability to psychological and physical triggers for a binge [44].

Despite emphasis on regular eating as a fundamental component of CBT for BN [45], there has been limited empirical investigation into its effectiveness as a singular component. Shah, Passi, Bryson and Agras [46] reported the consumption of three meals and one snack daily resulted in the highest abstinence from binge eating and purging in a sample of 158 BN patients receiving either CBT or interpersonal psychotherapy (IPT). Additionally, high adherence to regular eating has also been shown to lower weekly binge frequency in a sample of 38 university students presenting with regular binge eating [44].

The current study endeavours to expand upon the preliminary research examining self-monitoring and regular eating to investigate their joint effectiveness in a modified CBT treatment program. In an attempt to enhance the efficacy of online CBT and consequently improve treatment outcomes for people with BN, the current study explores the therapeutic effectiveness of food monitoring and the "three-hour rule" via an online, low-intensity CBT program known as Binge Eating eTherapy (BEeT), recently developed by the Centre for Eating and Dieting Disorders (CEDD) at the University of Sydney.

Firstly, it was hypothesised that following Stage 1 low-intensity CBT (online self-monitoring and "three-hour rule" training), participants will display a significant reduction in OBEs, LOC and compensatory behaviours. Secondly, in line with prior findings of 'binge drift', we hypothesise an increase in SBE pre-post treatment measures.

BN possesses the highest psychiatric comorbidity of the ED's [47], with up to 94.5% of sufferers meeting criteria for at least one DSM-IV disorder axis I diagnosis [48] and evidence suggests this comorbidity can be linked to more severe BN psychopathology [49,50] and symptom persistence [51]. For this reason, consideration of these factors was also considered pertinent in the current study. Specifically, we expected that a preliminary exploratory analysis of participants with comorbid mood disorders and/or severe bulimic behaviours in this cohort will display lower treatment compliance and poorer therapeutic outcomes.

2. Materials and Methods

2.1. Participants

Participants were recruited from the general Australian community using online advertisements on health websites, social media announcements, referrals from health professionals and paper advertisements placed on the grounds of the University of Sydney. The study was approved by the Sydney Local Health District Ethics Review Committee, Royal Prince Alfred Hospital Zone (Ethics Approval Number: X14-0302).

Of the 69 individuals who expressed interest, 26 females entered the study (See Figure 1). Participants were eligible for this study if they were aged between 16 to 65 years of age and met a full DSM-5 [52] diagnostic criteria for BN (purging or non-purging type). Participants below 18 years of age were required to provide parental consent. As assessed by the Eating Disorder Examination Questionnaire (EDE-Q) [53], participants must have engaged in OBEs and inappropriate compensatory behaviours (inclusive of vomiting, excessive laxative or diuretic use, extreme exercise or severe dietary restriction) at least once per week in the preceding 28 days from when the questionnaire was taken. The presence of such behaviours across the preceding three months was confirmed by a senior clinical psychologist with experience in treating ED patients who discussed symptom presentation with the patient in a thorough phone interview. As part of the interview, participants' self-evaluation due to shape and weight, as assessed on the EDE-Q, was also confirmed.

Exclusion criteria included a body mass index (BMI) below 18.5 and current participation in a CBT psychological treatment specifically for their eating disorder. Individuals engaging in general psychological or pharmacological treatment were not excluded from the study, neither were participants with a comorbid psychiatric disorder. If a safety plan and regular monitoring of risk could not be established for participants with self-harm and suicide behaviours, they were excluded from the study. Monitoring of risk included follow-up phone calls if participants' displayed thoughts of self-harm or suicide in their weekly questionnaires or Food Diary entries. In this phone call, the severity of these thoughts was clarified and regular contact of the participant with an informed health professional was confirmed. Previous or acute active suicidality or self-harm behaviours did not obviate inclusion.

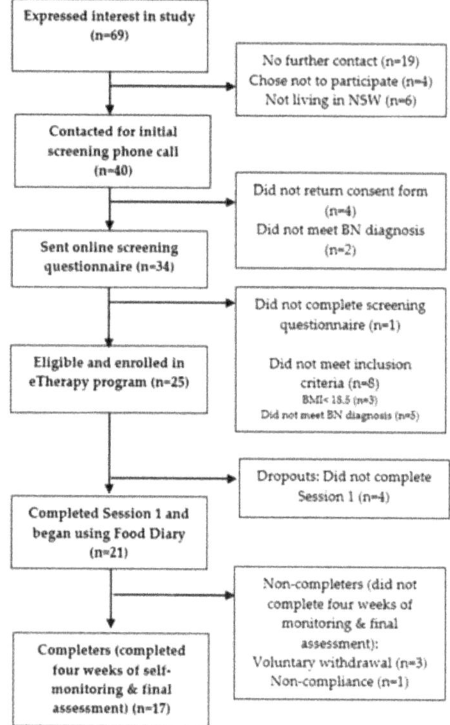

Figure 1. Flowchart of study participants.

2.2. Materials

2.2.1. Binge Eating eTherapy Program (BEeT)

The BEeT program consists of ten, one-hour interactive, multi-media sessions employing low-intensity CBT delivered by a pre-recorded therapist. Session 1 addresses the regular eating according to the "three-hour rule" and self-monitoring of eating using the online Food Diary. Access to the Food Diary tool was provided upon completion of Session 1 of the online program. Specifically, participants were educated on the impact of severe dietary restriction and how "delayed eating" is linked to urges to binge. Participants were encouraged to offset this by structuring their eating around three planned meals and two to three planned snacks daily.

The Food Diary tool is based upon the self-monitoring procedure for recording of eating behaviours as specified in most eating disorder therapies, including all existing CBT programs for BN [42,43,54,55]. Participants were to log a separate diary entry for each meal recording the following details: meal type, type and quantity of food and beverage consumed, the time at which intake occurred, whether the meal was considered to be a binge or over-eating, any urge to binge, type and quantity or length of any compensatory behaviours and associated events or feeling. On participants' entry of their dinner record in the diary, end of day on-screen feedback is provided on the "three-hour rule" and on the presence of binges across that day. Importantly, the feedback encouraged participants to continue practising the behavioural activities.

2.2.2. SMS Reminders

A daily SMS is sent to participants' mobile phones at approximately 9 a.m. as a reminder to record their meals using the Food Diary tool throughout the day. An additional evening SMS is sent at approximately 6 p.m. to participants who had not completed a Food Diary entry for the preceding two days to prompt reengagement.

2.3. *Psychometric Measures*

All the psychometric measures listed below formed part of the pre- and post-treatment maxi eScreens. The mini eScreen weekly assessments consisted of a shortened version of the EDE-Q, the Kessler Psychological Distress Scale (K10) and the self-harm and suicidality risk assessment. All psychometric measures were self-report assessments administered online. There exists a high correspondence between the psychometric measures delivered using online and written formats [56].

2.3.1. Eating Disorder Examination Questionnaire (EDE-Q)

The 16th edition of the EDE-Q [53] is a 30-item self-report version of the interview-delivered EDE [26]. The EDE-Q examines the behavioural features of one's ED, including the frequency and days of OBEs and SBEs as well as the frequency of purging, laxative use and excessive exercise over the preceding 28 days. The EDE-Q also contains four subscales (Shape Concern, Weight Concern, Eating Restraint, and Eating Concern) assessing the cognitive and emotional aspects of the ED, which utilise a seven-point Likert scale ranging from scores of 0 to 6, with higher scores indicative of more severe symptomology.

The EDE-Q was used to validate a diagnosis of BN and determine the severity of patients' bulimic behaviours, with frequency of binging and compensatory behaviours constituting the primary outcome measures. The EDE-Q upholds good reliability (Cronbach's $\alpha = 0.90$) [57].

2.3.2. Kessler Psychological Distress Scale (K10)

The K10 [58] is a screening tool used to monitor psychological distress experienced by patients and comprises of ten questions, each consisting of five response options, which assess the degree of negative emotionality experienced across the past 28 days (pre- and post-treatment questionnaires) or 7 days (weekly questionnaires). The K10 has good reliability (Cronbach's $\alpha = 0.93$) [58].

2.3.3. Eating Disorder Quality of Life Questionnaire (EDQOL)

The EDQOL [59] consists of 25-items examining the quality of life experienced by individuals suffering with an ED. Four subscales assess the impairment upon four primary domains including Psychological, Physical/Cognitive, Work/School and Financial domains. The EDQOL has good reliability (Cronbach's $\alpha = 0.94$) [59].

2.3.4. Three-Factor Eating Questionnaire (TFEQ)

The TFEQ [60] consists of three subscales assessing dietary restraint, disinhibition or loss of control over eating and hunger perception. The self-report assessment consists of 36 items with a yes/no response option, 14 items using a 1–4 response scale and a single vertical rating item.

2.3.5. General Information and Demographics

This series of questions concerns the general demographic information including age, gender, occupation, cultural background/ethnicity and setting of residence.

2.3.6. General Mental Health

This series of questions gathers information regarding participants' current primary and secondary mental health concerns, such as eating/weight issues, anxiety, stress, depression or substance/alcohol issues, whether or not these mental health concerns are being treated and by which mental health service, such as psychiatrist, psychologist, mental health nurse, social worker, counsellor, medical doctor or self-help book, and the type of treatment they are accessing, such as CBT, general counselling, hypnosis, antipsychotics or antidepressants.

2.3.7. Self-Harm and Suicidality Risk Assessment

This assessment reviews the history of participants' suicidal and self-harming thoughts and actions. It explores whether participants have had thoughts of suicide, attempted suicide or tried to injure or harm themselves in the previous 12 months or 28 days prior to completing the assessment.

2.4. Procedure

A brief telephone assessment screened participants for suitability; those eligible completed written informed consent and were then administered a comprehensive online assessment. Participants were instructed to complete Session 1 of the program and upon completion to immediately begin recording subsequent meals and episodes of binging and/or compensation in the online Food Diary for the following 28 days (See Figure 2).

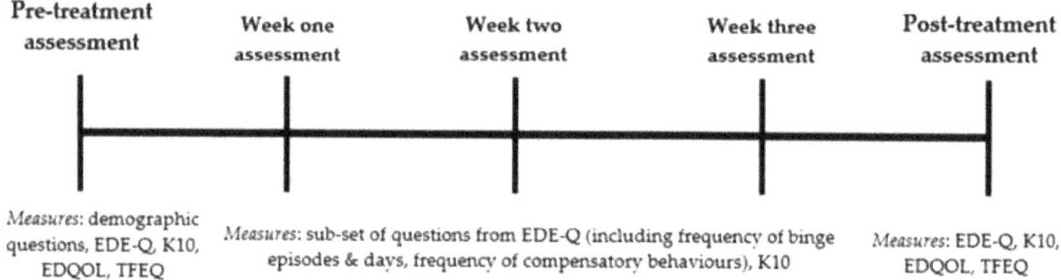

Figure 2. Schematic of the timing and sequence of assessments and included measures. Note: Week one, week two and week three assessments were identical. EDE-Q = Eating Disorder Examination-Questionnaire; K10 = Kessler Psychological Distress Scale; EDQOL = Eating Disorder Quality of Life Scale; TFEQ = Three Factor Eating Questionnaire.

On the 7th, 14th and 21st day following their first Food Diary entry, participants completed a mini eScreen questionnaire and received a 15- to 20-min check-in phone call from a research assistant trained by the CI (clinical psychologist). Each phone call was guided by a standardised set of questions and feedback developed by a clinical psychologist (S.M.) with over 15 years of experience using CBT for BN. Obstacles hindering participants' ability to adopt the Food Diary and three-hour rule were discussed, with a member of the treatment team presenting solutions in accordance with key CBT techniques of psychoeducation and positive reinforcement. Participants were sent an email the day prior to the scheduled phone call prompting completion of the mini eScreen questionnaire, followed by reminder text message on the day of the phone call.

On the 28th day of using the Food Diary, participants completed the final comprehensive online assessment (maxi eScreen) and received a final check-in phone call. Participants then gained access to remaining components of the BEeT program to engage in a pure self-help format independent of the study protocol.

2.5. Statistical Analysis

The data were cleaned and inspected for normality and baseline features of participants were examined. The statistical analysis was conducted in several stages, focusing on compliance then symptom outcome variance. First, attrition and compliance of participants with the treatment program was examined using the variables of mean number of days a Food Diary entry was made and the average number of daily Food Diary entries.

Secondly, linear regression analysis was used to test the statistical significance of differences between the pre- and post-treatment dependent variables of OBE frequency, OBE days, SBE days, LOC frequency, purge frequency, laxative frequency, exercise frequency, EDE-Q subscale scores, global EDE-Q score, global EDQOL score and global TFEQ score. Comparisons between groups were based upon a two-tailed Bonferroni-corrected α of 0.0036 (0.05/14). Linear regression analyses and pairwise comparisons were used to assess changes in OBE frequency, OBE days, purge frequency, laxative frequency, SBE frequency, dietary restriction and the number of days of Food Diary entries between the week one, two and three measures.

Finally, in order to determine if differences in participants' clinical and demographic features at baseline were associated with their treatment compliance, bulimic symptom severity and bulimic symptom improvement, these three outcome variables were converted into binary variables.

Treatment compliance variables (treatment completion, days of Food Diary entries, number of Food Diary entries) and treatment outcome variables (pre- to post-treatment change in binge frequency, purge frequency, laxative frequency, excessive exercise frequency, dietary restraint score) were converted into three binary distributions with the reference point (or cut-off) specified at 50%, 75% and 90% of the original variable value. Three distributions were created as a precautionary measure in the absence of any prior convention from previous BN treatment studies regarding the conversion of continuous dependent variables into binary variables.

A series of paired t-tests were used to examine differences between the binary variable levels in terms of the continuous variables of age and K10 score. Similarly, a Fisher's exact test examined differences between binary variable levels in terms of the categorical predictor variables of secondary mental health concerns, active/past suicidality and active/past self-harm. Analyses were conducted using the SPSS for Mac OS X version 22.0.

3. Results

3.1. Participant Characteristics

The mean age of the 25 female participants enrolled in the eTherapy program was 30.24 years (range 16–47 years, SD = 9.37) and the mean BMI was 25.1 (range 18.8–50.7, SD = 6.88). Only one participant was below 18 years of age. The sample included participants with normal weight BN and overweight BN. All participants met the DSM-5 criteria for BN at baseline [52]. Five participants (20.0%) satisfied the DSM-5 criteria for BN, non-purging type [52], the remainder met the purging type category. A high proportion of participants reported comorbid anxiety (32.0%) or depression (40.0%) as a secondary mental health concern. No participants were excluded on the basis of their self-harm or suicidality assessment. Nineteen participants (76.0%) reported engaging in another form of treatment at baseline. The most commonly reported treating professional was a psychologist or psychiatrist (56.0%), followed by GP (24.0%) and dietitian (12.0%). The sociodemographic variables of participants as reported at baseline are displayed in Table 1.

3.2. Attrition and Compliance

Of the 25 participants enrolled in the online program, four participants (16.0%) did not complete Session 1 and therefore did not access the Food Diary tool (dropouts). Four participants (16.0%) failed to complete the four weeks of monitoring and the final assessment (non-completers) and 17 participants (68.0%) engaged in the four-weeks of treatment and completed the final assessment (completers). The non-completers engaged in the Food Diary tool for an average of 18.8 days (SD = 2.06), that is approximately 2.5 weeks, prior to disengaging from the treatment program.

On average, the 17 completers logged at least one entry in the online Food Diary for 87.1% of the possible 28 days (range: 16–28 days, M = 24.4, SD = 4.76). The most common number of daily Food

Diary entries made by all participants was five per day. There was a significant difference in the mean number of days of self-monitoring (indexed by at least one Food Diary entry) between the four weeks of treatment, Wald χ^2 (3, N = 17) = 15.03, p = 0.002. Specifically, there was a significant decrease in the mean number of days monitored between week one (M = 6.7, SD = 0.86) and week two (M = 6.1, SD = 1.52, p = 0.042); week three (M = 6.06, SD = 1.89) and week four (M = 5.47, SD = 2.04, p = 0.05) and week one and week four (p = 0.002). Generally, the mean number of days monitored decreased each week, although at the end of treatment (week four) the average was still approximately 5.5 days of the 7. Participants' (n = 17) regularly monitored their food intake (indexed by five or more Food Diary entries) for an average of 21.2% of the possible 28 days (range: 0–28 days, M = 5.9 days, SD = 8.00).

Table 1. Baseline characteristics of participants (n = 25).

Participant Feature	Frequency (%)
Employed	60
Student	24
White/Caucasian	84
Asian	12
Metropolitan residence	64
Regional residence *	24
Rural residence	12
Comorbid anxiety	32
Comorbid depression	40
Comorbid substance/alcohol issues	16
Receiving concurrent treatment	76
Frequent alcohol consumption (4 or more times per week)	36
Past suicidality	60
Active suicidality (within previous 28 days)	20
Past self-harm	48
Active self-harm (within previous 28 days)	12

* NSW Health categorises regional residence as outside a major metropolitan city (e.g., Sydney) but not a rural location. Examples of regional locations include Wyong and Wagga Wagga.

Due to scheduling constraints, 13.2% of weekly phone calls were not completed at the exact seven-day mark. On average, these phone calls occurred 2.0 days (range: 1–8 days, SD = 2.35) later than the scheduled date and five phone calls did not take place. Moreover, 26.4% of the weekly questionnaires were not completed on time at the 7-day mark and were delayed by an average of 2.83 days (range: 1–11 days, SD = 2.81).

3.3. Treatment Outcomes

Table 2 provides the means and standard deviations for all dependent variables at each assessment period, as well as regression analysis results. Participants (n = 17) displayed a significant pre-post treatment decrease in the mean frequency of objective binge episodes, Wald χ^2 (1, N = 17) = 21.62, $p < 0.00$, mean number of days participants' experienced OBEs, Wald χ^2 (1, N = 17) = 12.99, $p < 0.001$ and frequency of perceived loss of control experienced during OBEs, Wald χ^2 (1, N = 17) = 12.47, $p < 0.001$. Pairwise comparisons revealed a significant increase in the mean number of objective binge days experienced in week one (M = 2.7, SD = 2.03) to week two (M = 3.5, SD = 2.07), p = 0.006.

There was no significant change in the number of days participants experienced subjective binge episodes between pre- and post-treatment measures, Wald χ^2 (1, N = 17) = 0.704, p = 0.401.

Using the Bonferroni correction, the decrease in the pre-post treatment frequency of purging episodes was no longer significant, Wald χ^2 (1, N = 13) = 4.30, p = 0.038. No significant differences were found in other compensatory behaviours of laxative use and excessive exercise.

There was a significant decrease from baseline to post-treatment in the mean global score on the EDE-Q, Wald χ^2 (1, N = 17) = 12.86, $p < 0.001$, as well as the mean scores on three EDE-Q subscales including dietary restraint, Wald χ^2 (1, N = 17) = 10.75, p = 0.001, eating concern, Wald χ^2 (1, N = 17) = 10.18, p = 0.001 and shape concern, Wald χ^2 (1, N = 17) = 9.92, p = 0.002.

The results of the Wilcoxon signed rank test (non-parametric sensitivity analysis) supported the respective statistical significance and non-significance of the preceding regression analyses examining the difference in bulimic symptomology between pre- and post-treatment measures.

Table 2. Treatment outcomes for Eating Disorder Examination-Questionnaire (EDE-Q), Eating Disorder Quality of Life Scale (EDQOL) and Three Factor Eating Questionnaire (TFEQ) Scores (n = 17).

Outcome	Pre-Treatment Means (*SD*)	Post-Treatment Means (*SD*)	*p* Value	Test Statistic Wald χ^2 (df = 1)
EDE-Q				
Objective binge frequency	23.7 (16.63)	14.9 (12.55)	$p < 0.001$ *	21.62
Objective binge days	17.9 (6.17)	10.8 (9.31)	$p < 0.001$ *	12.99
Loss of control frequency	21.0 (12.01)	14.1 (13.87)	$p < 0.001$ *	12.47
Subjective binge days (n = 16)	9.7 (9.60)	7.4 (6.26)	$p = 0.401$	0.70
Purge frequency (n = 13)	20.4 (20.45)	14.4 (18.85)	$p = 0.038$	4.30
Laxative use frequency (n = 7)	11.9 (11.45)	9.3 (10.61)	$p = 0.071$	3.25
Excessive exercise frequency (n = 11)	9.5 (10.58)	6.5 (8.42)	$p = 0.123$	2.38
Dietary restraint	4.1 (1.14)	2.9 (1.84)	$p = 0.001$ *	10.75
Eating concern	4.1 (1.11)	3.0 (1.41)	$p = 0.001$ *	10.18
Shape concern	5.3 (0.72)	4.5 (1.25)	$p = 0.002$ *	9.92
Weight concern	5.0 (0.60)	4.4 (1.48)	$p = 0.076$	3.14
Global score	4.6 (0.55)	3.7 (1.31)	$p < 0.001$ *	12.86
Other Outcomes				
EDQOL global score	1.9 (0.71)	1.8 (0.865)	$p = 0.564$	0.33
TFEQ global score	34.5 (4.91)	34.7 (4.61)	$p = 0.888$	0.02

* Statistically significant ($p < 0.0036$). Comparisons based upon Bonferroni-corrected α of 0.0036 (0.05/14). Note: EDE-Q = Eating Disorder Examination-Questionnaire; EDQOL = Eating Disorder Quality of Life Scale; TFEQ = Three Factor Eating Questionnaire.

3.4. *Predictors of Outcome and Dropout*

The Fisher's Exact Test revealed a significant association between the participants' level of bulimic severity and their degree of improvement in binge frequency, p = 0.002. Participants who displayed a 50% or greater reduction in binge frequency all were classed as less severe in bulimic presentation (defined by an average of 1–7 compensatory behaviours per week). In contrast, the majority (77.8%) of participants who displayed less than 50% reduction in binge frequency were classified as more severe in bulimic presentation.

Bulimic symptom severity was also associated with dietary restraint, p = 0.050. A statistical trend emerged whereby a larger number of participants who displayed a 50% or greater reduction in dietary restraint scores, had low bulimic severity (87.5%) as compared to high bulimic severity (12.5%). Conversely, more participants with high bulimic severity (66.7%) displayed less than 50% reduction in restraint scores as compared to those with low bulimic severity (33.3%).

Overall, treatment compliance and degree of improvement in compensatory behaviours were not significantly associated with participants' age, secondary mental health concern, K10 score, active/past suicidality, active/past self-harm and bulimic symptom severity.

4. Discussion

The findings of this study provide preliminary support for the food monitoring and regular eating techniques of CBT delivered online. Four weeks of guided, online stage 1 CBT resulted in a significant decrease in the frequency of OBEs, number of OBE days and frequency of associated LOC from baseline to post-treatment measures. There was also a significant decrease in both global EDE-Q scores and the EDE-Q subscales of dietary restraint, eating concern and shape concern. No change was observed in frequency of SBEs and compensatory behaviours including purging, laxative use and excessive exercise.

4.1. Attrition and Compliance

The current study has a considerably lower dropout rate (16%) than other online CBT studies (35% to 82%) [20]. Treatment compliance remained high with the Food Diary being entered at least once for an average of 87.1% of the possible 28 days. The food-monitoring compliance reported by previous studies is varied, ranging from 100% compliance for six to seven days of self-monitoring [9,34] to 46% compliance for 56 days of self-monitoring [41] The compliance achieved by the present study fits within the range reported by others and suggests that 28 days of food-monitoring may be an appropriate compromise between harnessing the technique's therapeutic potential and maintaining motivation to engage. Furthermore, many participants reported that the repetitive and tiresome nature of food monitoring was largely offset by the motivating nature of the weekly phone calls, with such anecdotal feedback suggesting an important role for therapeutic contact treatment compliance. However, due to the absence of appropriate control groups, the role of regular therapeutic contact and digital access to the Food Diary in producing heightened treatment compliance is yet to be elucidated.

Inaccuracies in the logging of meals in the Food Diary prevented accurate evaluation of participants' compliance with the "three-hour rule". The absence of such valuable information is due to the inaccurate recording of meal time or meal type, with most participants not adjusting the default settings of 7:00 a.m. and Breakfast when entering in the Food Diary. Consequently, an analysis of this data was not conducted. We recommend future studies adopt more stringently formatted systems to ensure accurate timing of meals is recorded [44].

4.2. Treatment Outcomes

The brief four week intervention achieved key symptom improvement comparable to the treatment outcomes of considerably longer online CBT self-help programs lasting for two to four months on average [16–19,21,61]. The preliminary results here contradict a recent review reporting that people with EDs do not find self-monitoring beneficial in practice [27] and rather supports the potential for concise, online self-monitoring programs. It is possible, however, that the observed improvements may possess short-term therapeutic effect, necessitating self-monitoring be examined over an extended time period which may cause the task to become burdensome.

The absence of a significant reduction across compensatory behaviours, despite an observed improvement in binging measures, may be due to several features of the current study. These include the short intervention period of four weeks and the small subset of participants having reported engaging in purging (n = 13), laxative use (n = 7) and excessive exercise (n = 11) as compensatory behaviours. Alternatively, given that the primary objective of food monitoring and the "three-hour rule" is to establish a regular eating pattern [42], it would appear logical for earlier change to be observed in binge frequency prior to compensatory behaviours. The paucity of evidence regarding the therapeutic effect of regular eating upon compensatory behaviours [46] necessitates future replication using larger sample sizes to confirm such suggestions. Additionally, considering early treatment response is known to predict short and long term BN treatment outcomes [38,39], the significant improvement observed in OBEs, LOC and dietary restraint following the use of only two behavioural techniques from Fairburn's 20-week program [42] may be indicative of future improvement.

Although participants' displayed an overall reduction in the number of OBE days from pre- to post-treatment measures, there was an unexpected increase in OBE days from week one (2.65 days) to week two (3.53 days). Given that the week two questionnaire was completed at the mid-point of treatment, perhaps the observed trend represents participants' initial motivation for recovery becoming later overpowered by the strength and habitual nature of their disordered eating behaviours. Alternatively, having people with BN closely review their egodystonic symptoms in the form of a Food Diary may prompt a decrease in mood and increase the likelihood of binges to regulate the distress and shame surrounding their eating behaviours [62]. More simply, participants may have developed heightened awareness regarding their behaviours in the second week of monitoring or perhaps documented their binges more truthfully once they became more comfortable with the treatment process. Further research is required to clarify whether an initial rise in OBE days is a typical BN treatment response or an anomaly of the current study.

Contrary to Hypothesis 2, no significant change was found in the number of days participants' recorded experiencing SBEs, and this challenges Hildebrandt and Latner's [34] 'binge drift' observation. The theoretical justification for 'binge drift' as the inability of self-monitoring to adjust dysfunctional cognitions [34] is also challenged by the observed decrease in the EDE-Q measures of attitudinal eating disorder psychopathology. Self-help CBT programs consisting of a longer two month treatment program have been unable to achieve such attitudinal change, similarly claiming that additional treatment time and greater focus upon cognitive elements are required [63,64]. Thus, the attitudinal improvement brought about by a considerably shorter behaviourally-based program alludes to suggestions that cognitive adjustments can be prompted by engaging in behavioural activities [30]. For example, persistence in implementing the "three-hour rule" allows for first-hand experience of the benefits of regular eating and provokes correction of certain fears or maladaptive cognitions regarding their shape. In a similar manner to the component analyses of CBT for depression [65], the ability of behavioural techniques to harness improvement in cognitive measures must be validated through direct comparison of the cognitive and behavioural components of CBT-BN.

4.3. Predictors of Treatment Compliance and Outcome

Participants with a more severe clinical presentation of BN displayed a smaller improvement in both OBE frequency and dietary restraint as compared to participants with less severe BN symptomology. Differential treatment responses as a function of one's clinical severity is mirrored in similar studies of guided self-help treatment [13,15] and fits within the "stepped-care" structure of treatment allocation [14]. Online stage 1 CBT appears to approach the therapeutic effectiveness of face-to-face treatment for a sub-set of less severe BN patients, whilst overcoming the barriers of cost, accessibility and duration of a treatment format, which may be unnecessarily excessive for their condition [8]. However, given the small sample size, it is possible that the statistical trend observed between dietary restraint and bulimic severity may represent a Type 2 error and requires replication in larger samples.

In contrast with existing literature on CBT treatment for BN [49,66,67], in this sample treatment compliance and bulimic symptom improvement was not significantly associated with baseline measures of depression or the presence of comorbid mood or anxiety disorders. The absence of such association may be due to the heavy concentration of behavioural techniques within the current study. Behavioural activities provide a practical and "hands-on" approach to treatment that is likely to enhance self-efficacy and offset the hopelessness brought upon by depressive traits and the bulimic symptoms [65,68,69]. Specifically, self-monitoring allows for direct observation of one's efforts to adhere to the "three-hour rule" and provides objective evidence of their attempts. Taken together with the encouragement provided by a therapeutic assistant, behavioural activities provide direct, observable change in depressed participants which may shift their external locus of control [66] and offset poor treatment compliance. Such justification is supported by recent suggestions regarding the importance of motivation as a predictor of BN treatment success [70] and should be included as a baseline measure in future studies. Additionally, the equivalent treatment compliance and therapeutic effectiveness across participants aged between 16 to 47 years, once more broadens the scope of candidates suitable for this treatment.

4.4. Strengths, Limitations and Future Research

The current study provides a novel contribution to the literature on BN treatment by offering preliminary pilot study evidence for the clinical effectiveness of an online, stage 1 CBT program.

The BEeT program employed in the study is a highly structured and sophisticated program, professionally developed by team of ED specialists and constructed based upon relevant empirical research on CBT-BN. Additionally, therapeutic guidance was provided by a non-expert trained in how to deliver the behavioural components of CBT treatment, offering promise as a method that could be used broadly by non-experts. The present study improves upon methodological limitations in the existing literature [71] having recruited a pure clinical sample of BN patients. Additionally, all communication took place via email and the telephone, maintaining the largely anonymous nature of online treatment and increasing the accessibility for patients who are busy with work, study or carer commitments as face-to-face interviews were not required.

Due to the relatively small sample size, these findings must be considered tentative until an adequately powered study is conducted. The absence of a waitlist control condition also limits the conclusions regarding the causal role of the treatment program and necessitates other robust research designs be conducted. A randomised controlled trial will also allow for comparison of online, stage 1 CBT against conventional CBT programs, with the presence of control arms providing further clarity regarding the role of therapeutic guidance techniques, such as reminder text messages and weekly phone calls, in provoking the greatest change in one's behaviours.

Given that 56% of participants reported receiving additional treatment, other than CBT, for their ED, it is possible that improvement observed may be partly attributed to their concurrent treatment program. However, seeing as all participants were engaged in their additional treatment prior to entering the current study, it appears that the self-monitoring and regular eating techniques enforced may have been instrumental in bringing about change.

Future research should control for concurrent treatment to isolate the effects of behavioural techniques and strengthen claims regarding its therapeutic effectiveness. Furthermore, considering previous research [72] suggests that the reactive effects of self-monitoring are limited to the time period for which the individual actively engages in self-monitoring, future studies should include a follow-up.

5. Conclusions

The present study provides preliminary evidence for the clinical effectiveness of brief behavioural self-monitoring and regular eating training (BEeT) delivered online which, if replicated in a larger sample, may result in the development of shorter, yet equally effective, forms of treatment. Concise programs would make treatment accessible for a much broader range of people with BN for whom their work or study commitments and financial constraints make it extremely difficult for them to engage in three months of one-hour weekly therapy sessions [14]. Additionally, the digital format of treatment delivery overcomes the barriers of accessibility and cost inherent in the treatment of EDs and which are of particular concern for rural and regional residents. The current findings provide the justification for a randomised controlled trial to elucidate the clinical benefits of emphasising behavioural techniques which form part of typical CBT-BN delivery by online modalities.

Acknowledgments: The development of the Binge Eating eTherapy program was funded by NSW Health.

Author Contributions: Sarah Barakat, Sarah Maguire, Phillipa Hay and Stephen Touyz conceived and designed the experiments; Sarah Barakat and Sarah Maguire performed the experiments; Sarah Barakat analyzed the data; Sarah Barakat, Sarah Maguire, Lois Surgenor, Brooke Donnelly, Blagica Miceska, Kirsty Fromholtz, Janice Russell, Phillipa Hay and Stephen Touyz contributed reagents/materials/analysis tools; Sarah Barakat wrote the paper.

Conflicts of Interest: The authors declare no conflict of interest. The founding sponsors had no role in the design of the study; in the collection, analyses, or interpretation of data; in the writing of the manuscript, and in the decision to publish the results.

References

1. Hay, P.; Chinn, D.; Forbes, D.; Madden, S.; Newton, R.; Sugenor, L.; Touyz, S.; Ward, W. Royal Australian and New Zealand College of Psychiatrists clinical practice guidelines for the treatment of eating disorders. *Aust. N. Z. J. Psychiatry* **2014**, *48*, 977–1008. [CrossRef] [PubMed]

2. National Collaborating Centre for Mental Health. *Eating Disorders: Core Interventions in the Treatment and Management of Anorexia Nervosa, Bulimia Nervosa and Related Eating Disorders*; NICE guideline (CG9); British Psychological Society: Leicester, UK; Royal College of Psychiatrists: London, UK, 2004.
3. Hart, L.M.; Granillo, M.T.; Jorm, A.F.; Paxton, S.J. Unmet need for treatment in the eating disorders: A systematic review of eating disorder specific treatment seeking among community cases. *Clin. Psychol. Rev.* **2011**, *31*, 727–735. [CrossRef] [PubMed]
4. National Eating Disorders Collaboration (NEDC). *Eating Disorders Prevention, Treatment and Management: An Evidence Review*; Commissioned by the Commonwealth Department of Health and Aging; National Eating Disorders Collaboration: Canberra, Australia, 2010.
5. Tobin, D.L.; Banker, J.D.; Weisberg, L.; Bowers, W. I know what you did last summer (and it was not CBT): A factor analytic model of international psychotherapeutic practice in the eating disorders. *Int. J. Eat. Disord.* **2007**, *40*, 754–757. [CrossRef] [PubMed]
6. Waller, G. Evidence-based treatment and therapist drift. *Behav. Res. Ther.* **2009**, *47*, 119–127. [CrossRef] [PubMed]
7. Stuhldreher, N.; Konnopka, A.; Wild, B.; Herzog, W.; Zipfel, S.; Löwe, B.; König, H.H. Cost-of-illness studies and cost-effectiveness analyses in eating disorders: A systematic review. *Int. J. Eat. Disord.* **2012**, *45*, 476–491. [CrossRef] [PubMed]
8. Williams, C. New technologies in self-help: Another effective way to get better? *Eur. Eat. Disord. Rev.* **2003**, *11*, 170–182. [CrossRef]
9. Latner, J.D.; Wilson, G.T. Self-monitoring and the assessment of binge eating. *Behav. Ther.* **2002**, *33*, 465–477. [CrossRef]
10. Hay, P.; Bacaltchuk, J.; Stefano, S. Psychotherapy for bulimia nervosa and binging. *Cochrane Database Syst. Rev.* **2004**, *1*, 1–73.
11. Fairburn, C.G. *Overcoming Binge Eating*, 1st ed.; Guilford Press: New York, NY, USA, 1995.
12. Palmer, R.L.; Birchall, H.; McGrain, L.; Sullivan, V. Self-help for bulimic disorders: A randomised controlled trial comparing minimal guidance with face-to-face or telephone guidance. *Br. J. Psychiatry* **2002**, *181*, 230–235. [CrossRef] [PubMed]
13. Thiels, C.; Schmidt, U.; Troop, N.; Treasure, J.; Garthe, R. Binge frequency predicts outcome in guided self-care treatment of bulimia nervosa. *Eur. Eat. Disord. Rev.* **2000**, *8*, 272–278. [CrossRef]
14. Treasure, J.; Schmidt, U.; Troop, N.; Tiller, J.; Todd, G.; Turnbull, S. Sequential treatment for bulimia nervosa incorporating a self-care manual. *Br. J. Psychiatry* **1996**, *168*, 94–98. [CrossRef] [PubMed]
15. Agras, W.S.; Crow, S.J.; Halmi, K.A.; Mitchell, J.E.; Wilson, G.T.; Kraemer, H.C. Outcome predictors for the cognitive behavior treatment of bulimia nervosa: Data from a multisite study. *Am. J. Psychiatry* **2000**, *157*, 1302–1308. [CrossRef] [PubMed]
16. Carrard, I.; Rouget, P.; Fernández-Aranda, F.; Volkart, A.C.; Damoiseau, M.; Lam, T. Evaluation and deployment of evidence based patient self-management support program for bulimia nervosa. *Int. J. Med. Inform.* **2006**, *75*, 101–109. [CrossRef] [PubMed]
17. Fernández-Aranda, F.; Núñez, A.; Martínez, C.; Krug, I.; Cappozzo, M.; Carrard, I.; Rouget, P.; Jiménez-Murcia, S.; Granero, R.; Penelo, E.; et al. Internet-based cognitive-behavioral therapy for bulimia nervosa: A controlled study. *Cyberpsychol. Behav.* **2009**, *12*, 37–41. [CrossRef] [PubMed]
18. Mitchell, J.E.; Crosby, R.D.; Wonderlich, S.A.; Crow, S.; Lancaster, K.; Simonich, H.; Swan-Kremeier, L.; Lysne, C.; Myers, T.C. A randomized trial comparing the efficacy of cognitive–behavioral therapy for bulimia nervosa delivered via telemedicine versus face-to-face. *Behav. Res. Ther.* **2008**, *46*, 581–592. [CrossRef] [PubMed]
19. Pretorius, N.; Arcelus, J.; Beecham, J.; Dawson, H.; Doherty, F.; Eisler, I.; Gallagher, C.; Gowers, S.; Isaacs, G.; Johnson-Sabine, E.; et al. Cognitive-behavioural therapy for adolescents with bulimic symptomatology: The acceptability and effectiveness of internet-based delivery. *Behav. Res. Ther.* **2009**, *47*, 729–736. [CrossRef] [PubMed]
20. Ruwaard, J.; Lange, A.; Broeksteeg, J.; Renteria-Agirre, A.; Schrieken, B.; Dolan, C.V.; Emmelkamp, P. Online cognitive–behavioural treatment of bulimic symptoms: A randomized controlled trial. *Clin. Psychol. Psychother.* **2013**, *20*, 308–318. [CrossRef] [PubMed]

21. Sánchez-Ortiz, V.C.; Munro, C.; Stahl, D.; House, J.; Startup, H.; Treasure, J.; Williams, C.; Schmidt, U. A randomized controlled trial of internet-based cognitive-behavioural therapy for bulimia nervosa or related disorders in a student population. *Psychol. Med.* **2011**, *41*, 407–417. [CrossRef] [PubMed]
22. Ljotsson, B.; Lundin, C.; Mitsell, K.; Carlbring, P.; Ramklint, M.; Ghaderi, A. Remote treatment of bulimia nervosa and binge eating disorder: A randomized trial of Internet-assisted cognitive behavioural therapy. *Behav. Res. Ther.* **2007**, *45*, 649–661. [CrossRef] [PubMed]
23. Robinson, P.H.; Serfaty, M.A. The use of e-mail in the identification of bulimia nervosa and its treatment. *Eur. Eat. Disord. Rev.* **2001**, *9*, 182–193. [CrossRef]
24. Bauer, S.; Okon, E.; Meermann, R.; Kordy, H. Technology-enhanced maintenance of treatment gains in eating disorders: Efficacy of an intervention delivered via text messaging. *J. Consult. Clin. Psychol.* **2012**, *80*, 700–706. [CrossRef] [PubMed]
25. Schmidt, U.; Andiappan, M.; Grover, M.; Robinson, S.; Perkins, S.; Dugmore, O.; Treasure, J.; Landau, S.; Eisler, I.; Williams, C. Randomised controlled trial of CD–ROM-based cognitive–behavioural self-care for bulimia nervosa. *Br. J. Psychiatry* **2008**, *193*, 493–500. [CrossRef] [PubMed]
26. Fairburn, C.G.; Cooper, Z. The Eating Disorder Examination (12th ed.). In *Binge Eating: Nature, Assessment and Treatment*; Fairburn, C.G., Wilson, G.T., Eds.; Guilford Press: New York, NY, USA, 1993; pp. 317–360.
27. Walsh, S.; Golden, E.; Priebe, S. Systematic review of patients' participation in and experiences of technology-based monitoring of mental health symptoms in the community. *Br. Med. J. Open* **2016**, *6*, e008362. [CrossRef] [PubMed]
28. Tregarthen, J.P.; Lock, J.; Darcy, A.M. Development of a smartphone application for eating disorder self-monitoring. *Int. J. Eat. Disord.* **2015**, *48*, 972–982. [CrossRef] [PubMed]
29. Geller, J.; Srikameswaran, S. What effective therapies have in common. *Adv. Eat. Disord. Theor. Res. Pract.* **2015**, *3*, 191–197. [CrossRef]
30. Longmore, R.J.; Worrell, M. Do we need to challenge thoughts in cognitive behavior therapy? *Clin. Psychol. Rev.* **2007**, *27*, 173–187. [CrossRef] [PubMed]
31. Fairburn, C.G.; Jones, R.; Peveler, R.C.; Carr, S.J.; Solomon, R.A.; O'Connor, M.E.; Burton, J.; Hope, R.A. Three psychological treatments for bulimia nervosa: A comparative trial. *Arch. Gen. Psychiatry* **1991**, *48*, 463–469. [CrossRef] [PubMed]
32. Korotitsch, W.J.; Nelson-Gray, R.O. An overview of self-monitoring research in assessment and treatment. *Psychol. Assess.* **1999**, *11*, 415–425. [CrossRef]
33. Wilson, G.T.; Vitousek, K.M. Self-monitoring in the assessment of eating disorders. *Psychol. Assess.* **1999**, *11*, 480–489. [CrossRef]
34. Hildebrandt, T.; Latner, J. Effect of self-monitoring on binge eating: Treatment response or 'binge drift'? *Eur. Eat. Disord. Rev.* **2006**, *14*, 17–22. [CrossRef]
35. Fairburn, C.G.; Agras, W.S.; Walsh, B.T.; Wilson, G.T.; Stice, E. Prediction of outcome in bulimia nervosa by early change in treatment. *Am. J. Psychiatry* **2004**, *161*, 2322–2324. [CrossRef] [PubMed]
36. Le Grange, D.; Doyle, P.; Crosby, R.D.; Chen, E. Early response to treatment in adolescent bulimia nervosa. *Int. J. Eat. Disord.* **2008**, *41*, 755–757. [CrossRef] [PubMed]
37. Raykos, B.C.; Watson, H.J.; Fursland, A.; Byrne, S.M.; Nathan, P. Prognostic value of rapid response to enhanced cognitive behavioral therapy in a routine clinic sample of eating disorder outpatients. *Int. J. Eat. Disord.* **2013**, *46*, 764–770. [CrossRef] [PubMed]
38. Thompson-Brenner, H.; Shingleton, R.M.; Sauer-Zavala, S.; Richards, L.K.; Pratt, E.M. Multiple measures of rapid response as predictors of remission in cognitive behavior therapy for bulimia nervosa. *Behav. Res. Ther.* **2015**, *64*, 9–14. [CrossRef] [PubMed]
39. Vall, E.; Wade, T.D. Predictors of treatment outcome in individuals with eating disorders: A systematic review and meta-analysis. *Int. J. Eat. Disord.* **2015**, *48*, 946–971. [CrossRef] [PubMed]
40. Cash, T.F.; Hrabosky, J.I. The effects of psychoeducation and self-monitoring in a cognitive-behavioral program for body-image improvement. *Eat. Disord.* **2003**, *11*, 255–270. [CrossRef] [PubMed]
41. Nichols, S.; Gusella, J. Food for thought: Will adolescent girls with eating disorders self-monitor in a CBT group. *Can. Child Psychiatry Rev.* **2003**, *12*, 37–39.
42. Fairburn, C.G. *Cognitive Behavior Therapy and Eating Disorders*; Guilford Press: New York, NY, USA, 2008.
43. Cooper, M.; Todd, G.; Wells, A. *Treating Bulimia Nervosa and Binge Eating: An Integrated Metacognitive and Cognitive Therapy Manual*; Routledge, Taylor & Francis Group: London, UK, 2009.

44. Zendegui, E.A.; West, J.A.; Zandberg, L.J. Binge eating frequency and regular eating adherence: The role of eating pattern in cognitive behavioral guided self-help. *Eat. Behav.* **2014**, *15*, 241–243. [CrossRef] [PubMed]
45. Telch, C.F.; Agras, S.W. The effects of short-term food deprivation on caloric intake in eating-disordered subjects. *Appetite* **1996**, *26*, 221–234. [CrossRef] [PubMed]
46. Shah, N.; Passi, V.; Bryson, S.; Agras, W.S. Patterns of eating and abstinence in women treated for bulimia nervosa. *Int. J. Eat. Disord.* **2005**, *38*, 330–334. [CrossRef] [PubMed]
47. Swanson, S.A.; Crow, S.J.; Le Grange, D.; Swendsen, J.; Merikangas, K.R. Prevalence and correlates of eating disorders in adolescents: Results from the national comorbidity survey replication adolescent supplement. *Arch. Gen. Psychiatry* **2011**, *68*, 714–723. [CrossRef] [PubMed]
48. Hudson, J.I.; Hiripi, E.; Pope, H.G.; Kessler, R.C. The prevalence and correlates of eating disorders in the National Comorbidity Survey Replication. *Biol. Psychiatry* **2007**, *61*, 348–358. [CrossRef] [PubMed]
49. Grilo, C.M.; Masheb, R.M.; Wilson, G.T. Subtyping binge eating disorder. *J. Consult. Clin. Psychol.* **2001**, *69*, 1066–1072. [CrossRef] [PubMed]
50. Grilo, C.M.; White, M.A.; Masheb, R.M. DSM-IV psychiatric disorder comorbidity and its correlates in binge eating disorder. *Int. J. Eat. Disord.* **2009**, *42*, 228–234. [CrossRef] [PubMed]
51. Stice, E.; Bohon, C.; Marti, C.N.; Fischer, K. Subtyping women with bulimia nervosa along dietary and negative affect dimensions: Further evidence of reliability and validity. *J. Consult. Clin. Psychol.* **2008**, *76*, 1022–1033. [CrossRef] [PubMed]
52. American Psychiatric Association. *Diagnostic and Statistical Manual of Mental Disorders*, 5th ed.; American Psychiatric Publishing: Arlington, VA, USA, 2013.
53. Fairburn, C.G.; Beglin, S.J. Eating Disorder Examination Questionnaire (6.0). In *Cognitive Behavior Therapy and Eating Disorders*; Fairburn, C.G., Ed.; Guildford Press: New York, NY, USA, 2008; pp. 309–315.
54. Fairburn, C.G.; Marcus, M.D.; Wilson, G.T. Cognitive-Behavioral Therapy for Binge Eating and Bulimia Nervosa: A Comprehensive Treatment Manual. In *Binge Eating: Nature, Assessment and Treatment*; Fairburn, C.G., Wilson, G.T., Eds.; Guildford Press: New York, NY, USA, 1993; pp. 361–404.
55. Fairburn, C.G.; Cooper, Z.; Shafran, R. Cognitive behaviour therapy for eating disorders: A "transdiagnostic" theory and treatment. *Behav. Res. Ther.* **2003**, *41*, 509–528. [CrossRef]
56. Luce, K.H.; Winzelberg, A.J.; Das, S.; Osborne, M.I.; Bryson, S.W.; Taylor, C.B. Reliability of self-report: Paper versus online administration. *Comput. Hum. Behav.* **2007**, *23*, 1384–1389. [CrossRef]
57. Peterson, C.B.; Crosby, R.D.; Wonderlich, S.A.; Joiner, T.; Crow, S.J.; Mitchell, J.E.; Bardone-Cone, A.M.; Klein, M.; Le Grange, D. Psychometric properties of the eating disorder examination-questionnaire: Factor structure and internal consistency. *Int. J. Eat. Disord.* **2007**, *40*, 386–389. [CrossRef] [PubMed]
58. Kessler, R.C.; Andrews, G.; Colpe, L.J.; Hiripi, E.; Mroczek, D.K.; Normand, S.L.; Walters, E.E.; Zaslavsky, A.M. Short screening scales to monitor population prevalences and trends in non-specific psychological distress. *Psychol. Med.* **2002**, *32*, 959–976. [CrossRef] [PubMed]
59. Engel, S.G.; Wittrock, D.A.; Crosby, R.D.; Wonderlich, S.A.; Mitchell, J.E.; Kolotkin, R.L. Development and psychometric validation of an eating disorder-specific health-related quality of life instrument. *Int. J. Eat. Disord.* **2006**, *39*, 62–71. [CrossRef] [PubMed]
60. Stunkard, A.J.; Messick, S. The three-factor eating questionnaire to measure dietary restraint, disinhibition and hunger. *J. Psychosom. Res.* **1985**, *29*, 71–83. [CrossRef]
61. Banasiak, S.J.; Paxton, S.J.; Hay, P. Guided self-help for bulimia nervosa in primary care: A randomized controlled trial. *Psychol. Med.* **2005**, *35*, 1283–1294. [CrossRef] [PubMed]
62. Williamson, D.A.; Muller, S.L.; Reas, D.L.; Thaw, J.M. Cognitive bias in eating disorders: Implications for theory and treatment. *Behav. Modif.* **1999**, *23*, 556–577. [CrossRef] [PubMed]
63. Cooper, P.J.; Coker, S.; Fleming, C. An evaluation of the efficacy of supervised cognitive behavioral self-help for bulimia nervosa. *J. Psychosom. Res.* **1996**, *40*, 281–287. [CrossRef]
64. Perkins, S.S.; Murphy, R.R.; Schmidt, U.U.; Williams, C. Self-help and guided self-help for eating disorders. *Cochrane Database Syst. Rev.* **2006**, *4*, 1–3.
65. Ilardi, S.S.; Craighead, W.E. The role of nonspecific factors in cognitive-behavior therapy for depression. *Clin. Psychol. Sci. Pract.* **1994**, *1*, 138–155. [CrossRef]
66. Steel, Z.; Jones, J.; Adcock, S.; Clancy, R.; Bridgford-West, L.; Austin, J. Why the high rate of dropout from individualized cognitive-behavior therapy for bulimia nervosa? *Int. J. Eat. Disord.* **2000**, *28*, 209–214. [CrossRef]

67. Chen, E.Y.; Le Grange, D. Subtyping adolescents with bulimia nervosa. *Behav. Res. Ther.* **2007**, *45*, 2813–2820. [CrossRef] [PubMed]
68. Bandura, A. Self-efficacy: Toward a unifying theory of behavioral change. *Psychol. Rev.* **1977**, *84*, 191–215. [CrossRef] [PubMed]
69. Cooper, P.J.; Coker, S.; Fleming, C. Self-help for bulimia nervosa: A preliminary report. *Int. J. Eat. Disord.* **1994**, *16*, 401–404. [CrossRef]
70. Steele, A.L.; Bergin, J.; Wade, T.D. Self-efficacy as a robust predictor of outcome in guided self-help treatment for broadly defined bulimia nervosa. *Int. J. Eat. Disord.* **2011**, *44*, 389–396. [CrossRef] [PubMed]
71. Hay, P.J.; Claudino, A.M. Bulimia nervosa: Online interventions. *Br. Med. J. Clin. Evid.* **2015**, *3*, 1–16.
72. Nelson, R.O.; Boykin, R.A.; Hayes, S.C. Long-term effects of self-monitoring on reactivity and on accuracy. *Behav. Res. Ther.* **1982**, *20*, 357–363. [CrossRef]

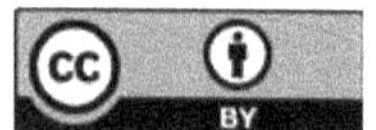

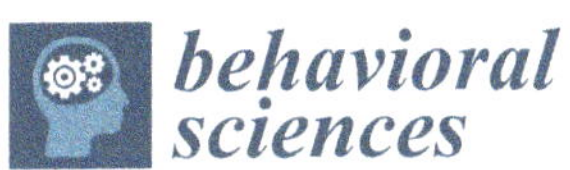
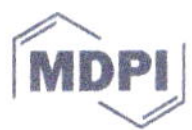

Review

Virtual Reality as a Promising Strategy in the Assessment and Treatment of Bulimia Nervosa and Binge Eating Disorder: A Systematic Review

Marcele Regine de Carvalho [1,2,*], Thiago Rodrigues de Santana Dias [3], Monica Duchesne [3], Antonio Egidio Nardi [2] and Jose Carlos Appolinario [3]

1 Institute of Psychology, Federal University of Rio de Janeiro, Avenida Pasteur, 250, Rio de Janeiro 22290-902, Brazil
2 LABPR, Institute of Psychiatry, Federal University of Rio de Janeiro, Rio de Janeiro 22290-140, Brazil; antonioenardi@gmail.com
3 Eating Disorders and Obesity Group, Institute of Psychiatry, Federal University of Rio de Janeiro, Rio de Janeiro 22290-140, Brazil; thiagorjdias.insight@gmail.com (T.R.d.S.D.); monica@duchesne.com.br (M.D.); jotappo@gmail.com (J.C.A.)
* Correspondence: marcelecarvalho@gmail.com; Tel.: +55-21-99658-7080

Received: 5 June 2017; Accepted: 6 July 2017; Published: 9 July 2017

Abstract: Several lines of evidence suggest that Virtual Reality (VR) has a potential utility in eating disorders. The objective of this study is to review the literature on the use of VR in bulimia nervosa (BN) and binge eating disorder (BED). Using PRISMA (Preferred Reporting Items for Systematic Reviews and Meta-Analyses) statement for reporting systematic reviews, we performed a PubMed, Web of Knowledge and SCOPUS search to identify studies employing VR in the assessment and treatment of BN and BED. The following search terms were used: "virtual reality", "eating disorders", "binge eating", and "bulimia nervosa". From the 420 articles identified, 19 were selected, nine investigated VR in assessment and 10 were treatment studies (one case-report, two non-controlled and six randomized controlled trials). The studies using VR in BN and BED are at an early stage. However, considering the available evidence, the use of VR in the assessment of those conditions showed some promise in identifying: (1) how those patients experienced their body image; and (2) environments or specific kinds of foods that may trigger binge–purging cycle. Some studies using VR-based environments associated to cognitive behavioral techniques showed their potential utility in improving motivation for change, self-esteem, body image disturbances and in reducing binge eating and purging behavior.

Keywords: virtual reality; systematic review; binge–purging eating disorders; bulimia nervosa; binge eating disorder

1. Introduction

Eating disorders (EDs) are widespread, disabling and often chronic mental disorders [1–3]. They are categorized, according to DSM-5 [4], as a group of conditions characterized by a persistent disturbance of eating or eating related behaviors resulting in altered consumption or absorption of food that impairs physical health and psychosocial functioning. The EDs diagnostic subgroup includes major discrete clinical entities such as anorexia nervosa (AN), bulimia nervosa (BN), binge eating disorder (BED) and their subthreshold syndromes. In general, patients with AN could be described by low body weight, food restriction, fear of becoming fat and an overvaluation of their weight/shape (body image (BI) concerns); in those with BN, the core symptomatology are the presence of recurrent binge eating (BE) episodes followed by inappropriate compensatory behaviors (self-induced vomits, fasting, etc.) to prevent weight gain and a self-evaluation unduly influenced by body shape/weight; and, subjects with BED also have recurrent BE but did not engage in compensatory behaviors as those seen in BN.

Based on several recent clinical and neurobiological findings a spectrum classification model has been proposed which distinguishes between eating disordered patients who restrict food intake without binging and those who binge and purge [5,6]. This distinction between restrictors and binge–purgers is thought to correspond to important phenomenological and etiological differences, including those related to predominant personality features, family-interaction styles, neurobiological abnormalities, and patterns of genetic transmission. Such differences imply that the restrictors versus binge–purgers distinction may delineate more homogenous subgroups of EDs in a more meaningful way regarding treatment [7].

Thus, BN and BED are classified as a binge–purging type of ED [6] and both are characterized by a unique phenomenon called BE, a pattern of disordered eating which consists of episodes of unusually large consumption of food associated with feelings of loss of control [4]. Moreover, even though body dissatisfaction was not included as a BED diagnostic criterion, several authors reported high levels of this symptomatology in this population [8]. Along with this core eating psychopathology, patients in binge–purging spectrum disorders usually displayed additional general psychopathology such as depression, anxiety, low self-esteem, and personality traits such as impulsivity.

Although, currently, the pathophysiology of BN and BED is not clearly understood, several hypotheses based on these emotional aspects have been proposed for the development and maintenance of these disorders [9,10] and may represent a potential path for the development of new interventions. In this perspective, BI disturbances/dissatisfaction may potentially lead to feelings of negative affect and attempts to reduce caloric intake, and in turn, negative affect and dietary restraint lead to BE [9]. More recently, certain personality traits as impulsivity have been implicated in triggering eating disordered eating. Impulsivity might be related to deficits in inhibitory control, i.e., the capacity to delay a response, to suppress inappropriate responses and to ignore distractions [11,12]. A growing body of evidence suggests that impulsivity and reduced inhibitory control are associated with overeating and binge-eating behavior [13,14].

BN and BED have a complex, multifactorial etiology, involving the interactions between genes and environment, with an interplay of biological, psychological and sociocultural factors. Although psychotherapeutic approaches (such as cognitive-behavior therapy (CBT)) are the most effective and recommended first-line treatment for those conditions, in general, currently available treatments have been shown only moderately effective. Thus, there is an urge to improve the understanding of EDs etiology and to develop a more efficacious and personalized forms of interventions [15].

Virtual reality (VR) is an emerging technology with a variety of uses ranging from clinical research to the assessment and treatment of several medical and psychological conditions [16]. A comprehensive definition for VR is "an advanced form of human–computer interface that allows the user to interact with and become immersed in a computer-generated environment in a naturalistic fashion" [17]. An important aspect of VR is that it induces a kind of "sense of presence", i.e., a feeling of "being there" in the middle of the virtual environment. This sensation of presence produces a setting where the subject can stay and live a specific experience, evoking emotional responses and a sense of self-reflectiveness [18]. Summarizing, VR reduces the gap between reality and imagination and have a potential utility in behavioral health for the assessment and treatment of mental disorders, because it allows the individual to face anxiogenic situations in a more controlled environment [19].

Initially designed for treatment of phobias, the use of VR in behavioral disorders has expanded for other mental health conditions [20]. Freeman and colleagues systematically reviewed the studies of VR in mental disorders and found that the main conditions investigated were anxiety disorders, schizophrenia, substance related disorders and EDs [16]. The authors pointed out that VR environments can be used to elicit psychiatric symptoms, manipulation of VR can inform the understanding of disorders, and simpler psychological treatments can be successfully administered in VR format.

Another systematic review focusing specifically on the potential use of VR in interventions for mental disorders [21] demonstrated that, overall, VR has been shown superior to treatment as usual or waiting lists and with similar efficacy as conventional CBT or in vivo exposure. However, it is important to mention that the effectiveness of VR-based interventions varied across diagnostic groups and the studies showed several methodological flaws. Both reviews [16,21] commented that EDs is a promising area for utilization of VR.

In general, VR is used in EDs studies exploring two main aspects of the EDs syndrome: BI distortions and uncontrolled eating. For the first aspect, it usually enables three-dimensional figures of the patient's body to be presented, helping him/her to reach an awareness of BI distortion and then providing the possibility to face and modify distortions, which results in a more realistic view of the body and a potential decrease in BI dissatisfaction. For the second topic, VR provides scenarios that simulate real-life situations and to encounter food cues known to trigger his/her disordered eating behavior. Riva and colleagues [20] pioneered the studies on the use of VR for the treatment of EDs as part of a collaborative network of the European VREPAR PROJECT (VR Environments for the Psychoneurophysiological Assessment and Rehabilitation Project). They developed the VEBIM (Virtual Environment for BI Modification), composed of five VR environments for the treatment of BI disturbance.

Ferrez-Garcia and colleagues [22] in 2013 summarized the available information regarding the use of VR for the treatment of EDs and obesity. From the 17 studies included in this systematic review, 11 investigated VR-based interventions specifically in patients with EDs. In terms of the diagnostic rubrics of the samples and designs of the studies, there were four case reports describing the effects of VR in AN subjects, two non-controlled and two controlled trials with patients with BED; two controlled studies with a mixed sample of AN and BN individuals; and one non-controlled study in an eating disorder not elsewhere specified (EDNOS) sample. In the same year, reviewing exposure therapy in the field of EDs, Koskina and colleagues [23] analyzed the existing evidences of food and BI exposure using VR environments. Taking together, these reviews considered that treatment studies with VR in EDs are emerging. Although the authors are generally supportive of the potential usefulness of VR in EDs they highlighted several methodological limitations of the current studies that need to be overcame in the future research.

To update the current knowledge on the use of VR-based environments in a more homogenous subgroup of binge–purging EDs we performed this systematic review in order to summarize the current evidences of VR in the assessment and treatment of BN and BED.

2. Methods

Using the PRISMA statement for reporting systematic reviews, we performed a PubMed, Web of Knowledge and SCOPUS search to identify studies using VR in the assessment and treatment of BN, BED and their subthreshold syndromes published until June 2017. Two independent reviewers (M.R.C. and T.R.S.D.) performed study selection procedures and data extraction. The decisions on inclusion or exclusion of the reviewers were recorded. The results from the data abstraction were compared after completing the review of the articles. Any discrepancies or disagreements were resolved by consensus, with attention to the previously defined selection criteria. A third reviewer would decide upon inclusion or exclusion in the case of a persistent disagreement between the reviewers. We searched for original clinical studies (controlled and uncontrolled) investigating the utility of VR environments in samples that includes patients with the diagnosis of BN and BED. Thus, if the sample of the study along with BN and BED also included patients with other ED rubrics (such as AN or EDNOS) the paper was incorporated. We included also case-reports. The bibliography of review articles was used to find articles not retrieved by the electronic search. The following combination of search terms were used: "virtual reality AND eating disorders", "virtual reality AND binge eating", and "virtual reality AND bulimia nervosa". The selection of papers suitable for this review was restricted to articles published in peer-reviewed journals. Where a title or abstract seemed to describe a study eligible for inclusion, the full article was obtained and examined to assess relevance based on the inclusion criteria. Subsequently, the articles were divided according to the study design, data extracted and organized in tables.

3. Results

The initial electronic search identified 420 studies using VR-based environments in patients with BN and BED. Additionally, nine studies were identified by hand searching the references of the original and review articles retrieved. After a careful process of appraisal, 19 studies met the inclusion criteria and were selected and included in this review (see Figure 1). From these 19 studies using VR in BN and BED, nine were classified as *assessment studies* [24–32]—which includes studies of symptom assessment, identification of symptom markers, tests of putative causal factors and other studies investigating different aspects of the conditions—(see Table 1) and 10 as *treatment studies* [33–42]—reports and studies with includes VR-based environments as a therapeutic intervention—(see Table 2).

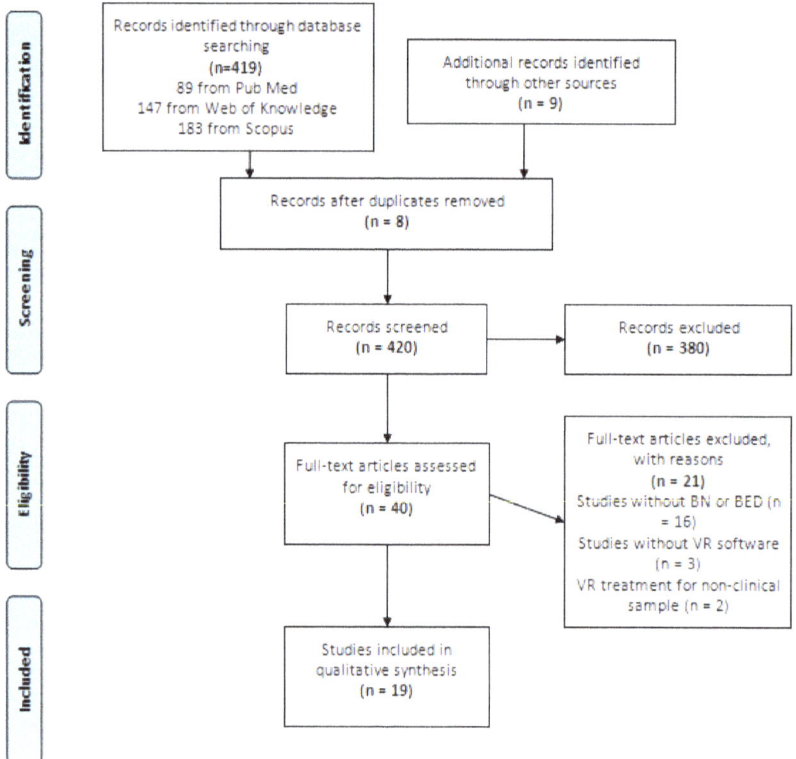

Figure 1. PRISMA Flow Diagram.

In general, an important aspect of those studies is that they have been conducted by basically three group of researchers using different VR-systems. Through six VR environments, which included exposure to food and social situations, assessment studies were mainly conducted by Gutiérrez-Maldonado et al. [24–26,28,30,31]; VEBIM developed by Riva et al. [38,43] with several updates such as VEBIM 2 or VREDIM (Virtual Reality for Eating Disorders Modification); and Virtual & Body developed by Perpiñá et al. [33], The latter two software packages were used in assessment and treatment studies. BI disturbance was the main target of the VR component in these interventions, and body dissatisfaction was the primary outcome variable assessed. Other outcomes often included were depression, self-esteem, assertiveness, and other symptoms related to ED. Considering the assessment studies from the nine studies included in this review, only two included a homogeneous sample of BN and BED individuals, while the others comprised mixed samples of restrictive and binge–purging type of EDs. Conversely, the treatment studies were less heterogeneous and, apparently, only two studies included mixed samples.

In the following paragraphs, we revised the selected studies in more detail.

3.1. VR in the Assessment of BN and BED

Among the umbrella of the assessments studies we found investigations trying to characterize the differential responses of EDs patient's symptomatology to BI and food related VR settings and to validate that these apparatuses really provide a real sense of presence. In this sense, Gutiérrez-Maldonado et al. [24] and Ferrer-García et al. [25] showed that ED patients presented higher anxiety when exposed to high-calorie food situations and to locations such as a swimming-pool when compared to a neutral environment. In another study, Gutiérrez-Maldonado et al. [26] reported that ED patients showed more BI distortions and body dissatisfaction facing high-calorie food environments when compared with in low calorie food environments. In relation to the sense of presence, a group of studies [27–29] have demonstrated that, while exposed to the virtual environments, ED patients experienced satisfactory sense of presence. Gorini et al. [27] confirmed this impression and reported that the higher sense of presence experienced in VR settings by a group of patients with AN and BN was associated with higher levels of anxiety.

More recently, assessment studies have investigated virtual food environments (food-cues) in terms of triggering, maintaining and/or relapsing mechanisms associated to BN and BED. They showed that exposure to virtual food could induce similar reactions as exposure to real food, and that VR environments relevant to ED were able to elicit emotional, cognitive and behavioral responses in these patients. Perpiñá et al. [29] exposed ED patients to a virtual kitchen where they could prepare and eat food. Before eating, patients displayed moderate to high scores of urge to eat, fear, and avoidance; and low desire to eat. After eating, they reported feelings of putting on weight, urge to eat and being upset; and some behavioral aspects such as pressure to exercise as a compensatory measure, to continue eating, and to purge. Gorini et al. [27] verified that virtual food was as effective as real food, and more effective than photographs, in producing psychological and physiological responses in ED patients. Ferrer-García et al. [30] and Pla-Sanjuanelo et al. [31] used a software with four VR scenarios that contained foods chosen by the participants as the ones that produced the highest level of craving, and verified that VR was useful for inducing food craving in BN and BED patients. Participants with higher levels of trait and state-craving showed a greater desire to eat during exposure to virtual foods [31].

Ferrer-García et al. [30] and Ferrer-García and Gutiérrez-Maldonado [28] reported that high-calorie food settings and certain social situations produced the highest levels of subjective discomfort. In the study of Perpiñá et al. [29], patients showed a high reality judgment and sense of presence and scored higher on emotional involvement and attention when compared to controls. Perpiñá and Roncero [32] also reported that the highest scores on emotional involvement, attention, reality judgment and presence were obtained by the ED group. They also remark that the level of emotional reactivity to VR proportionally increased the sense of presence in the virtual environment. In contrast with those findings, Ferrer-García and Gutiérrez-Maldonado [28] reported a low sense of presence experienced in ED patients. However, considering those patients that reported greater sense of presence they displayed a higher level of subjective discomfort in food related situations.

Table 1. Studies using virtual reality in the assessment of bulimia nervosa and binge eating disorder.

Study	Sample Size (M/F)	Diagnostic	Study Design	Intervention	Software Characteristics	Sessions	Follow-up	Instruments	Outcomes
Gutiérrez-Maldonado et al. (2006) [24]	30 (0/30) AN: 17 (0/17) BN:11 (0/11) EDNOS: 2 (0/2)	AN BN EDNOS	NCAS	Exposure to food and people.	6 VR environments: living-room, kitchen with high calorie food, a kitchen with low-calorie food, a restaurant with high-calorie food, a restaurant with low-calorie food, swimming-pool.	1	-	STAI, CDB, EDI-2, PQ.	Higher state anxiety in the high-calorie food situations and the swimming-pool than in the neutral environment. Higher depressed mood in the high-calorie food situations. Significant differences on the level of state anxiety and depression mood comparing low-calorie and high-calorie food environments; no differences were found between environments with people and those without. AN and BN patients responded with similar levels of emotional intensity to the different situations. VR was useful for eliciting emotional reactions
Ferrer-García et al. (2009) [25]	193 (0/193) CIG: 85 (0/85) (AN: 49, BN:22, EDNOS:14) CG: 108 (0/108)	AN BN EDNOS	CAS	Exposure to food and people.	6 VR environments: neutral, kitchen with high calorie food, a kitchen with low-calorie food, a restaurant with high-calorie food, a restaurant with low-calorie food, swimming-pool.	1	-	EAT, STAI, CDB.	ED patients showed significantly higher levels of anxiety and depressed mood in the high-calorie food environments and the swimming pool than in the neutral room. ED patients' anxiety increased when other people were present, but in high-calorie environments, their anxiety increased when they were alone. ED patients showed a more depressed mood after eating low-calorie food when other people were present. After eating high-calorie food, they felt more depressed when they were alone. VR was useful for eliciting emotional reactions.
Gutiérrez-Maldonado et al. (2010) [26]	193 (0/193) CIG: 85 (0/85) (AN: 49, BN:22, EDNOS:14) CG: 108 (0/108)	AN BN EDNOS	CAS	Exposure to food and people.	4 VR environments: kitchen with high calorie food, a kitchen with low-calorie food, a restaurant with high-calorie food, a restaurant with low-calorie food.	1	-	EAT, BIAS.	ED patients showed more BI distortion and body dissatisfaction in the high-calorie food environments than in the low calorie food environments. People variable was not significant. BN patients showed greater BI distortion when were alone after eating high-calorie food than after eating low-calorie food. Where the patient was accompanied, BI distortion levels were similar, regardless of the kind of food. AN and EDNOS patients presented higher levels of body distortion after eating high-calorie food than after eating low-calorie food, independently of the presence or absence of people. BI distortion and BI dissatisfaction can be influenced by VR situational factors.

Table 1. *Cont.*

Study	Sample Size (M/F)	Diagnostic	Study Design	Intervention	Software Characteristics	Sessions	Follow-up	Instruments	Outcomes
Gorini et al. (2010) [27]	CIG:20 (0/20) (AN:10, BN:10) CG:10 (0/10)	AN, BN (DSM-IV)	CAS	RF PH VR	Small restaurant with a buffet table, 6 foods.	1	-	EDI-2, STAI-S, VAS-A, ITC-SOPI.	Higher level of anxiety for patients compared to control. Patients felt more anxious when exposed to real and virtual food than to the pictures of food. Patients showed higher heart rate and skin conductance compared to control group. Their level of physiological anxiety was higher in the RF and VR condition, than in the PH condition. Higher sense of presence was associated with higher levels of anxiety. Virtual food was as effective as real food, and more effective than photographs, in producing psychological and physiological responses in ED patients.
Ferrer-García and Gutiérrez-Maldonado (2011) [28]	71 (0/71) (AN:49, BN:22)	AN, BN	NCAS	Exposure to food and people.	5 VR environments: neutral room, kitchen with high calorie food, a kitchen with low-calorie food, a restaurant with high-calorie food, a restaurant with low-calorie food.	1	-	EAT-26, PQ.	High-calorie environments and social situations produced the highest levels of subjective discomfort. Patients with severe symptomatology showed a higher subjective discomfort in all environments than with moderate symptoms. Reported sense of presence was low. Patients with high sense of presence showed the highest levels of subjective discomfort in all food situations.
Perpiñá et al. (2013) [29]	CIG:22 (0/22) (AN:11, BN:4, EDNOS:7) CG:37 (0/37)	AN, BN, EDNOS (DSM-IV-TR)	CAS	Exposure to food.	Kitchen with 2 areas: prep area and area with a table and a chair.	1	-	BDI-II, BAI, RS, RJPQ, ITC-SOPI.	Before eating patients showed moderate–high scores on control urge to eat, fear, avoidance; and low desire to eat. After eating, they reported feelings of putting on weight, urge to continue eating, of being upset etc.; and reported wanted actions: to do exercise to "compensate", to continue eating, to continue with their daily routine, to purge. Patients showed a high reality judgment and sense of presence and scored higher on emotional involvement, attention and negative effects. VR software was clinically meaningful to patients.
Ferrer-García et al. (2015) [30]	CIG: 40 (10/30) (BN:23, BED:17) CG: 78 (9/69)	BN, BED (DSM-5)	CAS	Exposure to food.	4 VR scenarios (kitchen, dining room, bedroom, and bakery/café) + 10 foods (of 30 available foods that elicit craving).	1	-	DEBQ.	BN and BED patients showed higher levels of emotional, external and restrictive eating and food craving than controls. External eating was associated with food craving both in patients and controls. VR was useful for inducing food craving in BN and BED patients.

Table 1. *Cont.*

Study	Sample Size (M/F)	Diagnostic	Study Design	Intervention	Software Characteristics	Sessions	Follow-up	Instruments	Outcomes
Pla-Sanjuanelo et al. (2015) [31]	118 (19/99) CIG: 40 (10/30) (BED: 17 BN:23) CG: 78 (9/69)	BED (DSM-5) BN (SCID-I)	CAS	Exposure to Food.	4 VR scenarios + 10 foods (of 30 available foods that elicit craving).	1	-	FCQ-T, FCQ-S.	Participants with higher levels of trait and state-craving showed a greater desire to eat during exposure to virtual foods. State-craving was associated with perceived craving experience in both groups during VR exposure. VR-CET model may be helpful in improving the treatment of BE and BN patients.
Perpiñá and Roncero (2016) [32]	62 (0/62) ED: 20 (0/20) (AN:10, BN:4, EDNOS:6) Obese: 19 (0/19) CG:23 (0/23)	AN, BN, EDNOS (DSM-IV-TR) Obesity	CAS	Exposure to food.	Kitchen with 2 areas: prep area and area with a table and a chair.	1 (30 min.)	-	RJPQ, ITC-SOPI.	ED group had the highest scores on emotional involvement, attention, reality judgment and presence, negative effects. Obese group had the lowest scores on reality judgment and presence, satisfaction, sense of physical space in VE experience. Attribution of reality to the virtual eating was predicted by engagement and belonging to the ED group. The palatability of a virtual food was predicted by attention capturing and belonging to the obese group. The level of emotional reactivity to VR proportionally increased the sense of presence. VR was useful for assessing and measuring ED patients' responses in a naturalistic setting.

Note: Participants—AN: Anorexia Nervosa; BED: Binge Eating Disorder; BN: Bulimia Nervosa; ED: Eating disorder; EDNOS eating disorder not otherwise specified; **Intervention**—CET: Cue Exposure Therapy; PH: Photograph slide show; RF: Real Food view; **Study Design**—AS: Assessment Study; CAS: Controlled Assessment Study; **Instruments**—BAI: Beck Anxiety Inventory; BDI II: Beck Depression Inventory; BIAS: Body Image Assessment Software; CDB: The Barcelona Depression Questionnaire; DEBQ: Dutch Eating Behavior Questionnaire; EAT: Eating Attitudes Test; EDI 2: Eating Disorders Inventory 2; FCQ-T, FCQ-S: State and Trait Food Cravings Questionnaires; ITC-SOPI: Sense of Presence Inventory; PQ: Presence Questionnaire; RJPQ: The Reality Judgment and Presence Questionnaire; RS: Restraint Scale; STAI: Sate-Trait Anxiety Inventory; VAS-A: Visual analogue scale for anxiety.; **Other:** CG: Control Group; CIG: Clinical Group; F: Female; M: Male.

3.2. VR in the Treatment of BN and BED

3.2.1. Case Report

Roncero and Perpiñá [41] described a case of a 17-year-old woman with BN and assessed the effect of VR as a therapeutic tool to normalize eating patterns as part of a CBT treatment. The patient was treated for seven weeks using VR sessions and Fairburn's CBTC protocol [44] for BN. The VR software consisted of a kitchen with two areas that contained elements to cook, drink and eat. The patient could access the foods freely or block them if desired. She could also perform alternative behaviors in the virtual environment (for example, making a phone call). At the end of the treatment, the patient showed a reduction in BE, purges and food avoidance. In addition, after VR exposure, the patient showed an overall improvement, such as a decrease in drive for thinness, bulimia measures and in general psychopathology. The authors concluded that VR was an effective complement to CBT treatment in this bulimic patient.

3.2.2. Non-Controlled Clinical Trials

Riva et al. [35] conduct two studies with female participants, one of them with an obese group and other with BED patients, to evaluate a VR-based treatment to be used in the assessment and treatment of those patients. VEBIM 2 software was used, which includes cognitivebehavioral and visualmotorial methods. VR first session aimed to assess stimulus that elicit abnormal eating behavior, focusing on patient's concerns about food, eating, shape and weight. The other four sessions intended to assess and modify the symptoms of anxiety related to food exposure and the patient's body experience. For these purposes, different zones are used, such as sitting-room, dining-room, kitchen, bedroom and working environments. In both studies, patients who ate 1200 kcal per day, besides VR intervention, also participated in bi-weekly psycho-nutritional groups held by dietitians. In both groups, results showed a reduced level of body dissatisfaction, an improvement on social activities and a reduced use of disguising clothes. BI change was associated to a reduction in problematic eating. The authors concluded that the obtained data were promising, but controlled and follow-up studies are needed to test this VR approach. Riva et al. [34], in another paper, reported again both clinical trials of the previous study Riva et al. [35] with obese and BED patients and extended the sample conducting another non-controlled clinical trial, with the same objective and design, with EDNOS patients. The results pointed out to a reduction on body dissatisfaction, but it was slighter than the observed in other samples. The patients improved on social activities and reduced disguising clothes' use. Again, authors concluded that VR-based treatment could be useful to BI modification in obesity, BED and EDNOS; however, more studies are needed.

3.2.3. Randomized Controlled Trials

Perpiñá et al. [33] conduct a randomized controlled trial with AN and BN female patients to measure the effectiveness of the treatment of BI through VR. Patients were assigned to two conditions: cognitive-behavioral treatment plus VR exposure or cognitive-behavioral treatment plus relaxation. The VR software consisted of six areas where the patients could experience discrepancies about weight and BI: an accommodation zone; a food area with a virtual balance (to discuss the discrepancies about subjective, desired and healthy weight; and to address overestimation of weight after eating); a room with posters showing different body shapes (to help the patient understand that weight is a relative concept); a room with mirrors (to deal with the representation of BI); a doorframe with strips (to deal with the estimated body size); and another zone to contrast body areas (to contrast subjective body shape, desired body shape and body shape that the patient thought that a significant person would have of her). The patients moved through the VR settings according to their progress. CBT plus VR group showed significantly improvement in general psychopathology, ED related symptoms and BI aspects (less weight fear, higher satisfaction with their bodies in social contexts, less thoughts and negative attitudes about their bodies, and less fear of achieving a healthy weight) when compared to

CBT plus relaxation group. The results showed that greater improvement was achieved through the addition of VR to the treatment of BI.

To evaluate the efficacy of a VR-based multidimensional approach in the treatment of BI disturbances, Riva et al. [36] conduct a randomized controlled trial with female BED patients involved in a residential weight control treatment, which included a low-calorie diet (1200 Kcal/day) and physical training. Patients were assigned to two conditions: VR-based treatment and a psycho-nutritional intervention. VREDIM software was used, an enhanced version of the VEBIM environment, that includes cognitive-behavioral and visual-motorial methods. The software consists of different zones: room with balance, drawing room, kitchen, dining room, bathroom, office, beach, supermarket etc. Initially the focuses of the intervention were patient's concerns about food, eating, shape, and weight. Then, patients had to answer the "miracle question"; that is, they were asked to imagine what life would be like without their complaint. They built their solution, which was used to guide the therapeutic process. Next, the focuses are to manage anxiety symptoms related to food exposure and body experience. The psycho-nutritional group was also based on a cognitive-behavior approach, applied with the purpose of teaching methods for stress management, problem-solving and eating behavior. Results for VR treatment showed an overall psychological status improvement, reduced level of body dissatisfaction and anxiety, increased self-efficacy and motivation for change, reduced concern about social judgment and reduced overeating. The control group presented anxiety reduction on the Assertion Inventory (AI), but it was not confirmed by the State-Trait Anxiety Inventory (STAI) score. VREDIM was more effective than psycho-nutritional group on body satisfaction improvement, overeating and anxiety level reduction. Patients of both groups had remission of BE episodes at the end of the treatment. VR-based therapy improved BI (and its associated behaviors) treatment of patients involved in a weight control program with physical training.

Riva et al. [37] in a randomized controlled trail with female BED patients compared the efficacy of three interventions (ECT: experiential cognitive therapy, CBT, and NG: nutritional group) with a waiting list, and also observed the outcomes over a six-month follow-up period. ECT used VREDIM software and included nutritional intervention and physical training. CBT was based on Fairburn's [45,46] protocol and included group sessions to improve assertiveness and motivation to change, as well as nutritional intervention and physical training. Nutritional group included a low-calorie diet (1200 Kcal/day), prescribed by dieticians, and physical training. Results showed that ECT helped with the decrease of anxiety and depression levels and improved assertive behavior. CBT decreased patients' depression level and NG decreased anxiety level. Patients of all interventions groups improved on self-esteem, eating control, eating self-efficacy and weight loss. They also reduced binge episodes. ECT was more effective than CBT in improving overall psychological state, BI, body satisfaction and resistance to social pressure. At a six-month follow-up, ECT improved body satisfaction and self-esteem and reduced the frequency of binge episodes of BED patients when compared to CBT and NG. VR-based therapy improved BED patient's treatment when compared to other conditions.

Riva et al. [38] reported a clinical trial with female patients with obesity, BED, BN and EDNOS comparing ECT, CBT, nutritional group and a control group. ECT used VREDIM software and also included nutritional intervention and physical training. CBT was delivered with a nutritional intervention and physical training. Nutritional group included psychological support and physical training. For ED patients, at post-treatment, ECT decreased anxiety and depression levels and improved assertive behavior. CBT decreased depression level and NG intervention decreased anxiety. Otherwise, the waiting list group had increased anxiety level and weight gain. All interventions groups improved patients' self-esteem, eating control, eating self-efficacy and weight loss. When all groups were compared, ECT was the best intervention for eating control improvement. ECT and CBT were better on improving body satisfaction and body perception. ECT was better than CBT on BI and self-efficacy improvement. Besides, for obese patients, at post-treatment, ECT and CBT decreased depression levels and improved self-esteem and assertive behavior. All interventions helped to decrease patients' anxiety and improved eating control and eating self-efficacy. When compared, all interventions groups had body satisfaction and body perception improvement. ECT was the best intervention for eating control improvement. ECT and CBT were better in improving motivation to change. ECT was better than CBT in BI improvement. The authors concluded that ECT was more effective than the others approach in the treatment of obese, BED, BN and EDNOS patients.

Perpiñá et al. [42] examined the evolution of the results of a previous study carried out by her research group [33] over six-month and one-year follow-up periods. The group that received CBT plus relaxation in the first study received VR sessions after that treatment, so in this follow-up study the entire sample had completed the treatment in the VR condition. The results at post-treatment were maintained at one-year follow-up, and for some measures such as appearance-related schemas and ED related components the improvement continued along the follow-up period. General psychopathology improved from pre-treatment to one-year follow-up, and The Brief Symptom Inventory (BSI) score was always below the pre-treatment level, but it rose between 6 and 12 months. VR was useful in the treatment of BI and can enhance the efficacy of the standard CBT.

To compare CBT treatment for ED with a CBT protocol focused on BI treatment plus VR, Marco et al. [39] enrolled AN, BN and EDNOS female patients to two randomized groups over a one-year follow-up study. CBT for AN followed Garner et al. [47] protocol, CBT for BN was based on Wilson et al. [48], and CBT for EDNOS followed one of these two protocols, according to each patient needs. CBT for BI treatment was adapted from Butters and Cash [49] and Perpiñá et al. [50]. VR software consisted of five situations: virtual scale and a kitchen, a room with posters, a room with mirrors, a doorframe with strips and a zone to contrast body areas. The purposes of the exposure to each environment were described above Perpiñá et al. [33] VR treatment group showed more BI improvement than CBT and greater improvement in the behavior clinical measures. At post-treatment, VR group improved on body attitudes, frequency of negative automatic thoughts on BI, body satisfaction, discomfort caused by body-related situations and BN symptoms (measured by Bulimic Investigatory Test; BITE). These results were maintained or continued to improve (body attitudes, frequency of negative automatic thoughts on BI) at one-year follow-up. All participants improved in the ED measures and it was maintained at follow-up. The authors analyzed the clinical effectiveness of both treatment conditions. Patients of VR group showed clinically significant improvement on post-treatment and follow-up and all BI and ED scores were similar to those of the healthy population. Their Eating Attitudes Test (EAT) scores were better than the healthy population. In addition, BITE normalization was achieved at follow-up. Otherwise, patients of CBT group did not show clinically significant improvement at post-treatment or follow-up. In conclusion, CBT focused on BI treatment plus VR improved CBT standard treatment for ED.

Cesa et al. [40] in a randomized controlled trial with a one-year follow-up, tested the efficacy of CBT including a VR protocol (ECT) in morbidly obese patients with BED compared with CBT alone and an inpatient multimodal treatment (IP), that included psycho-nutritional groups, a low-calorie diet (1200 Kcal/day), and physical training. In fact, both other groups also received the IP. CBT protocol was based on Fairburn et al. [44] and Ricca et al. [51]. NeuroVR software was used, which includes 14 virtual environments that present situations related to maintaining and relapse mechanisms (Home, Supermarket, Pub, Restaurant, Swimming Pool, Beach, Gymnasium) and BI comparison areas. All patients had a reduction in weight, BE episodes (decreased to zero) and improved body satisfaction. Only patients of ECT improved on BI concerns. ECT and CBT were more effective than IP alone in preventing weight regain at follow-up, and only ECT was effective in patients' further weight loss. At follow-up BE episodes were reported in all groups, but ECT and CBT groups were successful at maintaining them at a low rate. VR based therapy showed some advances when compared to other groups at post and follow-up treatment.

Table 2. Studies using virtual reality in the treatment of bulimia nervosa and binge eating disorder.

Study	Sample Size (M/F)	Diagnostic	Study Design	Intervention	Software Characteristics	Sessions	Follow-Up	Instruments	Outcomes
Treatment									
Perpiñá et al. (1999) [33]	13 (0/13) AN: 7 (0/7) BN: 6 (0/6)	AN, BN (DSM-IV)	RCCT	SBIT+VR SBIT + Relaxation	6 situations: Accommodation zone, food area with a virtual balance, room with posters, room with mirrors, a doorframe with strips and a zone to contrast body areas.	SBIT: 8 (3 h, weekly, group) Relaxation: 6 (1 h, weekly) VR: 6 (1 h, weekly).	-	BDI, PANAS, EAT, RS, BITE, EDI-2, BSQ, BIAQ, BAT, BES, BIATQ, ASI, SIBID, BASS.	VR condition participants showed a greater improvement in specific BI variables, depression and anxiety when compared to non-VR group. VR was a helpful tool for confronting the patients with BI distortions.
Riva et al. (2000) [34]	43 (0/43) Obese: 18 (0/18) BED: 25 (0/25)	Obesity (BMI>35) BED (DSM-IV)	NCCT	VEBIM 2 (ECT)	VEBIM 2 Different zones (Sitting-room, dining-room, kitchen, bedroom, working environments etc.).	5 (biweekly).	-	MMPI-2, EDI-2, BSS, BIAQ, FRS, CDRS.	In both groups, results showed a reduced level of body dissatisfaction, an improvement on social activities and a reduced use of disguising clothes. Obtained data were promising, but controlled and follow-up studies are needed to test this VR approach.
Riva et al. (2000) [35]	57 (0/57) Obese: 18 (0/18) BED: 25 (0/25) EDNOS: 14 (0/14)	Obesity (BMI>35) BED, EDNOS (DSM-IV)	NCCT	VEBIM 2	VEBIM 2 Different zones (Sitting-room, dining-room, kitchen, bedroom, working environments etc.).	5 (biweekly).	-	BSS, BIAQ, FRS, CDRS.	All groups showed a reduced level of body dissatisfaction, an improvement on social activities and a reduced use of disguising clothes. In the EDNOS group the reduction in body dissatisfaction was slighter than in other samples. VR-based treatment could be useful to BI modification in obesity, BED and EDNOS; but more studies are needed.
Riva et al. (2002) [36]	20 (0/20)	BED (DSM-IV)	RCCT	VR (+LCD+PT) PN (+LCD +PT)	VREDIM Different zones (Room with balance, drawing room, kitchen, dining room, bathroom, office, beach, supermarket etc.).	VR: 7 (50 min.) LCD: daily PT: NR (at least 30 min. walk/twice a week) PN: NR (3 times a week).	-	DIET, STAI, AI, WELSQ, URICA, BSS, BIAQ, FRS, CDRS.	VR treatment showed reduced level of body dissatisfaction and anxiety, increased self-efficacy and motivation for change, reduced concern about social judgment and reduced overeating. PN group presented anxiety reduction on the AI, but it was not confirmed by the STAI score. VR was more effective than PN on body satisfaction improvement, overeating and anxiety level reduction. VR-based therapy improved BI treatment.

Table 2. *Cont.*

Study	Sample Size (M/F)	Diagnostic	Study Design	Intervention	Software Characteristics	Sessions	Follow-Up	Instruments	Outcomes
Treatment									
Riva et al. (2003) [37]	36 (0/36)	BED (DSM-IV)	RCCT	ECT (+NG+PT) CBT (+NG +PT) NG (+PT) WL	VREDIM Different zones (Room with balance, drawing room, kitchen, dining room, bathroom, office, beach, supermarket etc.).	ECT: 15 (over 6 weeks) 10 VR sessions CBT: 15 (over 6 weeks) NG: 5 (weekly).	6 months	DIET, STAI, BDI II, RAS, RSEQ, WELSQ, URICA, BSS, BIAQ, CDRS.	ECT decreased anxiety and depression and improved assertive behavior. CBT decreased depression. NG decreased anxiety. All interventions groups improved patients' self-esteem, eating control, eating self-efficacy, weight loss. They also reduced binge episodes. ECT was more effective than CBT on improving overall psychological state, body image, body satisfaction and resistance to social pressure. At follow-up, ECT improved body satisfaction and self-esteem and reduced the frequency of binge episodes when compared to CBT and NG. VR-based therapy improved BED patients' treatment.
Riva et al. (2004) [38]	120 (0/120) Obese: 68 (0/68) BED: 36 (0/36) BN: 12 (0/12) EDNOS: 3 (0/3)	Obesity, BED, BN, EDNOS	RCCT	ECT (+NG+PT) CBT (+NG+PT) NG (+PT+PI) WL	VREDIM Different zones (Room with balance, drawing room, kitchen, dining room, bathroom, office, beach, supermarket etc.).	ECT: 15 (10 VR sessions of 15 min.) CBT: 15 NG: 4–6 PI: NR.	-	STAI, BDI, RSEQ, RAS, DIET, WELSQ, URICA, BSS, BIAQ, CDRS.	**ED:** ECT was the best intervention for eating control improvement. ECT and CBT were better on improving body satisfaction and body perception. ECT was better than CBT on BI and self-efficacy improvement. **Obesity:** All intervention groups helped on improving body satisfaction and body perception. ECT was the best intervention for eating control improvement. ECT and CBT were better to improve motivation to change. ECT was better than CBT on BI improvement. ECT was more effective than the others approaches.

Table 2. *Cont.*

Study	Sample Size (M/F)	Diagnostic	Study Design	Intervention	Software Characteristics	Sessions	Follow-Up	Instruments	Outcomes
Treatment									
Perpiñá et al. (2004) [42]	12 (0/12) AN: 7 (0/7) BN: 5 (0/5)	AN, BN (DSM-IV)	RCCT	SBIT+VR SBIT + Relaxation + VR	6 situations: Accommodation zone, food area with a virtual balance, room with posters, room with mirrors, a doorframe with strips and a zone to contrast body areas.	SBIT: 8 (3 h, weekly, group) Relaxation: 6 (1 h, weekly) VR: 6 (1 h, weekly).	6 months, 1 year	BIATQ, SIBID, ASI, BAT, EDI-2, EAT, BSI.	Improvement in all measures. Post-treatment results were maintained at follow-up, and for some measures like appearance-related schemas and ED related components the improvement continued along the follow-up period. General psychopathology improved from pre-treatment to one-year follow-up, and BSI score was always below the pre-treatment level, but it rose between 6 and 12 months. VR was useful in the treatment of BI and capable of enhancing the efficacy of the standard CBT.
Marco et al. (2013) [39]	18 (0/18)	BN, AN, EDNOS (DSM-IV-TR)	RCCT	CBT CBT (BI)+VR	5 situations: Virtual scale and kitchen, room with posters, room with mirrors, a doorframe with strips and a zone to contrast body areas.	CBT for BN:19 (Group, 2 h, weekly) CBTC for AN:23 (individual) CBT: 15 (group) + VR: 8 (1 h, weekly).	1 year	BAT, BIATQ, BASS, SIBID, BITE, EAT.	CBT+VR showed more BI improvement than CBT; CBT+VR showed more body attitudes and frequency of negative automatic thoughts on BI improvement at post-treatment and this continued to rise at follow-up; more body satisfaction, discomfort caused by body-related situations and BN symptoms (BITE) improvement at post-treatment and follow-up; greater improvement in the behavior clinical measures. All participants improved in the ED measures and it was maintained at follow-up. CBT+VR post-treatment and follow-up showed clinically significant improvement and all BI and ED scores were similar to healthy population. CBT+VR also showed EAT better scores than healthy population. BITE normalization was achieved at follow-up. CBT focused on BI plus VR improved CBT standard treatment for ED.

Table 2. *Cont.*

Study	Sample Size (M/F)	Diagnostic	Study Design	Intervention	Software Characteristics	Sessions	Follow-Up	Instruments	Outcomes
Treatment									
Cesa et al. (2013) [40]	66 (0/66)	Obesity + BED (DSM-IV-TR)	RCCT	ECT (+IP) CBT (+IP) IP	Neuro-VR 14 environments (Home, Supermarket, Pub, Restaurant, Swimming Pool, Beach, Gymnasium, BI comparison areas).	ECT: 15 (5 weeks, 10 biweekly VR sessions) CBT:15 (5 weeks) IP (6 weeks).	1 year	EDI-Symptom Checklist, BSS, BIAQ, CDRS.	Weight decreased, number of binge eating episodes decreased to zero, body satisfaction improved in all groups. BI concerns improved only in ECT. ECT and CBT were more effective than IP alone in preventing weight regain at follow-up. Only ECT was effective in further weight loss. Binge eating episodes were reported at follow-up, ECT and CBT were successful in maintaining them at a low rate.
Roncero and Perpiñá (2015) [41]	1 (0/1)	BN (DSM-IV-TR)	CR	CBT+VR	Kitchen with two areas that included elements to cook, drink and eat.	CBT:7 VR:7 (60 min/weekly or biweekly).	-	EDI-2, BITE, ACTA, BDI-2, BAI.	Reduction in binges, purges and food avoidance; development of the ability to make decisions over impulses.

Note: Participants—AN: Anorexia Nervosa; BED: Binge Eating Disorder; BN: Bulimia Nervosa; ED: Eating disorder; EDNOS eating disorder not otherwise specified; **Intervention**—CBT: Cognitive Behavior Therapy; ECT: Experiential Cognitive Therapy; IP: Integrated multimodal medically managed inpatient program; LCD: Low-calorie Diet; PI: Psychological support; PN: Psycho-nutritional intervention; SBIT: standard BI treatment; VEBIM: Virtual Reality for Body Image Modification; VREDIM: Virtual Reality for Eating Disorders Modification; WL: Waiting List Group; **Study Design**—CR: Case Report; NCCT: Non-Controlled Clinical Trial; RCCT: Randomized Controlled Clinical Trial; **Instruments**—ACTA: Attitudes Toward Chance in eating disorders; AI: Assertion Inventory; ASI: Appearance Schemas Inventory; BAI: Beck Anxiety Inventory; BAT: Body Attitudes Test; BASS: Body Areas Satisfaction Scale; BDI II: Beck Depression Inventory; BIAQ: Body Image Avoidance Questionnaire; BIATQ: Body Image Automatic Thoughts Questionnaire; BITE: Bulimic Investigatory Test; BSI: The Brief Symptom Inventory; BSS: Body Satisfaction Scale; CDRS: Contour drawing rating scale; DIET: Dieter's Inventory of Eating Temptations; EAT: Eating Attitudes Test; EDI 2: Eating Disorders Inventory 2; EDI-Symptom Checklist: Eating Disorder Inventory-Symptom Checklist; FRS: Figure rating scale; MMPI 2: Minnesota Multiphasic Personality Inventory 2; PANAS: Positive and Negative Affect Schedule; RAS: Rathus Assertiveness Schedule; RSEQ: Rosenberg Self-Esteem Questionnaire; SIBID: Situational Inventory of Body Image Dysphoria; STAI: Sate-Trait Anxiety Inventory; URICA: University of Rhode Island Change Assessment Scale; WELSQ: Weight Efficacy Life-Style Questionnaire; **Other**—BMI: Body Mass Index; BI: Body Image; CG: Control Group; ClG: Clinical Group; F: Female; M: Male; NG: Nutritional Group; PT: Physical Training; SCID-I: Structured Clinical Interview for DSM-IV Axis I Disorders.

4. Discussion

This systematic review on the use of VR based environments in the assessment and treatment of BN and BED expanded the information provided by previous reviews [16,21,52] by focusing in a more homogenous group of binge–purging EDs and adding more recent investigations in the area [30–32,41]. From the 18 studies selected, nine were characterized as assessment studies because they investigated different aspects of these syndromes using VR-related settings, and nine were considered treatment studies by exploring the usefulness of VR as a potential therapeutic strategy in BN and BED. Based on the studies selected, the use of VR in EDs is an evolving area and, although in an early stage, the results of current studies are promising. First, the overall findings support the idea that patients with BN and BED immersed in VR environments felt a sense of presence, improving the ecological validity of this procedure in this group of individuals. Secondly, considering the available evidences the use of VR in the assessment of BN and BED showed some promise to identify: (1) how those patients experienced their BI; and (2) and environments or specific kind of foods that may trigger binge–purging cycle. Finally, the studies using VR technologies associated to cognitive behavioral procedures demonstrate their potential utility in improving eating related (binge-eating, urge to eat, etc.), general psychopathology and other aspects of these binge–purging conditions. Studies showed that VR assessment tools provide novelty features when compared to available psychometric tests. Through VR systems it is possible to manipulate the size and shape of body areas and to compare the visualization of the differences between the actual, perceived and desired body weight or shape of ED patients [27]. Psychometric instruments can collect information through patients reporting, but VR can turn these reports into concrete perceptions. Other advantage is that the perception of presence in the virtual environments can elicit compulsive behaviors in a way like reality, and this is a benefit when studying the triggers of BE and the response to them.

VR treatment can present some advantages over reality, but its objective is not to substitute real experiences. Virtual exposure has been considered an alternative for imaginary exposure and an intermediate step for in vivo exposure. If experienced anxiety is too high, receiving a virtual exposure treatment can increase patients' possibilities of accepting an in vivo exposure program in the future [53]. In addition, exposures could be detailed customized by the therapist in the VR exposure condition, which can help patients to cope with stimulus or complex environments in a more feasible and controlled way. The possibility of monitoring the responses of the patient also offers an advantage over real exposure [54,55]. It was already argued that patients may progress more rapidly in their VR exposure hierarchy due to a perception of increased control and safety [55]. Besides these advantages, these VR based apparatus are accessible and have a good cost-effectiveness ratio. Just to give an example, the VR systems used in BN BED studies used affordable equipment such as a basic computer hardware (1 GB RAM, 256 Mb graphic card, and 17-in) sold for about USD 500,00 (unit); and VR glasses, with an approximate value of USD 700,00 (unit). In addition, the Neuro VR [40] software is available for free download at http://www.neurovr2.org/.

The rationale of the use of VR exposure is that it is supposed to work according emotion-processing model. The confrontation with a threatening stimuli (which elicits the fearful responses) activates the fear network. The processes of habituation and extinction aid modification of the fear structure, making its meaning less threatening, as new and incompatible information is added into the emotional network [20]. Thus, VR exposure can reduce eating-related anxiety during and after exposure to virtual foods and environments, helping to disrupt the reconsolidation of adverse food/situations related memories [23,31]. For the exposure therapy, the hierarchy is created in the software, and patients are first exposed to stimuli that elicit the lowest levels of craving until they can reach the ones that elicit the highest levels. During the exposure, the level of craving is assessed, and the patient must stay in the situation until the levels of craving and anxiety diminish sufficiently. Then, the patient can cope with the following stimuli in the hierarchy.

Another reason for the use of VR is related to the Allocentric Lock Theory, which suggests that ED may be associated with impairment in the ability to update a stored negative allocentric (offline) representation of one's body with real-time (online/egocentric) perception-driven inputs [56,57]. The addition of VR sensory training to unlock the body memory (body image rescripting protocol) by increasing the contribution of new egocentric/internal somatosensory information directly related to the existing allocentric memory was able to improve the efficacy of CBT at one-year follow-up, supporting its rationale [40,58]. In addition, Riva et al. [54] emphasizes the role of VR in transforming external and internal experience. External experience can be modified by focusing on the personal efficacy and self-reflectiveness, and both can be achieved through the sense of presence and emotional engagement that the exposure to virtual environments can provide. Besides, inner experience can be modified by structuring, altering, and/or replacing bodily self-consciousness.

It is important to register that, after a first phase of immaturity (published between 1999 and 2004) with studies showing several methodological flows the field has evolved. The more recent studies, in particular the ones published in the last five years follow the guidelines required by high level RCTs. Two different randomized, controlled trials [39,40] have shown at one-year follow-up that VR had a higher efficacy than the gold standard in the field, i.e., cognitive behavioral therapy (CBT).

In line with the theoretical framework mentioned previously, the rationale behind the VR systems currently used in the ED studies incorporated environments to deal with BI distortions [59] and regulation of emotions [25]. More recently, settings offering exposure with response prevention of bingeing have been also included [30]. The novelty of this proposal is the addition of VR to cue-exposure procedures. Food cue-exposure therapy (CET) has been proposed as an effective treatment for binge–purging syndromes, eliminating or significantly reducing binging and purging behaviors [60].

Future recommendations included the need for more high-quality RCTs, [61], with robust sample sizes and long-term follow-ups to investigate the effects of VR-based interventions in BN and BED. Forthcoming studies should also compare VR-based interventions in more homogenous groups of BN and BED patients (and not in mixed samples as observed in this review) with waiting lists and active interventions such as psychotherapy and pharmacotherapy. To facilitate comparability of treatments, standardized outcome measures (instruments to assess eating-related and general psychopathology) should be used in line with current available literature on other interventional studies in BN and BED.

A limitation of this study was the impossibility to report separately the results related to binge–purging EDs. The objective of the review was to exclude studies with AN-only subjects, as this subgroup of restrictive type of eating disorders have a distinctive pathophysiology. However, currently, as there are few studies with BN and BED-only samples, mixed samples were incorporated. Unfortunately, specific information related with binge–purging EDs were not possible to be selected because of the lack of report and analysis of each group of patients separately in the primary studies results.

5. Conclusions

In conclusion, based on the current available data VR-based environments may be considered a promising strategy for the assessment and treatment of BN and BED. Considering the available evidence, the use of VR in the assessment of those conditions showed some promise in identifying: (1) how those patients experienced their body image; and (2) environments or specific kind of foods that may trigger binge–purging cycle. VR-based environments associated to cognitive behavioral techniques showed their potential utility in improving motivation for change, self-esteem, body image disturbances and in reducing binge eating and purging behavior.

Author Contributions: Marcele Regine de Carvalho was the primary investigator, was responsible for electronic search, and wrote the manuscript. She implemented the PRISMA method. Jose Carlos Appolinario contributed theoretically to the content, wrote the manuscript, and revised the paper. He also contributed with manual search and offered advice regarding content. Thiago Rodrigues de Santana Dias conducted the electronic and manual search, wrote the manuscript and contributed with tables and figures. Monica Duchesne assisted with tables and figures and revised the paper. Antonio Egidio Nardi revised the paper. All authors agreed to be listed and approved the submitted version of the manuscript.

Conflicts of Interest: The authors declare no conflict of interest.

References

1. Whiteford, H.A.; Ferrari, A.J.; Degenhardt, L.; Feigin, V.; Vos, T. The Global Burden of Mental, Neurological and Substance Use Disorders: An Analysis from the Global Burden of Disease Study 2010. *PLoS ONE* **2015**, *10*, 1–14. [CrossRef] [PubMed]
2. Whiteford, H.; Degenhardt, L.; Rehm, J.; Baxter, A.; Ferrari, A.; Erskine, H.; Charlson, F.; Norman, R.; Flaxman, A.; Johns, N.; et al. Global burden of disease attributable to mental and substance use disorders: Findings from the Global Burden of Disease Study 2010. *Lancet* **2013**, *382*, 1575–1586. [CrossRef]
3. Smink, F.; Hoeken, D.; Hoek, H. Epidemiology of Eating Disorders: Incidence, Prevalence and Mortality Rates. *Curr. Psychiatry Rep.* **2012**, *14*, 406–414. [CrossRef] [PubMed]
4. American Psychiatric Association. *Diagnostic and Statistical Manual of Mental Disorders*, 5th ed.; (DSM-5); American Psychiatric Association Publishing: Arlington, VA, USA, 2013.
5. Brooks, S.; Rask-Andersen, M.; Benedict, C.; Schiöth, H. A debate on current eating disorder diagnoses in light of neurobiological findings: Is it time for a spectrum model? *BMC Psychiatry* **2012**, *12*, 76. [CrossRef] [PubMed]
6. Vervaet, M.; Van Heeringen, C.; Audenaert, K. Personality-Related Characteristics in Restricting Versus Binging and Purging Eating Disordered Patients. *Compr. Psychiatry* **2004**, *45*, 37–43. [CrossRef] [PubMed]
7. Pennesi, J.-L.; Wade, T.D. A systematic review of the existing models of disordered eating: Do they inform the development of effective interventions? *Clin. Psychol. Rev.* **2016**, *43*, 175–192. [CrossRef] [PubMed]
8. Ahrberg, M.; Trojca, D.; Nasrawi, N.; Vocks, S. Body image disturbance in binge eating disorder: A review. *Eur. Eat. Disord. Rev.* **2011**, *19*, 375–381. [CrossRef] [PubMed]
9. Mason, T.B.; Lewis, R.J. Assessing the roles of impulsivity, food-related cognitions, BMI, and demographics in the dual pathway model of binge eating among men and women. *Eat. Behav.* **2015**, *18*, 151–155. [CrossRef] [PubMed]
10. Stice, E. Interactive and Mediational Etiologic Models of Eating Disorder Onset: Evidence from Prospective Studies. *Annu. Rev. Clin. Psychol.* **2016**, *12*, 359–381. [CrossRef] [PubMed]
11. Claes, L.; Robinson, M.D.; Muehlenkamp, J.J.; Vandereycken, W.; Bijttebier, P. Differentiating bingeing/purging and restrictive eating disorder subtypes: The roles of temperament, effortful control, and cognitive control. *Pers. Individ. Dif.* **2010**, *48*, 166–170. [CrossRef]
12. Lezak, M.D.; Howieson, D.B.; Loring, D.W.; Hannay, H.J.; Fischer, J.S. *Neuropsychological Assessment*, 4th ed.; Oxford University Press: Oxford, UK, 2004.
13. Wu, M.; Hartmann, M.; Skunde, M.; Herzog, W.; Friederich, H.C. Inhibitory control in bulimic-type eating disorders: A systematic review and meta-analysis. *PLoS ONE* **2013**, *8*, e83412. [CrossRef] [PubMed]
14. Racine, S.E.; Culbert, K.M.; Larson, C.L.; Klump, K.L. The possible influence of impulsivity and dietary restraint on associations between serotonin genes and binge eating. *J. Psychiatr. Res.* **2009**, *43*, 1278–1286. [CrossRef] [PubMed]
15. Schmidt, U.; Campbell, I.C. Treatment of eating disorders can not remain "brainless": The case for brain-directed treatments. *Eur. Eat. Disord. Rev.* **2013**, *21*, 425–427. [CrossRef] [PubMed]
16. Freeman, D.; Reeve, S.; Robinson, A.; Ehlers, A.; Clark, D.; Spanlang, B.; Slater, M. Virtual reality in the assessment, understanding, and treatment of mental health disorders. *Psychol. Med.* **2017**, *22*, 1–8. [CrossRef] [PubMed]
17. Schultheis, M.T.; Rizzo, A.A. The application of virtual reality technology in rehabilitation. *Rehabil. Psychol.* **2001**, *46*, 296–311. [CrossRef]
18. Baños, R.M.; Botella, C.; Guerrero, B.; Liaño, V.; Alcañiz, M.; Rey, B. The third pole of the sense of presence: Comparing virtual and imagery spaces. *Psychnol. J.* **2005**, *3*, 90–100.
19. North, M.M.; North, S.M. Virtual Reality Therapy. In *Computer-Assisted and Web-Based Innovations in Psychology, Special Education, and Health*; Academic Press: London, UK, 2016; pp. 141–156.
20. De Carvalho, M.R.; De Freire, R.C.; Nardi, A.E. Virtual reality as a mechanism for exposure therapy. *World J. Biol. Psychiatry* **2010**, *11*, 220–230. [CrossRef] [PubMed]
21. Valmaggia, L.R.; Latif, L.; Kempton, M.J.; Rus-Calafell, M. Virtual reality in the psychological treatment for mental health problems: A systematic review of recent evidence. *Psychiatry Res.* **2016**, *236*, 189–195. [CrossRef] [PubMed]
22. Ferrer-Garcia, M.; Gutierrez-Maldonado, J.; Riva, G. Virtual reality based treatments in eating disorders and obesity: A review. *J. Contemp. Psychother.* **2013**, *43*, 207–221. [CrossRef]

23. Koskina, A.; Campbell, I.C.; Schmidt, U. Exposure therapy in eating disorders revisited. *Neurosci. Biobehav. Rev.* **2013**, *37*, 193–208. [CrossRef] [PubMed]
24. Gutiérrez-Maldonado, J.; Ferrer-García, M.; Caqueo-Urízar, A.; Letosa-Porta, A. Assessment of Emotional Reactivity Produced by Exposure to Virtual Environments in Patients with Eating Disorders. *Cyberpsychol. Behav.* **2006**, *9*, 507–513. [CrossRef] [PubMed]
25. Ferrer-Garcia, M.; Gutierrez-Maldonado, J.; Caqueo-Urizar, A.; Moreno, E. The Validity of Virtual Environments for Eliciting Emotional Responses in Patients with Eating Disorders and in Controls. *Behav. Modif.* **2009**, *33*, 830–854. [CrossRef] [PubMed]
26. Gutiérrez-Maldonado, J.; Ferrer-García, M.; Caqueo-Urízar, A.; Moreno, E. Body Image in Eating Disorders: The Influence of Exposure to Virtual-Reality Environments. *Cyberpsychol. Behav. Soc. Netw.* **2010**, *13*, 521–531. [CrossRef] [PubMed]
27. Gorini, A.; Griez, E.; Petrova, A.; Riva, G.; Pull, C.; Gorini, A.; Riva, G.; Gregg, L.; Tarrier, N.; Barfield, W.; et al. Assessment of the emotional responses produced by exposure to real food, virtual food and photographs of food in patients affected by eating disorders. *Ann. Gen. Psychiatry* **2010**, *9*, 30. [CrossRef] [PubMed]
28. Ferrer-Garcia, M.; Gutierrez-Maldonado, J. Virtual reality exposure in patients with eating disorders: influence of symptom severity and presence. *Stud. Health Technol. Inform.* **2011**, *167*, 80–85. [PubMed]
29. Perpiñá, C.; Roncero, M.; Fernández-Aranda, F.; Jiménez-Murcia, S.; Forcano, L.; Sánchez, I. Clinical validation of a virtual environment for normalizing eating patterns in eating disorders. *Compr. Psychiatry* **2013**, *54*, 680–686. [CrossRef] [PubMed]
30. Ferrer-Garcia, M.; Gutiérrez-Maldonado, J.; Pla-Sanjuanelo, J.; Vilalta-Abella, F.; Andreu-Gracia, A.; Dakanalis, A.; Fernandez-Aranda, F.; Fuste-Escolano, A.; Ribas-Sabate, J.; Riva, G.; et al. ExternalEating as a PredictorofCue-reactivitytoFood-related Virtual Environments. *Stud. Health Technol. Inform.* **2015**, *219*, 117–122. [PubMed]
31. Pla-Sanjuanelo, J.; Ferrer-Garcia, M.; Gutiérrez -Maldonado, J.; Vilalta-Abella, F.; Andreu-Gracia, A.; Dakanalis, A.; Fernandez-Aranda, F.; Fuste-Escolano, A.; Ribas-Sabate, J.; Riva, G.; et al. TraitandStateCraving as IndicatorsofValidityof VR-based Software for BingeEatingTreatment. *Stud. Health Technol. Inform.* **2015**, *219*, 141–146. [PubMed]
32. Perpinã, C.; Roncero, M. Similarities and differences between eating disorders and obese patients in a virtual environment for normalizing eating patterns. *Compr. Psychiatry* **2016**, *67*, 39–45. [CrossRef] [PubMed]
33. Perpiñá, C.; Botella, C.; Baños, R.; Marco, H.; Alcañiz, M.; Quero, S. Body image and virtual reality in eating disorders: Is exposure to virtual reality more effective than the classical body image treatment? *Cyberpsychol. Behav.* **1999**, *2*, 149–155. [CrossRef] [PubMed]
34. Riva, G.; Bacchetta, M.; Baruffi, M.; Rinaldi, S.; Vincelli, F.; Molinari, E. Virtual reality-based experiential cognitive treatment of obesity and binge-eating disorders. *Clin. Psychol. Psychother.* **2000**, *7*, 209–219. [CrossRef]
35. Riva, G.; Bacchetta, M.; Baruffi, M.; Cirillo, G.; Molinari, E. Virtual Reality Environment for Body Image Modification: A Multidimensional Therapy for the Treatment of Body Image in Obesity and Related Pathologies. *Cyberpsychol. Behav.* **2000**, *3*, 421–431. [CrossRef]
36. Riva, G.; Bacchetta, M.; Baruffi, M.; Molinari, E. Virtual-reality-based multidimensional therapy for the treatment of body image disturbances in binge eating disorders: A preliminary controlled study. *IEEE Trans. Inf. Technol. Biomed.* **2002**, *6*, 224–234. [CrossRef] [PubMed]
37. Riva, G.; Bacchetta, M.; Cesa, G.; Conti, S.; Molinari, E. Six-Month Follow-Up of In-Patient Experiential Cognitive Therapy for Binge Eating Disorders. *Cyberpsychol. Behav.* **2003**, *6*, 251–258. [CrossRef] [PubMed]
38. Riva, G.; Bacchetta, M.; Cesa, G.; Conti, S.; Molinari, E. The use of VR in the treatment of eating disorders. *Stud. Health Technol. Inform.* **2004**, *99*, 121–163. [PubMed]
39. Marco, J.H.; Perpiñá, C.; Botella, C. Effectiveness of cognitive behavioral therapy supported by virtual reality in the treatment of body image in eating disorders: One year follow-up. *Psychiatry Res.* **2013**, *209*, 619–625. [CrossRef] [PubMed]
40. Cesa, G.L.; Manzoni, G.M.; Bacchetta, M.; Castelnuovo, G.; Conti, S.; Gaggioli, A.; Mantovani, F.; Molinari, E.; Cardenas-López, G.; Riva, G. Virtual reality for enhancing the cognitive behavioral treatment of obesity with binge eating disorder: Randomized controlled study with one-year follow-up. *J. Med. Internet Res.* **2013**, *15*, 1–13. [CrossRef] [PubMed]
41. Roncero, M.; Perpiñá, C. Normalizing the eating pattern with virtual reality for bulimia nervosa: A case report. *Rev. Mex. Trastor. Aliment.* **2015**, *6*, 152–159. [CrossRef]

42. Perpiñá, C.; Marco, J.H.; Botella, C.; Baños, R. Tratamiento de laimagen corporal enlostrastornosalimentarios mediante tratamiento cognitivo-comportamental apoyadoconrealidad virtual: Resultados al año de seguimiento. *Psicol. Conductual* **2004**, *12*, 519–537.
43. Riva, G.; Bolzoni, M.; Carella, F.; Galimberti, C.; Griffin, M.J.; Lewis, C.H.; Luongo, R.; Mardegan, P.; Melis, L.; Molinari-Tosatti, L.; et al. Virtual Reality Environments for Psycho-Neuro-Physiological Assessment and Rehabilitation. *Stud. Health Technol. Inform.* **1997**, *39*, 34–45. [PubMed]
44. Fairburn, C.G.; Marcus, M.D.; Wilson, G.T. Cognitive-behavioral therapy for binge eating and bulimia nervosa: A comprehensive treatment manual. In *Binge Eating: Nature, Assessment, and Treatment*; Weill Cornell Medical College: New York, NY, USA, 1993; pp. 361–404.
45. Fairburn, C.; Garner, D.; Garnfinkel, P. Cognitive-Behavioral Treatment for Bulimia. In *Handbook of Psychotherapy for Anorexia and Bulimia*; Gamer, D.M., Garnfinkel, P.E., Eds.; Guilford Press: New York, NY, USA, 1985; pp. 160–192.
46. Fairburn, C. *Overcoming Binge Eating*; Guilford Press: New York, NY, USA, 1995.
47. Garner, D.; Vitousek, K.; Pike, K. Cognitive-Behavioral Therapy for AN. In *Handbook of Treatment for Eating Disorders*; Garner, D., Garfinkel, P., Eds.; Guilford Press: New York, NY, USA, 1997; pp. 94–145.
48. Wilson, T.; Fairburn, C.; Agras, W. Cognitive-Behavioral Therapy for Bulimia Nervosa. In *Handbook of Treatment for Eating Disorders*; Garner, D., Garfinkel, P., Eds.; Guilford Press: New York, NY, USA, 1997; pp. 67–93.
49. Butters, J.; Cash, T. Cognitive-behavioral treatment of women's body-image dissatisfaction. *J. Consult. Clin. Psychol.* **1987**, *55*, 889–897. [CrossRef] [PubMed]
50. Perpiñá, C.; Botella, C.; Baños, R. Imagen Corporal em Los Trastornos Alimentarios. In *Evaluación y Tratamiento por Medio de Realidad Virtual*; Promolibro: Valencia, Spain, 2000.
51. Ricca, V.; Mannucci, E.; Zucchi, T.; Rotella, C.M.; Faravelli, C. Cognitive-behavioural therapy for bulimia nervosa and binge eating disorder. A review. *Psychother. Psychosom.* **2000**, *69*, 287–295. [CrossRef] [PubMed]
52. Wiederhold, B.K.; Riva, G.; Gutiérrez-Maldonado, J. Virtual Reality in the Assessment and Treatment of Weight-Related Disorders. *Cyberpsychol. Behav. Soc. Netw.* **2016**, *19*, 67–73. [CrossRef] [PubMed]
53. Botella, C.; Villa, H.; Garcia-Palacios, A.; Baños, R.; Perpiñá, C.; Alcañiz, M. Clinically significant virtual environments for the treatment of panic disorder and agoraphobia. *Cyberpsychol. Behav.* **2004**, *7*, 527–535. [CrossRef] [PubMed]
54. Riva, G.; Baños, R.; Botella, C.; Mantovani, F.; Gaggioli, A. Transforming Experience: The Potential of Augmented Reality and Virtual Reality for Enhancing Personal and Clinical Change. *Front. Psychiatry* **2016**, *7*, 164. [CrossRef] [PubMed]
55. Powers, M.; Emmelkamp, P. Virtual reality exposure therapy for anxiety disorders: A meta-analysis. *J. Anxiety Disord.* **2008**, *22*, 561–569. [CrossRef] [PubMed]
56. Riva, G.; Gaudio, S.; Dakanalis, A. The Neuropsychology of Self Objectification. *Eur. Psychol.* **2015**, *20*, 34–43. [CrossRef]
57. Riva, G. Out of my real body: Cognitive neuroscience meets eating disorders. *Front. Hum. Neurosci.* **2014**, *8*, 236. [CrossRef] [PubMed]
58. Manzoni, G.; Cesa, G.; Bacchetta, M.; Castelnuovo, G.; Conti, S.; Gaggioli, A.; Riva, G. Virtual Reality-Enhanced Cognitive-Behavioral Therapy for Morbid Obesity: A Randomized Controlled Study with 1 Year Follow-Up. *Cyberpsychol. Behav. Soc. Netw.* **2016**, *19*, 134–140. [CrossRef] [PubMed]
59. Ferrer-garcía, M.; Gutiérrez-maldonado, J. The use of virtual reality in the study, assessment, and treatment of body image in eating disorders and nonclinical samples: A review of the literature. *Body Image* **2012**, *9*, 1–11. [CrossRef] [PubMed]
60. Bohon, C.; Stice, E. Negative affect and neural response to palatable food intake in bulimia nervosa. *Appetite* **2012**, *58*, 964–970. [CrossRef] [PubMed]
61. Moher, D.; Jones, A.; Lepage, L.; CONSORT Group. Use of the CONSORT Statement and Quality of Reports of Randomized Trials. *JAMA* **2001**, *285*, 1992–1995. [CrossRef] [PubMed]

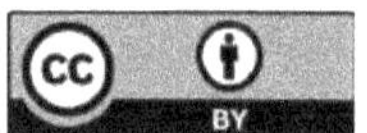

MDPI
St. Alban-Anlage 66
4052 Basel, Switzerland
Tel. +41 61 683 77 34
Fax +41 61 302 89 18
http://www.mdpi.com

Behavioral Sciences Editorial Office
E-mail: behavsci@mdpi.com
http://www.mdpi.com/journal/behavsci

www.ingramcontent.com/pod-product-compliance
Lightning Source LLC
Chambersburg PA
CBHW051851210326
41597CB00033B/5856
* 9 7 8 3 0 3 8 4 2 8 5 3 4 *